++Clinical General Practice

VOLUME 1

For Butterworth-Heinemann:

Senior Commissioning Editor: Heidi Allen
Development Editor: Kim Benson
Production Manager: Yolanta Motylinska
Design/Production: Kneath Associates and Helius

For Update:

Editor: Andrew Baxter

++Clinical General Practice

VOLUME 1

Edited by **Mary Selby**

GENERAL PRACTITIONER, NEWMARKET, SUFFOLK

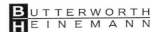

EDINBURGH   LONDON   NEW YORK   OXFORD   PHILADELPHIA   ST LOUIS   SYDNEY   TORONTO
2004

BUTTERWORTH-HEINEMANN
An imprint of Elsevier Limited

First edition 2004

ISBN 0 7506 8787 8

British Library Cataloguing in Publication Data
A catalogue record for this book is available from the British Library

Library of Congress Cataloging in Publication Data
A catalog record for this book is available from the Library of Congress

Note
Medical knowledge is constantly changing. As new information becomes available, changes in treatment, procedures, equipment and the use of drugs become necessary. The author/contributors and the publishers have taken great care to ensure that the information given in this text is accurate and up to date. However, readers are strongly advised to confirm that the information, especially with regard to drug usage, complies with the latest legislation and standards of practice.

 your source for books,
journals and multimedia
in the health sciences
www.elsevierhealth.com

The
publisher's
policy is to use
**paper manufactured
from sustainable forests**

Printed in Spain

Contents

Contents

Contents

Contents

VOLUME 2

Contents

Contents

Contributors

Kesh Baboolal MD, FRCP   Consultant Nephrologist, University Hospital of Wales, Cardiff, UK

Alvin Bodner MA, MB, ChB, FRCGP   General Practitioner and Vocational Training Scheme Organiser, Castleton Health Centre, Rochdale, Lancashire, UK

David Brooks MD, FRCGP, DRCOG   General Practitioner, Middleton, Manchester, UK

Christopher H Buller MMedSc, MRCPsych   Senior Registrar in Adult Psychiatry, Professorial Unit, High Royds Hospital, Ilkley, West Yorkshire, UK

John Coope MBE, MB ChB, FRCGP   General Practitioner, Bollington, Cheshire, UK

Alun Cooper BSc, MRCGP   General Practitioner Principal, Bridge Medical Centre, Crawley, West Sussex, UK

Michael Coren BSc, MB BS, MRCP, MRCPCH   Consultant Paediatrician, Paddington Green Children's Unit, St. Mary's Hospital, London, UK

Aeron G Davies FRCP   Consultant Physician, Bronglais General Hospital, Aberystwyth, Ceredigion, UK

John S Duncan DM, FRCP   Professor of Neurology, The National Hospital for Neurology and Neurosurgery, London, UK; Medical Director, The National Society for Epilepsy, London, UK

Cosmo Hallstrom MD, MRCP, FRCPsych, DPM   Honorary Consultant Psychiatrist, Charing Cross Hospital, London, UK; Florence Nightingale Clinic, London, UK; Senior Lecturer, Imperial College, London, UK

W Iain F Henderson MB ChB, DRCOG, DPD   General Practitioner, Kingsway Medical Practice, Scotstoun, Glasgow; Hospital Practitioner in Dermatology, Western Infirmary, Glasgow, UK

Nigel Higson MA, BM, BCh, DRCOG   General Practitioner, Goodwood Court Medical Practice, Hove, East Sussex, UK

Graham Jackson FRCP, FESC, FACC   Consultant Cardiologist, Cardiothoracic Department, Guy's and St Thomas' Hospital Trust, London, UK

Sarah Jarvis BM BCh, FRCGP, DRCOG   General Practitioner, Richford Gate Medical Practice, London, UK

Barry Lewis MB ChB, DRCOG, MRCGP   General Practitioner, Rochdale, Lancashire, UK; Associate Adviser in GP Education, Manchester University, Manchester, UK

Wayne Lewis MB, BCh, BA, MA, MRCGP, DRCOG   General Practitioner, Carreg Wen Surgery, Bleanavon, Pontypool, Gwent, UK

Francisco Machado BSc, MB BS, MRCP, DCH, DRCOG, MRCGP, Dip Med Ed   General Practitioner, Abersychan Surgery, Pontypool, Gwent, UK

Mike McGhee BSc, MMEd, MB BS, MRCGP, DRCOG   General Practitioner, The Surgery, Castle Donington, Derby, UK

Carol Manson McLeod BComm, RN, MScN   Patient Care Coordinator, Brandon Regional Health Authority, Brandon, Manitoba, Canada

Mike Mead MB BS, DCH, DRCOG, FRCGP   General Practitioner, Leicester, UK

Contributors

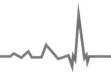

David Morris MB BChir, DCH, DRCOG, MRCP, MRCGP, PhD   General Practitioner, Bridgnorth Medical Practices, Bridgnorth, Shropshire, UK

Peter O'Kane BSc, MRCP   Specialist Registrar in Cardiology, Cardiothoracic Centre, Guy's and St Thomas' Hospital Trust, London, UK

Thomas Poyner FRCP(Lond), FRCP(Glasg), MRCGP, DPD   General and Hospital Practitioner, Stockton-on-Tees, UK

Greg Rubin FRCGP   Professor, Centre for Primary and Community Care, University of Sunderland, Sunderland, UK

Mary Selby MA, MB BChir, MRCGP   General Practitioner, Newmarket, Suffolk, UK

Robert J Simister MRCP   Research Fellow, The MRI Unit, The National Society for Epilepsy, Chalfont St Peter, Buckinghamshire, UK

Michael Tarlow FRCPH, FRCP   Senior Lecturer in Paediatrics, Institute of Child Health, Birmingham, UK; Honorary Consultant Paediatrician, Birmingham Children's Hospital, Birmingham, UK

Jill E Thistlethwaite BSc, MMedEd, MB BS, MRCGP, DRCOG   General Practitioner, Calderdale NHS Trust Mytholmroyd Health Centre, Thrush Hill Road, Hebden Bridge, Halifax; Senior Lecturer, Community-based Education, Leeds School of Medicine, Leeds, UK

Andrew Thornett   Mental Health Group, University of Southampton, Royal South Hants Hospital, Southampton, UK

Edward Warren FRCGP   General Practitioner, Sheffield, West Yorkshire, UK; Trainer, Barnsley Vocational Training Scheme, Barnsley, UK

Preface

Clinical General Practice is written by, edited by and intended for practising GPs, trainers and registrars. It is therefore about clinical general practice, written by those who do it.

The basis for the text is the rolling 3-year programme of curriculum articles, published in the GP educational journal *Update*. These have been widely praised for their excellence, and I was therefore delighted to be asked to edit the best of them into two volumes, the target of which is a place not just in the practice library but on the consulting room shelf. The division of the text into two volumes was born out of convenience rather than any need to divide the material itself.

As a practising GP myself, I have tried to include those articles that I thought most useful, most helpful and most easily digestible, and those from which I learned the most. Volume 1 includes heart disease, endocrinology and paediatrics, together with urology, mental health, neurology, dermatology and gastroenterology. Volume 2 covers chest disease, rheumatology, care of the elderly, obstetrics, gynaecology, contaception, ENT, ophthalmology and oncology/palliative care.

Of course, it would be impossible to incorporate all of clinical general practice into these volumes, as the remit of the GP is potentially infinite. Nevertheless, most GPs are able to identify the core clinical conditions and syndromes that make up the bulk of their daily work. Many of these are the areas that are least well covered during the hospital component of GP training.

The books therefore aim to offer comprehensive coverage of the 'bread and butter' of general practice, offering the complete GP 'take' on those diseases and presentations which require the bulk of our time. Some of the conditions featured, such as meningococcal disease, will be encountered rarely by the average GP – but their importance means we consider them disproportionately often. Others, such as hypertension control and otitis media, are daily features of our working lives.

Each individual chapter retains most of its original references, for those who want more information, together with a set of key points extracted form the text either by the original author or by myself. The material has been updated where necessary to incorporate the most recent published research and guidelines. However, although medical practice changes every day, the essentials of the way we assess and treat our patients are slower to change, and it is hoped that these books will remain up to date for many years to come.

I hope the books' straightforward, applicable and approachable style will make them a useful learning resource and reference for GP registrars, and an essential teaching resource for trainers. Indeed, they would be an excellent starting point both for the GP constructing his or her personal development plan and for the registrar preparing for the membership exam.

Mary Selby

1. Diabetes

E Warren

THIS CHAPTER REVIEWS

- The presentation of diabetes.
- How to explain diabetes to patients and how to deliver the information they need.
- The treatment and complications of diabetes.
- How to monitor patients.

Prevalence

About 2% of people in the UK have diabetes, although a third of these cases are undiagnosed.[1,2] The typical GP deals with two or three new diabetics each year, and has a further 20–30 diagnosed cases on his or her list.[2]

The incidence of all types of diabetes is steadily increasing. Type 2, non-insulin dependent, disease accounts for about 85% of all diabetes, and the prevalence has risen by 50% in the past 20 years.[3] Prevalence rises with age and also with obesity, so the ageing and increasingly obese population account for much of this.[2,3]

There is no known cure for any type of diabetes, so management is concerned mainly with minimizing the risks of the illness. A diagnosis of diabetes signals the beginning of a lifelong relationship between patient and healthcare advisers.

Presentation

Diabetes may present with acute or subacute symptoms, or may be diagnosed on routine testing on at-risk groups such as pregnant women.

Typical symptoms are thirst, polyuria and weight loss, but tiredness, pruritis, blurred vision, foot ulceration, candida and recurrent sepsis are common.

The criteria for confirming the diagnosis are:[4]

- random plasma glucose 11.1 mmol/l or more
- fasting plasma glucose 7.0 mmol/l or more
- plasma glucose 11.1 mmol/l or more 2 hours after 75 g oral glucose.

Treatment goals

Treatment aims for risk minimization, but without making life intolerable for the patient. Goals are:

- minimal symptoms
- normoglycaemia
- blood pressure control
- minimal complications
- reduced risk of cardiovascular disease.

Minimizing symptoms

Diabetes is often diagnosed at a stage when symptoms are not particularly severe, and it is unreasonable to institute a treatment that makes the patient feel worse.

Symptoms occur if blood sugar is too high or too low. Hypoglycaemia causes particular problems because it tends to come on suddenly, and can lead to implications for the patient's fitness to drive.

Attempting normoglycaemia

Keeping blood sugars as near the normal range as possible reduces microvascular complications in both type 1 and type 2 diabetes.[5,6] However, tighter blood glucose results in greater weight gain and more episodes of hypoglycaemia.[7,8] Patients who monitor their blood sugars properly achieve better glycaemic control.[9]

There is a continuous relationship between glycaemic control and microvascular complications, so it is not clear what the target blood sugar should be.[10]

Recommended targets are:[11]

- HbA$_{1c}$ 7.0% or less (rarely achieved and maintained, even in trials)
- fasting blood glucose 4–7 mmol/l
- self-monitored blood glucose before meals 4–7 mmol/l.

Blood pressure control

About 40% of diabetics have raised blood pressure. Reducing blood pressure reduces microvascular complications, diabetes-related deaths and stroke, although not myocardial infarction or all-cause mortality.[12]

It does not seem to matter which medication is used to reduce blood pressure,[12] but angiotensin-converting enzyme (ACE) inhibitors may protect against neuropathy and retinopathy independently of their effects on blood pressure, and are probably the first-choice agents.[10]

At least a third of diabetic patients need three or more drugs to achieve satisfactory control.[6]

The British Hypertension Society suggests target blood pressures of less than 140/80 (audit standard) and less than 130/75 (optimal pressure) for patients with diabetes (see p. 9).[13]

Minimizing complications

Through regular monitoring of feet, nerves, kidneys and eyes, the health professional can make sure the best treatment is given if complications do occur.

Reducing cardiovascular risks

Diabetes is an extra risk factor for cardiovascular disease, and needs to taken into account when assessing overall risk.

Treatment options

Diet

All patients with diabetes should be advised on their diet, and the involvement of a specialist dietician is essential.[14]

The diet should be tailored to the individual and aims for steady and gradual release of dietary sugars into the blood. Even sophisticated regimens of insulin injection cannot approach the efficiency of a normally functioning pancreas, whereas hypoglycaemic therapies can achieve only an even rate of removal of sugar from the blood. This therefore needs to be matched by an even supply to avoid wide fluctuations in blood sugar levels.

The diet should derive 50–60% of calories from complex carbohydrates, while simple sugars should be restricted. Fibre content should be high, as this slows absorption of sugars from the gut.[14]

A low-fat diet is a good general principle, and patients with elevated lipid levels will need special attention.[14] Three-quarters of newly diagnosed type 2 diabetics are obese.[15] Overweight patients need calorie restriction to reduce the body mass index, ideally to 25 kg/m^2 or less and certainly to below 27 kg/m^2.

Diabetics who do shift work, have heavy manual jobs or are involved in sport will need special attention from the dietetic team.

Hypoglycaemic medication

Less than 20% of people with type 2 diabetes are controlled after 3 months on diet alone. Drug therapy should then be considered.[16]

Metformin

Metformin reduces glucose absorption from the gut, and increases insulin sensitivity.[17] It is the only diabetic treatment that reduces circulating insulin, bringing a theoretical reduction in the risk of coronary heart disease, and does not cause weight gain. It is the first-choice treatment for overweight diabetics.[12] It does not cause hypoglycaemic episodes.

Diarrhoea is the most common side-effect. Metformin should not be used in patients with severe heart failure, renal or hepatic failure or in heavy users of alcohol because of the rare risk of lactic acidosis, which carries a mortality of up to 50%.[18]

Sulphonylureas

Sulphonylureas work mainly by boosting the insulin output of the failing pancreas. They are the first-choice treatment for patients of normal weight.[12] All sulphonylureas may cause rashes and weight gain.

Glitazones

The glitazones (pioglitazone (Actos), rosiglitazone (Avandia)) are recommended for use in combination with either a sulphonylurea or metformin when a combination of these two is unsuccessful. Patients using a glitazone need additional monitoring with periodic liver function tests.[19]

Acarbose

Acarbose (Glucobay) is an α-glucosidase inhibitor that reduces blood sugar when used with diet alone or with

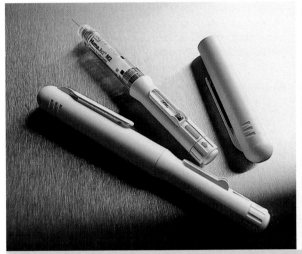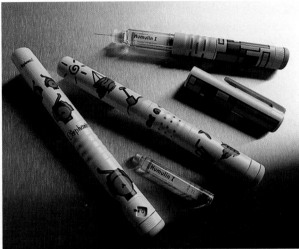

Figure 1.1 Equipment for injection of insulin (pen devices). Reproduced with permission from Rudnicka & Birch, *Diabetic Eye Disease*, Butterworth-Heinemann, 2000.

other hypoglycaemics. It can cause flatulence and diarrhoea, and its effects may decrease with time.

Prandial glucose regulators
Nateglinide (Starlix) and repaglinide (Novonorm) can be taken just before the main meal, and stimulate the release of insulin from the pancreas.

Insulin
The prime indications for insulin therapy are:[19]

- inadequate control by diet, exercise and maximal oral agents, especially if associated with unintentional weight loss
- intercurrent events such as severe infection, surgery or myocardial infarction
- renal impairment
- diabetic complications.

Box 1.1 Relative risks in diabetic patients[10]

Blindness	20
End-stage renal disease	25
Amputation	40
Myocardial infarction	2–5
Stroke	2–3

Some pen devices for the injection of insulin are shown in Figure 1.1.

Complications

Diabetics bear considerable excess morbidity and mortality (Box 1.1), mostly mediated through the effects of diabetes on large and small blood vessels.

In general, it is the microvascular complications of diabetes that cause morbidity and disability, and the macrovascular complications that kill.

Diabetic eye disease

A fifth of type 2 diabetics already have retinopathy when their diabetes is diagnosed.[10] Ten years after diagnosis, 10% of type 1 and 50% of type 2 diabetics have retinopathy. After 25 years, 90% of all diabetics are affected.[20]

A combination of fundoscopy and retinal photography through dilated pupils appears to be the best way of detecting pathology. Simply looking at the optic fundi through undilated pupils will miss up to two-thirds of cases of retinopathy.[21] Opticians are as good as doctors at finding retinopathy.[22]

Non-proliferative (background) retinopathy is a relatively benign condition: only 3% of patients have any visual impairment after 5 years. Laser treatment has markedly improved the outlook in more severe diabetic retinopathy. ▶

Diabetic renal disease

Fifteen percent of diagnosed diabetics have proteinuria. If they live long enough, 75% develop renal failure.[2]

Microalbuminuria is a marker for a high risk of progression to frank nephropathy: diagnosis and treatment of diabetic renal disease are discussed in Chapter 2.

Diabetic nerve problems

Sensory neuropathy affects half of diabetics.[10] Twenty-five percent are at risk of foot disease and half of diabetic men have erectile dysfunction.[2]

The combination of neuropathy with poor circulation may lead to persistent lesions that can be dealt with only by amputation.

Cardiovascular problems

About 75% of diabetes patients die of an arteriosclerotic complication, such as a heart attack or stroke, and 3% have intermittent claudication.[2,23] Known cardiovascular risk factors, such as hypertension, obesity, raised cholesterol and lack of exercise, tend to cluster in diabetics, and people with diabetes are just as likely to smoke as anyone else.[24]

For any given risk factor, the diabetic faces 2–4 times the cardiovascular risk of the non-diabetic.[23]5This may be the result of diabetic cardiomyopathy.[26] A diabetic patient who has a heart attack is twice as likely to die as a non-diabetic patient.[10]

Tight blood pressure and cholesterol control are therefore an important part of management.[27] There is no clear consensus on the age at which raised cholesterol and lipid profiles should first be sought and treated in those diabetic from childhood. The recommended cholesterol target for diabetic patients with a 15% 10-year coronary heart disease (CHD) risk should be the same as for patients who already have CHD.[27]

Getting the message across

Telling the patient

Diabetes is an incurable disease carrying implications of loss of health, potential restrictions on lifestyle, and increased likelihood of disability and premature death. Patients often experience a sense of loss and grief at diagnosis similar to that of bereavement. Nevertheless, the patient will need information about their diabetes. Essentials should be dealt with first, and not too much information should be offered at one time. The speed with which information must be imparted depends on individual circumstances – the patient presenting in hospital in ketoacidosis may need more initial information than the well patient, in whom dietary control is first attempted.

As with any condition that requires lifestyle changes, care must be taken not to blame the patient for the illness. Cooperation, not conflict, is more likely to secure the best outcome.

Information for the patient

Ultimately, patients need to know what diabetes is, the treatment options, and when and how to seek advice, in addition to being offered information on the complications of the condition and how to reduce them.

Health professionals should miss no opportunity to check how much a diabetic knows about the condition, and to offer information. The time immediately after diagnosis is particularly sensitive, and there may be denial, guilt, anger and anxiety. Education should be tailored to the patient, and all members of the care team should have a consistent approach.

It takes time to share information. The risks may be difficult to discuss, partly because the information is unwelcome, but also because patients may still be trying to adjust to their diagnosis.

Literature can be a valuable resource, and Diabetes UK (formerly the British Diabetic Association) has a lot of patient literature. Diabetes UK can also advise patients in a variety of areas, such as insurers to cover holiday travel for diabetics, special holidays for diabetic children, and alert bracelets for children and adults giving information on their condition.

Key points

- Keeping blood sugars as near the normal range as possible reduces microvascular complications.
- Tighter blood glucose results in greater weight gain.
- Reducing blood pressure reduces microvascular complications, diabetes-related deaths and stroke, although not myocardial infarction or all-cause mortality.
- Less than 20% of people with type 2 diabetes have their diabetes controlled after 3 months on diet alone.
- Microalbuminuria is a marker for a high risk of progression to frank nephropathy.

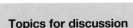

Topics for discussion
- The best way for patients to deal with diabetes psychologically is to forget about it and get on with living.
- Why do most diabetics 'cheat' on their diet?
- Diabetics who continue to smoke are not worth bothering with.
- It is more important to control diabetics' blood pressure than their blood sugar.

- **After 25 years, 90% of all diabetics have retinopathy.**
- **Non-proliferative retinopathy is a relatively benign condition: only 3% of patients have any visual impairment after 5 years.**
- **A diabetic patient who has a heart attack is twice as likely to die as a non-diabetic patient.**
- **There is no clear consensus on the age at which raised cholesterol and lipid profiles should first be sought and treated in those diabetic from childhood.**
- **It is unreasonable to institute a treatment that makes the patient feel worse.**

Resources

Diabetes UK (formerly British Diabetic Association), 10 Queen Anne Street, London W1M 0BD. Tel. 0207 323 1531. Publishes self-help material for people with diabetes.

References

1. O'Rahilly S. Non-insulin dependent diabetes mellitus: the gathering storm. BMJ 1997; 314:955–959.

2. Fry J. Diabetes. Update 1993; 46:695–699.

3. Williams G. Diabetes black spots and death by postcode. BMJ 2001; 322:1375–1376.

4. Expert Committee on the Diagnosis and Classification of Diabetes Mellitus. Report of the Expert Committee on the Diagnosis and Classification of Diabetes Mellitus. Diabetes Care 1997; 20:1183–1197.

5. Diabetes Control and Complications Trial Research Group. The effects of intensive treatment of diabetes on the development and progression of long-term complications in insulin-dependent diabetes mellitus. N Engl J Med 1993; 329:977–986.

6. UK Prospective Diabetes Study Group. Intensive blood-glucose control with sulphonylureas or insulin compared with conventional treatment and risk of complications in patients with type 2 diabetes (UKPDS 33). Lancet 1998; 352:837–853.

7. Hermann WH. Glycaemic control in diabetes. BMJ 1999; 319:104–106.

8. Amiel SA. Diabetic control and complications. BMJ 1993; 307:881–882.

9. Evans JMM, Newton RW, Ruta DA, et al. Frequency of blood glucose monitoring in relation to glycaemic control: observational study with diabetes database. BMJ 1999; 319: 83–86.

10. Donnelly R, Emslie-Smith AM, Gardner ID, et al. ABC of arterial and venous disease. Vascular complications of diabetes. BMJ 2000; 320:1062–1066.

11. British Diabetic Association. UKPDS. Implications for the care of people with type 2 diabetes. London: BDA; 1998.

12. Reducing long-term complications of type 2 diabetes. Drug Therapeut Bull 1999; 37:84–87.

13. British Hypertension Society. Available at: http://www.hyp.ac.uk/bhs/resources/guidelines.htm

14. Waine C, Tasker P, Gedney J, et al. Guidelines for the care of patients with diabetes. London: Royal College of General Practitioners; 1993.

15. Non-insulin-dependent diabetes mellitus (part 2). MeReC Bulletin 1996; 7:29–32.

16. Singh D. Obesity in NIDDM. Geriatric Medicine 1996; 26:42–45.

17. Amiel SA. Non-insulin-dependent diabetes mellitus. Update 1994; 48:256–265.

18. Non-insulin-dependent diabetes mellitus (part 1). MeReC Bulletin 1996; 7:21–24.

19. National Institute for Clinical Excellence. Summary of guidance issued to the NHS in England and Wales. Vol 2. London: TSO; 2001.

20. Mills KB. Diabetic retinopathy. Romford: Smith and Nephew Pharmaceuticals; 1990.

21. Ryder R. Screening for diabetic retinopathy. BMJ 1995; 311:207–208.

22. Flanagan D. Screening for diabetic retinopathy. Practitioner 1994; 238:37–42.

23. Kenny CJ, Koperski M, Page M, et al. GP pocket guide to NIDDM. London: Medical Imprint; 1995.

24. Minerva. BMJ 1997; 314:1634.

25. Close C. Take action against diabetes. Medical Monitor 1997; 10:54–56.

26. Minerva. BMJ 2001; 322:564.

27. British Cardiac Society, British Hyperlipidaemia Association, British Hypertension Society, British Diabetic Association. Joint British recommendations on prevention of coronary heart disease in clinical practice: summary. BMJ 2000; 320:705–708.

2. Diabetic nephropathy

THIS CHAPTER REVIEWS

- The significance of microalbuminuria.
- The natural history and causes of nephropathy.
- The management of patients with microalbuminuria and nephropathy.
- The links between hypertension and nephropathy.
- The management of renal failure in patients with diabetes.
- The prevention of nephropathy.
- Prevalence.

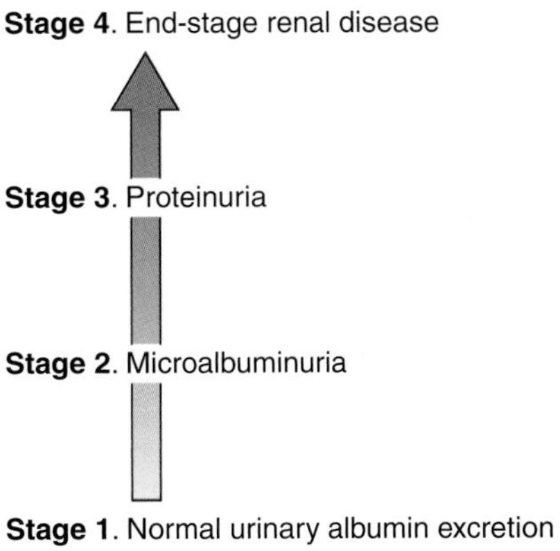

Stage 4. End-stage renal disease

Stage 3. Proteinuria

Stage 2. Microalbuminuria

Stage 1. Normal urinary albumin excretion

Figure 2.1 The four stages of nephropathy.

Microalbuminuria (incipient diabetic nephropathy), proteinuria and end-stage renal disease (ESRD) are related to the length of time that a patient has had diabetes – the longer the duration of the condition the higher the prevalence. The four stages of nephropathy are illustrated in Figure 2.1.

About a third of patients with type 1 diabetes have proteinuria after 20 years, while there is a cumulative incidence of incipient diabetic nephropathy with persistent microalbuminuria of 23% in white patients with type 2 diabetes.[1]

The likelihood of nephropathy varies with ethnic origin; black patients are more likely than white patients to have the condition. Patients with type 2 diabetes and nephropathy are less likely to progress to ESRD than are patients with type 1 diabetes.

Aetiology

Diabetic nephropathy is a microvascular complication of diabetes. It is caused by a thickening of the glomerular basement membrane, which eventually leads to a decrease in the ability of the kidney to filter and thus to a decline in

glomerular filtration rate. It can affect patients with both type 1 and type 2 diabetes and is the leading cause of ESRD in Europe and the USA. Optimal diabetes control significantly decreases the risk.

Presentation

The early stages of diabetic nephropathy have no warning symptoms or signs. At some point patients will develop microalbuminuria, which may be detected by estimating the urinary albumen/creatinine ratio. The presence of microalbuminuria is consistent with a urinary albumen excretion rate of between 30 and 299 mg every 24 hours. By the time proteinuria can be detected using a dipstick, there is more than 0.5 g/day of total protein in the urine. Proteinuria may initially be intermittent for several years, so regular tests are essential.

Patients with diabetes who attend for check-ups and monitoring should have urinalysis at least once a year. Patients presenting with type 1 diabetes should be tested ▸

7

for microalbuminuria within 12 months, as the condition may be detected only 1 year after diagnosis.[2]

Patients with type 2 diabetes should be screened for microalbuminuria at diagnosis and annually thereafter. Some will already have microalbuminuria at the time of diagnosis because the condition may have been present for many years before initial presentation.

False-positive results do occur. Temporary microalbuminuria can be precipitated by vigorous exercise and acute illness, as well as short-term hyperglycaemia and urinary tract infections. Infection should therefore be excluded by midstream urine culture, and a diagnosis of microalbuminuria should only be made conclusively after two or three positive tests for either microalbuminuria or macroalbuminuria over a period of 3–6 months.

Patients with proteinuria on dipstick testing, once a urinary tract infection has been excluded, should collect urine over a 24-hour period to help quantify the exact amount of protein excretion.

Significance and prognosis

Microalbuminuria shows that the patient is at increased risk of developing overt proteinuria. Patients are at increased risk of developing microangiopathy and macroangiopathy. They are also more likely to die prematurely than diabetic patients who do not have nephropathy: microalbuminuria is a marker for a greatly increased risk of death from ischaemic heart disease.

Most of the excess mortality linked to diabetes, as compared with the non-diabetic population, is related to proteinuria. About two-thirds of patients with proteinuria develop renal failure or ESRD, while the other third die from cardiovascular disease.[3]

As treatment and interventions for ischaemic heart disease become more effective it is likely that the incidence of ESRD will rise. Because nephropathy is linked to poor blood sugar control, patients with the condition are also likely to have widespread macrovascular disease, severe retinopathy and neuropathy. Patients who do not have hypertension initially will almost certainly develop high blood pressure as their renal function deteriorates.

Once overt nephropathy has occurred the glomerular filtration rate will fall at a rate that varies from individual to individual over the years.

Fifty percent of patients with type 1 diabetes and overt nephropathy will progress to ESRD within 10 years and

75% will do so within 20 years. Only 20% of patients with type 2 diabetes will progress to ESRD by 20 years.[4]

Contributory factors

Nephropathy is partly due to inadequate diabetes control, resulting in prolonged or persistent hyperglycaemia, and partly the result of a genetic disposition. Hypercholesterolaemia is also a risk factor for nephropathy. Increased blood pressure and smoking have been shown to be risk factors in patients with type 1 diabetes.[5] However, recent evidence suggests there is no link between development of nephropathy and obesity, pre-existing ischaemic heart disease, arterial blood pressure and a history of smoking in patients with type 2 diabetes.[1]

Follow-up

Once a patient has been found to have microalbuminuria it is important that the following investigations are carried out regularly:

- urinary albumin
- serum urea and electrolytes
- serum HBA_{1c}
- serum lipids.

A diabetic patient who attends for an annual check-up will have had these investigations performed at least once a year, but they should be carried out more regularly once there are signs of renal compromise.

Management

Optimum blood sugar control can help to prevent the progression of microalbuminuria to overt diabetic nephropathy in patients with both type 1 and type 2 diabetes.[4,6] Insulin treatment may be beneficial for some patients with type 2 diabetes (Fig. 2.2).[2]

Hyperlipidaemia should be controlled and other cardiovascular risk factors discussed with the patient. Those who smoke should be aware of the dangers, and overweight patients should be offered advice by a dietician. Although this information may have been offered at an earlier stage, the development of a complication like nephropathy can precipitate a change in lifestyle.

Without specific management, up to 40% of patients with type 2 diabetes and microalbuminuria will progress to overt nephropathy.

it is now standard practice to prescribe an ACE inhibitor in the early stages of nephropathy.

Patients with deteriorating renal function who are not already being looked after in secondary care should be referred to a diabetologist and possibly also a renal physician.

Hypertension and nephropathy

As both high systolic and diastolic blood pressure accelerate the progression of microalbuminuria to overt nephropathy, aggressive treatment of hypertension is fundamental in the management of these patients. In type 1 diabetes, hypertension is usually caused by underlying nephropathy, and is often diagnosed at the same time as microalbuminuria. About one-third of patients with type 2 diabetes are hypertensive when their diabetes is diagnosed, and this may be due to underlying nephropathy, essential hypertension or renal vascular disease.[10]

The most recent British Hypertension Society guidelines for the treatment of hypertension in patients with diabetes are given in Table 2.1. Many patients require a combination of an ACE inhibitor and one or more other drugs to control their blood pressure. Calcium channel blockers are useful add-on drugs that have been shown to slow deterioration in renal function; they may also be used alone if an ACE inhibitor is contraindicated.[11]

Renal failure

The serum creatinine level is an indication of the degree of renal failure. The level does not increase until the glomerular filtration rate has fallen by 50–70%. Increasing renal failure affects the renal clearance of drugs and insulin requirements will drop in patients with type 1 diabetes.

As metformin and most sulphonylureas are excreted by the kidneys, they begin to accumulate, causing renal failure, hypoglycaemia and other toxic effects. Therefore patients with uraemia and type 2 disease should be switched to insulin once their serum creatinine level is greater than 200 µg/l.

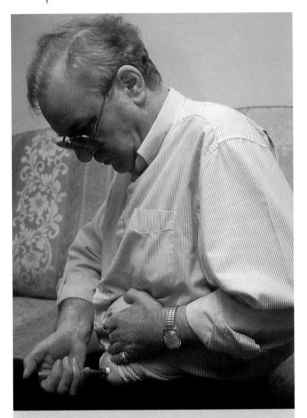

Figure 2.2 Patient injecting himself. Reproduced with permission from the Mike Wyndham Picture Library.

The drug treatment of choice for both microalbuminuria and proteinuria, whether or not there is associated hypertension, is an angiotensin-converting enzyme (ACE) inhibitor. Trial results have shown that ramipril can be beneficial.[7]

ACE inhibitors reduce urinary albumen excretion, and halt progression from microalbuminuria to frank proteinuria.[8,9] Although their long-term effect on renal function is unclear,

Table 2.1 The British Hypertension Society blood pressure targets for patients with diabetes

	Home monitoring	In clinic
Optimal pressure	<130/75	<140/85
Audit standard	<140/80	140/85

All patients with renal failure should be on low protein diets. Some patients with renal failure are suitable for treatment by haemodialysis, continuous ambulatory peritoneal dialysis (CAPD) or renal transplantation. Patients with co-existing ischaemic heart disease are usually managed by dialysis, as they respond poorly to kidney transplants. A renal transplant is usually only considered if the patient is under 60 years old and has a serum creatinine above 500 µg/l. CAPD is the treatment of choice for the elderly.

Conclusion

The United Kingdom Prospective Diabetes Study (UKPDS) has shown conclusively that intensive treatment and optimum glycaemic control can significantly reduce the risk of developing microalbuminuria and overt nephropathy, as well as other complications in patients with diabetes.[12] Similar results have been reported in patients with type 1 disease.[13]

Key points

- Patients with diabetes should be screened annually for microalbuminuria.
- Microalbuminuria is a marker of microvascular disease in patients with diabetes. It is also associated with a risk of developing ischaemic heart disease and a raised mortality.
- Microalbuminuria usually progresses to proteinuria and then end-stage renal disease unless treated.
- Patients with microalbuminuria or overt nephropathy should be started on an ACE inhibitor.
- Hypertension should be treated aggressively to prevent or slow nephropathy.

Resources

British Hypertension Society. Available at: http://www.hyp.ac.uk/bhs/gl2000.htm 2000

References

1. Gall M-A, Hougaard P, Boch-Johnsen K, et al. Risk factors for development of incipient and overt diabetic nephropathy in patients with non-insulin dependent diabetes mellitus: prospective, observational study. BMJ 1997; 314:783–788.

2. Bennett PH, Haffner S, Bertram, et al. Screening and management of microalbuminuria in patients with diabetes mellitus. Am J Kid Dis 1995; 25:107–112.

3. Williams G, Pickup JC. Handbook of diabetes. 2nd edn. Oxford: Blackwell Science; 1999.

4. American Diabetes Association. Clinical practice recommendations: diabetic nephropathy. Diabetes Care 2000; 23(suppl 1).

5. Microalbuminuria Collaborative Study Group, United Kingdom. Risk factors for the development of microalbuminuria in patients with insulin dependent diabetes. BMJ 1993; 306:1235–1239.

6. Wang PH, Lau J, Chalmers TC. Meta-analysis of effects of intensive blood glucose control on late complications of type 1 diabetes. Lancet 1993; 341:1306–1309.

7. Heart Outcomes Prevention Evaluation (HOPE) Study Investigators. Effects of ramipril on cardiovascular and microvascular outcomes in people with diabetes mellitus: results of the HOPE study and the MICRO-HOPE substudy. Lancet 2000; 355: 253–259.

8. Viberti GC, Mogensen CE, Groop L, et al. Effect of captopril on progression to clinical proteinuria in normotensive patients with microalbuminuria. JAMA 1994; 271:275–279.

9. Ravid M, Savin H, Jutrin I, et al. Long-term stabilizing effect of angiotensin-converting enzyme inhibition on plasma creatinine and on proteinuria in normotensive type 2 diabetic patients. Ann Intern Med 1993; 118:577–581.

10. Teuscher A, Egger M, Herman JB. Diabetes and hypertension: blood pressure in clinical diabetic patients and control population. Arch Intern Med 1989; 149:1942–1945.

11. Cooper ME. Pathogenesis, prevention and treatment of diabetic nephropathy. Lancet 1998; 352:213–218.

12. UK Prospective Diabetes Study Group. Intensive blood-glucose control with sulphonylureas or insulin compared with conventional treatment in patients with type 2 diabetes. Lancet 1998; 352:837–853.

13. The Diabetes Control and Complications Trial Research Group. The effect of intensive treatment of diabetes on the development and progression of long-term complications in insulin-dependent diabetes mellitus. New Engl J Med 1993; 329:977–986.

3. Obesity

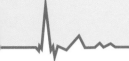

D Brooks

THIS CHAPTER REVIEWS

- The increasing prevalence of obesity.
- The known causative factors.
- The role of the primary healthcare team in addressing the problem.
- The range of possible interventions and the importance of follow-up.
- The role of other agencies.

Prevalence

Most adults in England are overweight and one in five is obese. The prevalence has trebled since 1980, and there is no sign that it is moderating. Each year, 30,000 premature deaths can be linked to obesity. It costs the NHS £500 million annually in patient care and £2 billion in sickness absence.

Obese people are at increased risk of serious disease, such as heart disease and diabetes, but even modest weight losses may produce important health benefits.

Definition

Obesity is most commonly defined in terms of body mass index (BMI):

$$BMI = weight\ (kg)/height^2\ (m^2)$$

Risks associated with different BMI values are given in Table 3.1.

Waist circumference is relevant, as it indicates the accumulation of abdominal fat. A high proportion of abdominal fat (apple, or male, pattern) is a risk factor. A high proportion of fat on the buttocks and thighs (pear, or female, pattern) does not appear to be a major risk factor. Men with a waist circumference greater than 94 cm and women with a waist circumference greater than 81 cm would benefit from losing weight. A waist/hip ratio of 0.95 or more for men and 0.85 or more for women indicates an increased risk of obesity-related diseases.

Epidemiology and risk factors

- Obesity develops as a result of an interaction between genetic disposition and lifestyle. Social, behavioural, cultural, psychological, metabolic and genetic factors are involved.

Table 3.1 Risk table: classification of different BMI values and their relationship with associated diseases[1]

BMI	Classification	Risk of disease
Over 20–25	Desirable range	Average
Over 25–30	Overweight	Increased
Over 30–35	Obese (class 1)	Moderate
Over 35–40	Obese (class 2)	Severe
Over 40	Morbidly obese (class 3)	Very severe

- Obesity in the population increases with age, although prevalence among schoolchildren is increasing.
- Lower socio-economic groups are at higher risk. The age-standardized prevalence of obesity in women is 21% in social class 5 compared with 12% in social class 1.
- Prevalence is higher in certain ethnic minority groups. South Asians are at greater risk when compared with Afro-Caribbeans and Caucasians.
- Risk is greater in people with learning difficulties, such as Down's syndrome.
- Smoking cessation is associated with higher risk.
- Children in families where one or more parents are overweight or obese are at greater risk of developing the condition.[1,2]

Health consequences

Cardiovascular disease

- Obesity increases the risk of cardiovascular disease, including stroke, left ventricular hypertrophy, arrhythmias, chronic heart failure, myocardial infarction, angina and peripheral vascular disease.
- Mortality as a result of cardiovascular disease is almost 50% higher in obese patients than in those of average weight, and is 90% higher in those with severe obesity.[3]
- Sixty percent of obese patients have hypertension. Weight loss reduces hypertension.[4]

Diabetes

- Prevalence of diabetes is 2.9 times higher in overweight patients.[3]
- About 80% of people with type 2 diabetes are obese.[1,2]
- Type 2 diabetes has recently been described in obese Caucasian teenagers, and had already been noted in Asian and African children.[5]

Arthritis and joint problems

- Prevalence of osteoarthritis increases with increasing weight.[6]
- Mechanical problems with hips and knees increase with weight.

Cancer

- Obese women have increased risk of cancer of the breast, uterus, cervix, ovary and gallbladder.

- Overweight men have an increased risk of colorectal and prostate cancers.[7]

Other problems

- Other problems include gallstones and obstructive sleep apnoea.[2]

Management of obesity

Diet and exercise

Diet alone is not helpful over the longer term; more than 90% of people who attempt to lose weight gain it back. Diet associated with exercise and behavioural and cognitive therapy may be more effective.[2]

Weight gain is dependent on a person's energy intake being greater than their energy expenditure. One pound (0.45 kg) is equal to 3500 calories; a person consuming 500 more calories than he or she expends daily will gain 0.45 kg each week.

Body weight tends to range within 10% of a set value. Weight alterations cause changes in energy expenditure that favour a return to the set point. This helps to explain the common problem of recidivism following attempted weight loss.[8]

A reasonable goal is to lose 10% of body mass over a 6-month period. People with a BMI in the range 27–35 should be encouraged to lose 0.25–0.5 kg a week at a daily calorie deficit of 300–500. People with a BMI above 35 should lose 0.5–1 kg a week at a daily calorie deficit of 500–1000. Total caloric intake is determined by calculating basic energy expenditure and activity, then subtracting 500 calories, to result in a weight loss of 0.45 kg a week.

This usually means a diet of 1000–1200 kcal/day for women and 1200–1500 kcal/day for men. Initial exercise goals should be moderate activity for 30–45 minutes each day. A long-term goal should be at least 30 minutes of activity each day.[8]

The diet recommended should be low in fat and total calories. A healthy diet contains 25% fat, 20% protein and 55% carbohydrates.[8]

Drugs

Various drugs have been used in the management of obesity. All must be considered as only part of a management plan.

Most of the drugs used are sympathomimetics, which are pharmacologically related to the amphetamines, and which suppress appetite centrally. They are not recommended, due to side-effects from central nervous system stimulation, abuse potential and problems with tolerance. They also raise blood pressure.

Older amphetamines and thyroxine are frequently prescribed by some private slimming clinics, and even patients with a normal BMI have been offered such prescriptions. Patients seeking to use such treatment should be strongly discouraged and advised on the risks entailed.

Two new agents, sibutramine (Reductil) and orlistat (Xenical), are available in England and Wales on the recommendation of the National Institute of Clinical Excellence (NICE).[9]

Sibutramine

Sibutramine is a serotonin/noradrenaline reuptake inhibitor, which enhances satiety. It is more effective than placebo at promoting weight loss in adults with a BMI between 25 and 40. It should be used as part of an overall treatment plan for the management of obesity for:

- people aged 18–65 years who have already made serious attempts to lose weight by dieting, exercise and/or changes in their behaviour, *and* who

- have a BMI of 27.0 or more as well as other significant disease (e.g. type 2 diabetes, high cholesterol) *or*

- have a BMI of 30.0 or more.

Treatment with sibutramine should continue beyond 4 weeks only if the patient has lost 2 kg in weight. They should continue on this treatment beyond 3 months only if they have lost at least 5% of their body weight from the start of the drug treatment. Sibutramine should be stopped if patients do not lose weight as described, and they should be considered non-responders. Treatment is not recommended for more than 12 months.

Sibutramine can lead to increases in blood pressure, so this should be checked regularly. It is not recommended for patients who already have high blood pressure (145/90 or above).

Orlistat

Orlistat is a lipase inhibitor. Mean weight loss achieved per year is 2–5 kg greater than that achieved with placebo. There is evidence that weight loss is sustained for over 12 months. The drug is licensed for use for up to 24 months.

Orlistat should be prescribed only to adults (18–75 years) who have a BMI of 28 and a significant disease, or who have a BMI of 30 without significant disease.

Before the drug is prescribed, the patient should have already lost at least 2.5 kg by diet and increased physical activity. Treatment should continue for more than 3 months only if the patient has lost at least 5% of his or her body mass from the start of drug treatment. It should continue for more than 6 months only if weight loss has been at least 10% of body weight. Other patients should be considered non-responders.

Surgery

Surgery has produced greater and more sustained weight loss than dietary or pharmacological therapy, although these methods have not been compared in randomized trials. Weight loss surgery is appropriate in people with class 3 obesity, or class 2 obesity with comorbid conditions, when diet, exercise and pharmacological therapy have failed and there is a high risk of obesity-related illness and death.

The most common gastric restriction procedure is the vertical banded gastroplasty, which involves partial partitioning of the stomach at the proximal segment. This narrows the lumen and causes early satiety. The most common gastric bypass procedure is the Roux-en-Y oesophagojejunostomy, in which a segment of jejunum is interposed between the oesophagus and the duodenum.

Joined-up management

As obesity is essentially a lifestyle problem, organizations other than those in the health sector must become involved if the problem is to be tackled effectively. The problem should be addressed in the young before obesity has developed. Diet and nutrition matter, especially in schools. Sponsorship deals with the fast-food industry may not be a good idea. Initiative pilots of free fruit in schools are an innovative idea.

The food industry and the food standards agency have an important role to play. What do 'low fat' and 'reduced fat' actually mean? Education is a priority. Sport and exercise facilities matter. Private health clubs are expensive. Facilities for cycling and walking are improving. The media have a role in providing information, encouragement and support. Poverty and obesity are linked in lower socio-economic groups and initiatives are needed here.

The NHS plan and the National Service Framework for Coronary Heart Disease include action to address the

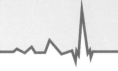

- Men with a waist circumference greater than 94 cm and women with a waist circumference greater than 81 cm would benefit from losing weight.
- Obesity is strongly linked to heart disease, type 2 diabetes, high blood pressure and osteoarthritis.
- Even modest weight losses may produce health benefits.
- Diet associated with exercise and behavioural and cognitive therapy may be more effective than diet alone.
- Surgery is effective in people with very severe obesity or obesity-associated diseases.

problem. The Health Survey for England provides information about trends in eating habits, height, weight and body shape.[1]

Follow-up

As relapse is so common, follow-up is very important. Longer term follow-up and the use of maintenance interventions to sustain weight loss are needed.

Role of the primary healthcare team

Members of the primary healthcare team may feel frustrated when dealing with patients with weight problems because treatment is long term and relapse common. Practice nurses, dieticians, health visitors and school nurses can play an important role in identifying patients with weight problems and providing support. Family therapy may be helpful in high-risk groups. Exercise-on-prescription programmes are being developed. Primary care trusts must ensure that the team is adequately resourced.

Key points

- **20% of English adults are obese and this is increasing.**
- **Obesity often begins in childhood, and more is needed to tackle it there.**

References

1. House of Commons. Select Committee on Public Accounts, 9th Report, Jan 2002.

2. NHS Centre for Reviews and Dissemination. The prevalence and treatment of obesity. Effective Health Care 1997; 3.

3. American Association of Clinical Endocrinologists Obesity Task Force on Obesity. Endocrine Practice 1998; 4:297–323.

4. Van Itallie TB. Health implications of overweight and obesity in the United States. Ann Intern Med 1985; 103:983–988.

5. Dyer O. First case of type 2 diabetes found in white UK teenagers. BMJ 2002; 324:506.

6. Huang Z, Willett WC, Manson JE, et al. Body weight. Weight change and risk for hypertension in women. Ann Intern Med 1998; 1–8:81–88.

7. Pi-Sunyer FX. Medical hazards of obesity. Ann Intern Med 1983; 119:655–660.

8. Wolf C, Tanner M. Best practice. Obesity. Western J Med 2002; 176:23–28.

9. Wise J. Obesity drug endorsed by NICE. BMJ 2001; 322:627.

4. Diabetes in children

M Selby

THIS CHAPTER REVIEWS

- The presentation of diabetes in children.
- The management of diabetes in children.
- The role of the GP in managing diabetes in children.
- Acute illness rules for diabetic children.

Prevalence

Diabetes mellitus affects 2 children per 1000 in the UK. Most are managed by hospital-based diabetic teams, but GPs should have a working knowledge of their management and a high index of suspicion for new presentations.

The prevalence of diabetes is increasing in children and increases with age.[1]

Almost all affected children have type 1 (insulin dependent) diabetes. There is a rare subgroup with maturity-onset diabetes of the young, an insulin-resistant non-ketotic form which has recently been described for the first time in Caucasian adolescents and has been seen in the past in adolescents of Asian descent.

Aetiology

Genetic and environmental factors play a part: there is 30–50% concordance in identical twins. A child with a diabetic mother has a 1 in 40–80 chance of developing diabetes, and for a child with a with a diabetic father the chance is 1 in 20–40.

Viral infections and dietary factors may trigger islet cell destruction in those affected, and there is an association with autoimmune disease.[2]

Presentation

Initial postprandial hyperglycaemia progresses to sustained hyperglycaemia. Presentation may be:

- subacute, with polydipsia, polyuria, weight loss, skin infections, enuresis/nocturia or tiredness and malaise
- late and acute with ketoacidosis, when there may be a precipitating concurrent illness.

Parents may have thought that weight loss is due to dieting or an eating disorder, and the whole picture may be of several months duration.

Ketoacidosis (Box 4.1) always requires urgent admission.

Diagnosis

Diagnosis is confirmed by a random blood glucose of more than 11.1.

A fasting plasma glucose >7.0 or a raised HbA_{1c} also confirms diabetes. Glucose tolerance testing is rarely necessary in children.

Any child in whom diabetes is suspected should be seen acutely in hospital for confirmation and initiation of treatment, even if well.

Box 4.1 Presentation of ketoacidosis

- Dehydration
- Vomiting bile
- Abdominal pain
- Hypovolaemia, shock
- Sighing (Kussmaul) breathing
- Impaired consciousness
- Ketotic breath (pear drops)
- Moderate/large ketonuria

News of the diagnosis is usually broken in hospital. Parents and children are often shocked and distressed, but it is extraordinary how quickly most get to grips with managing their disease.

Treatment: insulin regimens

Children are treated with insulin from the start. The usual regimen is twice daily subcutaneous insulin, with about two-thirds of the dose given in the morning, and one-third before tea (Box 4.2). Fixed mixtures of fast- (actrapid) and medium-acting (isophane) insulins are used, and these are available in various proportions of actrapid/isophane. Prepubertal children generally start on a 10/90 mix, with the proportion of actrapid being increased around puberty.

Older teenagers may move to a long-acting baseline insulin with actrapid three times daily. Actrapid is given 20 minutes before eating, but the recent development of rapid-acting insulins has made a big difference to some children. These preparations can be given during or even just after a meal, so that faddy eaters can have their insulin tailored to their appetite.

Blood testing

Children test their blood sugar four times daily until control is established. The aim is to keep blood glucose in the range 4–10.

Tests need to be more than 2 hours after the last snack, and children are given a glucometer with a memory store, and a diary to record readings. Many paediatric diabetic teams supply glucometers from donated funds, as they are not available on FP10.

Target of blood sugar control

An HbA_{1c} level of 6.5–7.5% is the aim in children. If it is higher than this, the child is getting either too little insulin or

too much food. Later the two factors are distinguishable by whether the child's weight gain is normal. Children who run high but fail to gain weight are getting insufficient insulin.

A low HbA_{1c} can mean that control is too tight. These children may become insensitive to hypos and there is the concern of cognitive impairment, particularly in the under fives.

Injecting: sites and technique

Injections are commenced by syringe, with emphasis on teaching self-reliance early. Parents and older children are taught to do injections and finger-prick testing. Children aged 7–8 years often do some of their injections and tests.

The optimal needle length is around 5 mm. Standard needles are 12.6 and 8 mm.

Injections are given perpendicular to the skin (Figs 4.1 and 4.2), without pinching, and injection sites must be rotated to avoid getting lumps. Injection into lumps or bruises should be avoided, although they may be less sensitive, as insulin is not released evenly from lumps. Rubbing skin briefly with ice may help with pain.

Pen devices are introduced early, as they have finer, shorter needles (5 mm). Pens are bulkier than syringes, so young children cannot usually hold them in one hand and depress the plunger. Injecting is less painful, but takes longer due to the fine bore of the needle.

Management

Lifestyle

Diet

Diet should be high in fibre, including five portions of fruit or vegetables a day, and low in sugary foods, to release carbohydrate as evenly as possibly throughout the day. This means three main meals and three snacks daily. A dietician will provide ongoing advice.

Exercise

Regular exercise improves cardiovascular fitness and diabetic control. Diabetic children should particularly be encouraged to exercise, because of the potential risks to their future health if they become unfit.

Clinic review

Children are usually reviewed three monthly for HbA_{1c}, growth check and insulin review. Annually, the team inspect the fundi and feet, check the urine albumin/creatinine ratio and blood pressure, and review management over the previous year. A coeliac screen is performed annually – children with coeliac disease and diabetes often have a history of unexplained hypos (Box 4.3), and around 1 in 40 diabetic children develop coeliac disease.

Troubleshooting

Illness and crisis management

The day to day management of variations in diabetic control passes to the child and their parents, who will soon see ▸

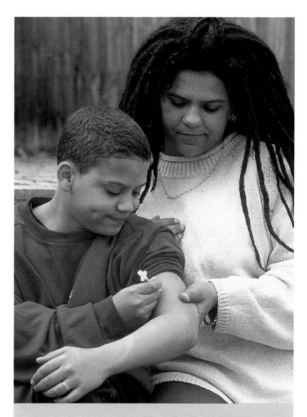

Figure 4.2 Pen injector devices, with their finer, shorter needles, cause less pain than standard syringes of the type shown here. Introduced early in child diabetes management, pen devices can now be prescribed on the FP10. Reproduced from Selby, *Update*, 16 August 2001.

Box 4.3 Hypos

- A hypo is defined as a blood sugar level <4.
- Typically, the patient feels sweaty, has 'jelly-legs', feels dizzy and has poor concentration.
- Parents may notice that the child is pale, bad tempered and confused.
- At night the child may wake or be heard thrashing around. Baby alarms may be useful.
- Children who feel hypo when their blood sugar is >4 are probably running high much of the time, and have become sensitive to small drops in blood sugar level.
- Children who are insensitive to true hypos are probably running too low.

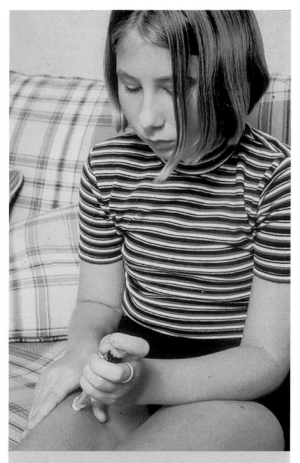

Figure 4.1 Injections are given perpendicular to the skin and injection sites must be varied to avoid causing lumps. The outer thighs are the most popular site, but the upper arms, bottom and lower abdomen may also be used. Reproduced from Selby, *Update*, 16 August 2001.

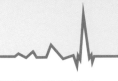

Box 4.4 Basic rules

1. **In the well child** hyperglycaemia is not dangerous. A well child without ketonuria can have their blood sugar brought down gradually, *ideally by extra exercise*. Get the child to increase their activity levels before the next test. If the blood glucose level is still >14, with the next dose of insulin give an additional 10% of the due dose as actrapid (20% if the blood sugar is >22).

2. **In the sick child** the rules are slightly different.

   (a) **In an unwell child who is not vomiting:**
   - Check the blood glucose at least 4 hourly and monitor urine for ketones. *Never omit the insulin in an ill child.*
   - If the blood sugar is <5 give half the usual insulin dose.
   - If the blood sugar is 5–14 give the usual insulin dose.
   - If the blood sugar is 14–22 continue the usual insulin dose and give an additional 5-10% of the total daily dose as actrapid before each meal and at bedtime.
   - For blood sugars >22, the regimen is as above,

   but give an additional 10–20% of the total daily insulin dose as actrapid before meals and at bedtime.
   - If bedtime actrapid is given, parents should check for hypo 2 hours later.

   (b) **In an unwell child who is vomiting:**
   - Push dioralyte. Even a vomiting child will absorb some by small sips.
   - If blood sugars are less than 14 in a vomiting child, give half the usual insulin dose.
   - Even if blood sugars are <5 still give the half the usual insulin, but add 1-2 teaspoons of sugar to each dioralyte sachet. If the blood sugar does not rise despite attempts to correct it with dioralyte and sugar, admit the child for intravenous fluids.
   - For blood sugar >14, follow the rules for non-vomiting.
   - Admit ill children with signs of diabetic ketoacidosis (DKA), increasing blood sugar or ketonuria.

---

that the same insulin dose may produce a different pattern of response on different days.

Blood sugar control is not a simple equation of matching insulin units to blood glucose. It depends on diet, health and recent control. For example, a day of heavy activity may deplete carbohydrate stores in the liver, causing apparently unexplained hypos the next day (if one does not consider the previous day's events). High blood sugars may be rebound high readings from an earlier hypo.

Parents should ideally use the diabetic team for advice on managing these day to day problems, but GPs may wish to know some simple crisis rules (Boxes 4.4 to 4.6).

Psychological problems and adolescence

Children may rebel against their diabetes at any age and in various ways. Fears of hypos are common, leading to running very high or repeated unnecessary testing.

Problems often occur in adolescence. This time of self-assertion and rebellion is difficult for children with chronic illness, and diabetes is particularly hard as there can be no day's respite. Puberty may be delayed, feeling different affects self-esteem, and fear of complications may surface as the child becomes more aware. Teenagers may discover

that there is no instant price for eating junk food and not altering their insulin, and may try to conform with their peers in this way. Eating disorders may be manifested by refusing to increase insulin in line with food intake, or by reducing food and insulin intake. If weight loss or gain is a problem, close liaison with a dietician is essential.

Many children will at some point read or hear about the late medical complications of diabetes, and become distressed and afraid. Sensitive handling and discussion about the importance of good control is essential.

Box 4.5 Tempting snacks for ill diabetic children

- Small glass of Lucozade
- Fruit yoghurt
- Thick soup with one slice of bread
- Cereal with milk
- Jelly with ice cream
- One slice of toast with jam
- Glass of milk with two biscuits

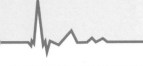

Box 4.6 Aims of management

Short-term aims
- Maintain blood sugar in the range 4–10 and HbA_{1c} in the range 6.5–7.5%
- Avoid hypos
- Educate
- Encourage self-reliance

Long-term aims
- Good control
- Normal growth
- Normal life
- Self-reliance
- Prevent complications
- Good health behaviour
- Good level of exercise

Diabetes UK offers help, support and information, with newsletters and information sheets, together with holidays for diabetic children and teenagers.

Key points
- **The prevalence of diabetes in children is 2% and increasing.**

- Most children are managed by hospital teams, but the GP needs to be aware of some simple illness rules.
- Diet, exercise and self-reliance are encouraged.
- Treatment is always with insulin.
- Children who consistently run high will feel hypo at normal blood sugar levels, exacerbating the problem.
- Children whose control is too tight may become insensitive to genuine hypos.
- Coeliac disease is common in diabetic children.
- Good control needs to be established in childhood to minimize complications in adulthood.

References

1. Metcalfe MA, Baum JD. Incidence of IDDM in children aged under 15 years in the British Isles during 1988. BMJ 1991; 302:443–447.

2. Saukkonen T, Savilahti E, Reijonen H, et al. Coeliac disease: frequent occurrence after onset of IDDM. Childhood Diabetes in Finland Study Group. Diabetic Medicine 1996; 13(5):464–470.

3. Lissauer T, Clayden G. Textbook of paediatrics, ch 22. Endocrine and metabolic disorders. London: Mosby; 1997.

4. Noble-Jamieson C, Rycroft N, Thompson AMS. Diabetes information sheets. Bury St Edmunds, Suffolk: West Suffolk Hospital; June 1998 (personal communication).

5. Thyroid disease

E Warren

Three forms of thyroid disease are seen in general practice: underactivity (hypothyroidism or myxoedema), overactivity (hyperthyroidism) and thyroid swellings, which may be associated with abnormal function of the gland.

Although hypothyroidism can usually be managed successfully in primary care, patients with an overactive thyroid should be referred. Thyroid swelling always calls for function testing.

Hypothyroidism

Hypothyroidism has a prevalence of 2% in women (0.2% in men).[1,2] This rises to 6% in women aged over 60 years and the peak incidence of new cases is at 70 years of age. The disease is rare before 30 years of age. The clinical features of the condition are outlined in Box 5.1.[3]

Causes

Most people in the UK now have enough iodine in their diet, so the main causes of primary hypothyroidism are chronic autoimmune thyroiditis (Hashimoto's thyroiditis or atrophic thyroiditis[3]) and destructive treatments for hyperthyroidism.[4] Drugs such as lithium and amiodarone can also cause primary thyroid failure.

Hypothyroidism secondary to pituitary failure is very much rarer, and is usually associated with panhypopituitrism

Box 5.1 Clinical features of hypothyroidism

- Lethargy
- Sleepiness
- Poor appetite
- Constipation
- Weight gain
- Dry skin, possibly with yellow tinge
- Dry hair and hair loss
- Puffiness around eyes
- Stiff or aching muscles
- Feeling the cold
- Hearing impairment
- Poor memory
- Associated disorders include carpal tunnel syndrome, ataxia, intellectual sluggishness
- Bradycardia
- Pericardial effusion with muffled heart sounds
- Thyroid gland may be palpable
- Menorrhagia is a rare presentation
- Many of the symptoms are non-specific (lack of energy, weight gain, stiff and aching muscles) and are also common in people who do not have thyroid disease

rather than just failure of thyroid stimulating hormone (TSH) production.

Investigation

Suspected hypothyroidism should be biochemically confirmed.[5] A low thyroxine (T4) level and an elevated TSH confirms primary hypothyroidism. Low levels of both confirm secondary hypothyroidism.

Individuals with TSH at the upper limit of normal or higher may feel better in a non-specific way if started on thyroxine.[6]

Treatment

Thyroxine is the treatment of choice.[5] Symptoms should improve within 3 weeks of starting treatment,[7] but can take up to 3 months. Improvement usually occurs when T4 is normal or a bit high, and TSH is normal or a bit low.[5] This represents slight overtreatment, but it appears to do no harm.[7]

A sizeable proportion of patients continue to report convincing symptoms of hypothyroidism despite being biochemicallly euthyroid. There is a school of thought advocating increasing thyroxine dose until symptoms resolve,[8] and one study reported maximal symptomatic benefit only when TSH is suprressed to <0.02 mU/l.[9] There remains, however, insufficient evidence to recommend this at present, due to the risks associated with an iatrogenic hyperthyroid state, including osteoporosis and atrial fibrillation.

When patients with angina start thyroxine, their angina may worsen, or they may suffer myocardial infarction or even sudden death. Start with low doses and increase slowly.

Start with a single daily dose of 50–100 µg (25 µg in elderly patients). Check the TSH again after 6 weeks. If it is still elevated, cautiously increase the daily dose.

Thyroxine treatment is usually lifelong, with thyroid function being checked every 12–18 months. However, the hypothyroid state may be transient in postpartum thyroiditis and after treatment for hyperthyroidism. In such cases, treat for 6 months, and then stop for a month before checking thyroid function.[7]

Patients on thyroxine treatment are entitled to free prescriptions and should apply for a medical exemption certificate using a form countersigned by their doctor.

Referral

Most cases of hypothyroidism can be managed without specialist involvement. The exceptions are:[5]

- children under 16 years old
- patients with evidence of pituitary disease (low TSH)
- newborn babies (congenital hypothyroidism has an incidence of 1 in 4000 and is associated with developmental delay)
- patients with complicating problems, such as ischaemic heart disease
- during pregnancy or postpartum.

Pregnant women need extra thyroxine (about 50 µg on top of their usual daily dose). Thyroid function should be checked each trimester.[6] Babies of hypothyroid mothers may suffer neurodevelopmental problems during gestation, even if they have no detectable thyroid abnormality at birth.

Subclinical hypothyroidism

Some patients (including up to 10% of women aged 55–60 years) have a normal T4 and an elevated TSH, and no symptoms. This is more common after iodine-131 treatment or surgery for hyperthyroidism.[5]

If a high TSH is found, check the thyroid peroxidase antibodies. If the test is positive for thyroid peroxidase, there is an autoimmune process going on and the patient's chance of developing overt hypothyroidism is over 5% a year. Start thyroxine.

If the test is negative, the conversion rate to overt hypothyroidism is under 3% a year and the elevated TSH may not last. Surveillance is appropriate. Start thyroxine if the TSH is above 10 mU/l.[5]

Hyperthyroidism

The prevalence of hyperthyroidism is 2% of women and 0.2% of men. The incidence of new cases is spread over all age groups.[1,2]

Box 5.2 Clinical features of hyperthyroidism

- Goitre: diffuse goitre suggests Grave's disease, nodular goitre suggests toxic nodular goitre
- Sinus tachycardia: atrial fibrillation and heart failure may occur
- Weight loss
- Sweating
- Palpitations
- Agitation
- Eyelid lag and retraction
- Pruritus
- Diarrhoea
- Hyperkinetic activity
- Ophthalmopathy (periorbital swelling, proptosis and diplopia are present in 50% of Graves disease patients and require prompt attention)
- Clubbing of fingers with periosteal new bone formation (Graves acropathy)
- High output heart failure
- Acute thyrotoxic storm (rare)
- Lethargy (common in the elderly hyperthyroid patient)

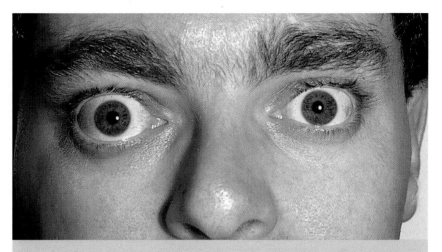

Figure 5.1 Hyperthyroidism. Exophthalmic eye signs of hyperthyroidism in 43-year-old man with 6-month history of hyperthyroidism. His family had noticed his increasingly staring eyes. He had proptosis and lid lag. Reproduced with permission from Burkitt & Quick, *Essential Surgery*, 3rd edn, Churchill Livingstone, 2001.

The clinical features of hyperthyroidism are outlined in Box 5.2.[4,10] The diagnosis is confirmed by an elevated T4 and a below normal TSH. It usually presents insidiously, and there is great individual variation in dominant features (Fig. 5.1).

A high index of suspicion is necessary in the elderly, where the classic presentation may be subtle or absent, but it may precipitate heart failure or atrial fibrillation or cause worsening angina.

Thyrotoxic storm is an abrupt and severe exacerbation of thyrotoxicosis presenting acutely with tremor, tachycardia, fever, agitation, nausea and altered mental status. It may be precipitated by stress, is deeply unpleasant for the patient and requires admission for intravenous treatment.

Causes

The most common causes of hyperthyroidism are Graves disease (75%) and toxic nodular goitre. Graves disease is an autoimmune disease caused by the presence of antibodies to TSH receptors on the thyroid follicular cells. It usually affects women aged 30–50 years and presents with diffuse thyroid enlargement, ophthalmopathy and, rarely, pretibial myoedema.

Hyperthyroidism is occasionally caused by an autonomous thyroxine-secreting thyroid adenoma. Confusingly, thyroiditis may give rise to overactivity of the thyroid, although this is usually transient.

Amiodarone can also cause thyroid overactivity as well as underactivity.[3]

Treatment options

Almost all cases of hyperthyroidism are successfully treated, although most patients are left hypothyroid as a result.

Carbimazole

Carbimazole is often used, at least at first. After a few months, this usually causes hypothyroidism requiring thyroxine replacement (the block–replace regimen). The typical dose is carbimazole 20 mg twice daily, with thyroxine added back in after a period of 6–8 weeks.

Pruritis and rash are common in patients using carbimazole, but usually pass with time. Agranulocytosis, a more serious adverse effect, usually occurs within 3 months of starting treatment. The drug must be stopped and an urgent blood count arranged if there is sore throat or other infection.[4]

Iodine-131

Iodine-131 damages the thyroid and is a definitive treatment for hyperthyroidism. The treatment takes 3 months to work. By 2 years, 20% of patients need thyroxine replacement.

Surgery

Surgery is the other definitive treatment. Most patients with toxic nodular goitre who undergo surgery are left permanently euthyroid. The success rate of surgery in Graves disease is 80%, but permanent hypothyroidism occurs in 5–40% of cases.

Referral

All patients with confirmed hyperthyroidism benefit from referral to a specialist.[6] However, GPs may be called upon to discuss proposed treatments with patients, and will need to carry out follow-up.

Acute thyroid storm and acute atrial fibrillation require admission. Patients with atrial fibrillation secondary to hyperthyroidism have a high risk of embolic disease, which may also resolve when the thyroid function has been corrected. Warfarin and cardioversion therapy may be appropriate.

Subclinical hyperthyroidism

This is defined as a persisting low TSH with normal levels of T4 and tri-iodothyronine (T3, the active metabolite of thyroxine).[5] About 3% of people have TSH levels below the normal range, and in 1% the hormone is biochemically undetectable.[4]

Patients with subclinical hyperthyroidism are at higher risk of atrial fibrillation in their seventh decade. They are also more prone to osteoporosis, but are not more likely to have an osteoporotic fracture.[5] Treatment is not recommended in the absence of symptoms.[5]

Thyroid swellings

Diffuse benign goitre is very common and is usually of no significance other than cosmetically (Fig. 5.2). The prevalence is highest in premenopausal women (around 25%) and declines with age. It is four times more common in women than in men. Some of the causes are outlined in Box 5.3.

Thyroid nodules and multinodular goitres are more common with increasing age, affecting 3% of elderly women and 1% of elderly men. They can be difficult to differentiate clinically from diffuse goitre.

Solitary thyroid nodules are always a worry. About 5% are malignant, although thyroid cancer is relatively rare, with about 1000 new cases each year in the UK.

A nodule that develops in a man over 70 years of age is particularly worrying.

Suspicious features include:[3,11]

- goitre development before 20 years or after 60 years of age
- history of neck irradiation
- rapid tumour growth
- family history of thyroid cancer
- male patient
- clinical features such as a firm, non-tender nodule, local lymphadenopathy or recurrent laryngeal nerve palsy.

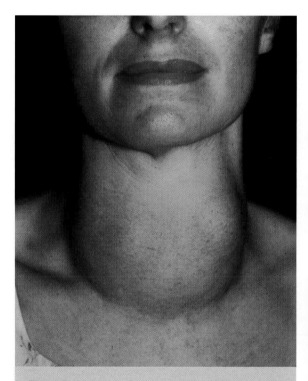

Figure 5.2 Longstanding multinodular goitre in a 40-year-old woman with a strong family history of thyroid disorders. The thyroid is multinodular on palpation and on ultrasound, there are multiple nodules of various sizes plus some small cysts. Any change in a multinodular goitre may herald malignancy. Reproduced with permission from Burkitt & Quick, *Essential Surgery*, 3rd edn, Churchill Livingstone, 2001.

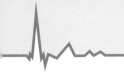

Box 5.3 Causes of benign goitre

- Simple colloid goitre
- Multinodular goitre
- Autoimmune thyroiditis
- Endemic iodine deficiency
- Goitrogens

Referral

Ultrasound of the thyroid will determine if enlargement is diffuse or nodular. A single nodule and/or a dominant or different nodule in a multinodular goitre are suspicious.[12]

All patients with thyroid swellings should have their thyroid function assessed.

Cold nodules (patient euthyroid) are more likely to be malignant than are toxic nodules, but a hot nodule can still be malignant.[11] Hard, fixed, growing or painful nodules are very suspicious. A definitive diagnosis can be fully confirmed only by fine-needle aspiration biopsy.

Most thyroid cancers have a good prognosis if treated promptly.

Diffuse thyroid enlargement does not need further investigation as long as there is no doubt that the goitre is benign, and the patient is happy with the management. If in doubt, refer.

Key points

- Hyperthyroidism and hypothyroidism are common disorders in general practice.
- Most hypothyroidism can be managed by the GP.
- Subclinical hypothyroidism may progress to overt disease. An estimate of thyroid peroxidase is helpful.
- Extra care is needed when using thyroxine in the elderly and those with angina.
- All hyperthyroidism should be referred.
- Most hyperthyroidism is due to Graves disease.
- Acute thyroid storm is rare but may present with agitation or psychosis.

- Consider thyroid disease in elderly patients with unexplained heart failure, atrial fibrillation or worsening angina.
- Up to a quarter of premenopausal women have a diffuse goitre.
- Clinical features suggesting thyroid cancer are a single or dominant nodule in a euthyroid patient.

References

1. Tunbridge WMG, Evered DC, Hall R, et al. The spectrum of thyroid disease in a community: the Whickham survey. Clin Epidemiol 1977; 7:481–493.

2. Vanderpump MPJ, Tunbridge WMG, French JM, et al. The incidence of thyroid disorders in the community: a 20 year follow-up of the Whickham survey. Clin Endocrinol 1995; 43:55–68.

3. Kendall-Taylor P. Thyroid disease: hypothyroidism and goitre. Update 1993; 46:757–763.

4. Tan T, Vanderpump M. Thyroid disease. General Practitioner 2000; 12 May:54–55.

5. Vanderpump MPJ, Ahlquist JAO, Franklyn JA, et al. Consensus statement for good practice and audit measures in the management of hypothyroidism and hyperthyroidism. BMJ 1996; 313:539–544.

6. Managing subclinical hypothyroidism. Drug Therapeut Bull 1998; 36:1–3.

7. Franklyn J. Prescribing thyroid hormones. Prescribers' J 996; 36:9–13.

8. Skinner GRB, Thomas R, Taylor M, et al. Thyroxine should be tried in clinically hyperthyroid but biochemically euthyroid patients. BMJ 1997; 314:1764.

9. Carr D, McLeod DT, Parry G, et al. Fine adjustment of thyroxine replacement dosage: comparison of the TRH test using a thyrotrophin assay with measurements of free thyroid hormones and clinical assessment. Clin Endocrinol 1988; 28:325–333.

10. Franklyn J. Thyroid disease. General Practitioner 1995; 3 Nov:53–56.

11. Jones MK. Management of thyroid nodular disease. BMJ 2001; 323:293–294.

12. Tan T, Vanderpump M. Thyroid disease. General Practitioner 2000; 19 May:54–55.

CORONARY HEART DISEASE

6. Hypertension

M Mead and JE Thistlethwaite

THIS CHAPTER REVIEWS

- The prevalence and diagnosis of hypertension.
- Which patients should be treated.
- How to assess a patient with hypertension.
- Measures for lowering blood pressure.
- Making a choice in drug treatment of hypertension.
- Follow-up of the patient with hypertension.
- Which patients should be referred.
- Involving the patient in their care.

Hypertension is one of the biggest killers in the UK today; it is a major risk factor for stroke, coronary heart disease (CHD) and heart failure. Hypertension is best thought of as a risk factor rather than a disease itself. Any patient with hypertension needs to be assessed for other CHD risk factors and the hypertension treated within the context of cardiovascular risk reduction.

We now know that the systolic blood pressure is a better guide to a patient's cardiovascular risk than is the diastolic blood pressure. In particular, isolated systolic hypertension (ISH) (systolic pressure 160 mmHg and diastolic pressure <90 mmHg) is worth treating in the elderly. For example, the SHEP trial of patients over the age of 60 years (average age 72 years) showed a 36% reduction in stroke incidence over 4.5 years as a result of diuretic treatment, which achieved an average drop of 12 mmHg in systolic blood pressure.[1] Trial evidence for treating hypertension in the elderly now extends beyond the age of 80 years.

Defining hypertension

We conventionally now define a 'normal' blood pressure in a non-diabetic adult as less than 140/90. This is an arbitrary cut-off point, since treatment even below these levels will reduce cardiovascular risk.

The audit standard of the British Hypertension Society guidelines (i.e. the minimum level to which blood pressure should be controlled) is less than 150/90, with the optimal target being less than 140/85. For patients with diabetes the audit standard is less than 140/85, with an optimal target of less than 140/80.[2]

Prevalence

The prevalence of high blood pressure within the community is alarming. In the Health Survey for England 1998,[3] 20% of adults (aged 16 years or over) had a systolic pressure >160 mmHg or a diastolic pressure >95 mmHg and 37% of adults had a systolic pressure >140 mmHg or a diastolic pressure >90 mmHg.

In older patients, hypertension is the rule rather than the exception. Over half of men and nearly two-thirds of women aged 70–79 years have a systolic pressure >160 mmHg or a diastolic pressure >95 mmHg.

Applying British Hypertension Society guidelines for treatment to the population of England, it has been estimated that 29.8% of the English population aged 35–74 years are candidates for antihypertensive therapy, of whom only 15.3% are currently being treated (i.e. an additional 14.5% of the English population aged 35–74 years need antihypertensive therapy).

Presentation

Hypertension is an asymptomatic condition. Even patients with severe hypertension are usually asymptomatic (except for the incredibly small number of patients with an hypertensive encephalopathy due to malignant hypertension). The most common presentation of undetected hypertension is a stroke or myocardial infarction, emphasizing the importance of screening in primary care.

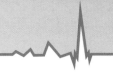

Diagnosis and treatment thresholds

GPs will be familiar with the diagnosis of hypertension. Remember that in cases of mild to moderate hypertension, the blood pressure must be taken accurately on several occasions before diagnosis is made. Up to 20% of patients with suspected mild hypertension may subsequently prove to have normal blood pressures when they measure their blood pressure at home or with ambulatory blood pressure monitoring, accounting for so-called 'white coat hypertension'.

Ambulatory blood pressure monitoring over 12–24 hours is particularly useful for patients with borderline hypertension or very labile blood pressure.[4] Repeated readings and home monitoring also help to exclude so-called 'white coat hypertension', where patients' blood pressure rises as a consequence of being assessed by a health professional. However, there is some evidence that 'white coat hypertension' is not as benign as was previously thought,[5] and patients who display this phenomenon may need follow-up.

Once blood pressure has been accurately assessed, we need to define what is to be treated (see Box 6.1). Note that these figures refer to sustained readings after a trial of non-drug measures.

Severe and malignant hypertension

Exceptions to the several-readings rule are the discovery of malignant hypertension (diastolic pressure >120 mmHg and symptoms or signs of retinopathy with fundal

---

Box 6.1 Who to treat: British Hypertension Society guidelines[2]

- Treat those patients with a sustained diastolic blood pressure ≥ 100 mmHg and those with a sustained systolic blood pressure ≥ 160 mmHg
- Treat those with a systolic pressure of 140–159 and/or a diastolic pressure of 90-99 who have evidence of target organ damage (e.g. stroke, heart failure, left ventricular hypertrophy, retinopathy, renal failure), evidence of established cardiovascular disease, who are diabetic or who have a CHD risk of >15% over 10 years.

Note: To calculate the CHD risk use the Joint British Societies Coronary Risk Prediction Chart[2] or as it appears in the British National Formulary. Many doctors now used computerized risk scoring systems.

Box 6.2 Examples of secondary causes of hypertension

- Drugs (e.g. combined oral contraceptives, NSAIDs, oral steroids)
- Renal disease (including diabetic renal disease)
- Renovascular disease
- Hormonal causes (Conn's syndrome, Cushing's syndrome, phaeochromocytoma)
- Coarctation of the aorta

---

haemorrhages, exudates, and papilloedema, neurological signs or proteinuria), when the patient is best admitted for assessment. Patients with severe hypertension (systolic pressure >220 mmHg or a diastolic pressure >120 mmHg) needs immediate treatment (and should be referred for it). In patients with a blood pressure in the rage 200–219 mmHg systolic and 110–119 mmHg diastolic should have their pressure confirmed over 1–2 weeks and then treated.

Assessment of the patient

There is a whole host of causes of hypertension (see Box 6.2), but in 95% of cases no cause is found (essential hypertension). The most common secondary cause is renal, both intrinsic renal disease and renovascular disease (i.e. due to disease narrowing the renal arteries).

Remember that non-steroidal anti-inflammatory drugs (NSAIDs) are a cause of hypertension, as these are commonly used drugs, particularly in the elderly.

Assessing a patient with hypertension in primary care involves answering four questions:

- Has the hypertension been adequately confirmed (see above)?
- Are there likely to be any causes?
- Are there any other major CHD risk factors (smoking, hyperlipidaemia, diabetes)?
- Is there already any target organ damage?

The patient's history should cover present and past medical events (including stroke, transient ischaemic attack, myocardial infarction, diabetes, renal impairment), current medication, smoking and family history. A family history of hypertension is common, since there is a strong genetic component.

Examination of the patient with mild hypertension in primary care is usually unhelpful. Textbooks list a long examination, including listening for loud aortic second sounds and renal bruits, but in reality most GPs will confine themselves to a standard cardiovascular examination, followed by some routine investigations (see Box 6.3). If you encounter patients with moderate or severe hypertension, however, these patients need a full examination, including ophthalmoscopy. Identification of retinal haemorrhages and exudates should ring alarm bells.

Investigations are aimed at identifying causes, CHD risk factors and target damage. Performing an ECG on every hypertensive patient may be unrealistic, but it does provide useful information, including identifying left ventricular hypertrophy (LVH) (although a normal ECG does not exclude it). LVH can increase mortality three- to four-fold, so patients with LVH require aggressive treatment to control blood pressure. An ECG may also reveal previously unrecognized myocardial ischaemia, or even infarction. It is worth checking a total/HDL cholesterol ratio as this is used to calculate (and is a better predictor of) CHD risk.

Management

Advise every patient with hypertension on lifestyle changes for lowering blood pressure. The Blood Pressure Association has a range of patient self-help material that may be useful.

Lifestyle modifications

- Weight reduction, if necessary.
- Reduction of alcohol intake to <21 units/week for men and <14 units/week for women.
- Stopping smoking.
- Restriction of sodium intake to 70–80 mmol/day (UK average 120–180 mmol/day) by reducing salt intake.

Box 6.3 Routine investigations for a patient with hypertension

- Urine test for blood, protein and sugar
- Serum creatinine, urea and electrolytes
- Serum total cholesterol/high density lipoprotein (HDL) cholesterol ratio
- Blood glucose
- Electrocardiogram (ECG)

- Increased exercise.
- Consumption of seven portions fruit and vegetables per day.

To reduce cardiovascular risk, also recommend:

- a reduced intake of saturated fat
- an increased consumption of fish oils.

Drug treatment

Modern drug therapy for patients with hypertension involves tailoring the therapy to the type of patient presenting, considering their age, race, renal status, presence of co-existing diseases and possible treatment side-effects.

If you need to combine antihypertensive agents (as you will in most patients), three useful combinations are:

- a diuretic with a beta blocker or ACE inhibitor or sartan
- a beta blocker with a dihydropyridine calcium channel blocker (*not* verapamil or diltiazem)
- an ACE inhibitor or sartan plus a dihydropyridine calcium channel blocker.

Moxonidine is a useful add-on to any of these combinations.

The main patient types and use of drug classes are listed in Table 6.1. The choice of antihypertensive is also governed by three other important considerations: the need for 24-hour control; contraindications to the different therapies and side-effects.

Treatment recommendations include:

- starting and stopping hypertension treatment slowly
- aiming for once or twice daily dosage
- not adding new drugs unless absolutely necessary
- changing drugs one at a time.

24-hour control

The most important requirement of treatment is a need for 24-hour control. Blood pressure rises in the morning with the onset of activity, and this early morning surge of blood pressure is associated with an increase in strokes, myocardial infarction and sudden cardiac death.[7] In addition, the risks of hypertension are an effect of a lifetime 'load' increasing left ventricular mass. Thus, clearly, if your blood pressure is only controlled for 18 hours a day you will be more at risk, both in the long term and in terms of early morning cardiovascular events, than if you have effective 24-hour control.

Table 6.1 Major classes of and indications for antihypertensive drugs[2]

Drug	Strong indication	Possible indication	Possible contraindication	Strong contraindication
Thiazides	Elderly	–	Dyslipidaemia	Gout
Beta blockers	Myocardial infarction, angina	Heart failure*	Heart failure* Dyslipidaemia Peripheral vascular disease	Asthma/chronic obstructive pulmonary disease Heart block
Alpha blockers	Prostatism	Dyslipidaemia	Postural hypotension	Urinary incontinence
Calcium antagonists (dihydropyridine)	Elderly isolated systolic hypertension	Elderly angina	–	–
Calcium antagonists (rate limiting)	Angina	Myocardial infarction	Combination with beta blocker	Heart failure Heart block
ACE inhibitors	Heart failure Left ventricular dysfunction Type 1 diabetic nephropathy	Chronic renal disease[†] Type 2 diabetic nephropathy	Renal impairment[†] Peripheral vascular disease[‡]	Pregnancy Renovascular disease
Angiotensin II antagonists	ACE inhibitor cough	Heart failure Intolerance of other drugs	Peripheral vascular disease[‡]	Renovascular disease Pregnancy

*Beta blockers can worsen heart failure, but in low doses are used to treat it.

[†]ACE inhibitors may be beneficial in chronic renal failure, but should be used with caution, close supervision and specialist advice when there is established renal impairment.

[‡]ACE inhibitors with caution due to risk of renovascular disease.

There are, however, considerable differences in half-lives between different antihypertensive agents within a given class. This must be taken into account when prescribing.

Side-effects

Side-effects are one of the major causes for patients stopping antihypertensive therapy. In a study of continuation rates in general practice after prescribing courses of beta blockers, diuretics, calcium channel blockers and ACE inhibitors it was found that by 6 months continuation rates were only 40–50% for all four classes of drug.[8] All the antihypertensive drug classes have a significant side-effect profile, except the sartans, where a comparative lack of side-effects is an advantage.

GPs need to make rational choices based on comparator trials of different drugs and drug classes. We already have recent evidence of the superiority of a sartan over a beta blocker in preventing cardiovascular morbidity and death for a similar reduction in blood pressure.[9] The future may well be in combining ACE inhibitors and sartans.

Follow-up

Patients with hypertension need lifelong monitoring. It is important to keep a check on attendance – you do not wish to see a poor attender or non-complier with a stroke several years after diagnosis but with no follow-up.

Make every effort to correct cardiovascular risk factors (smoking, hyperlipidaemia, obesity, etc) at each visit. In those successfully established on treatment, a 3–6 month measurement has been recommended. This workload can be eased by patients monitoring their own blood pressure and reporting back to the nurse or GP as required.

Those at risk of moving into the treatment range for hypertension (e.g. diabetics or those with a high normal blood pressure (135–139/85–89)) should be monitored annually.

Referral

The indications for specialist referral are listed in Box 6.4. With regard to 'resistant to treatment', much will depend on the GP's experience of using combination therapy. Using rational combinations of two or three (or sometimes four) drugs, the vast majority of patients should be manageable within primary care, although it should be remembered that even with multiple-drug therapy a few patients (5–10%) will not reach the required target blood pressure.

Involving the patient

Compliance is the key to conquering hypertension, and this can only be achieved by patients understanding the nature of hypertension and its treatment. It is essential that we provide our patients with up-to-date information and help answer their questions. It may be helpful to direct the patient to the Blood Pressure Association, who offer a wide range of resources for patients.

Resistant hypertension may be due to 'white coat hypertension', poor patient compliance with treatment, or genuine resistance. Poor compliance is often the prescriber's fault as much as the patient's, and should be

dealt with by understanding the patient's ideas and concerns. Patients with genuine resistant hypertension or target organ damage should be referred.

A patient whose blood pressure has been well controlled for many years may ask the practice nurse if it is possible to reduce the drug dose, or even discontinue the tablets altogether. An appointment with the GP should be advised. Absolute benefit from treatment is greater in the elderly (at least up to age 80 years) than in younger patients.[2]

Prevention

Education about the risks of smoking and obesity is needed to help prevent the development of hypertension among the general population, and should be started at an early age.

Individuals with normal blood pressure should be encouraged to maintain or adopt a healthy lifestyle. Just a 20-minute walk to work each day can reduce an the risk of developing high blood pressure.[6]

Involving the team

The management of hypertension in primary care is based on teamwork. All members of the primary care team need to be aware of the practice protocol on hypertension.

Practice nurses need to feel comfortable with their role. Their job can become extremely difficult if there is a lack of consensus in the practice, with partners holding a variety of views on opportunistic blood pressure readings and treatment.

District nurses may also be involved in measuring blood pressures in elderly housebound patients.

Although practice nurse clinics should release GPs' time for other tasks, patients who have been attending the surgery for years to have their blood pressure monitored may be reluctant to give up a cherished doctor's appointment.[10] Such patients should be encouraged to recognize the nurse's expertise in this area.

Primary care trusts

The primary care trust may wish to develop its own guidelines for the diagnosis and treatment of hypertension, based on existing advice. Ideally, the trust should have a formulary for prescribing antihypertensive therapy. The number of drugs available is huge, as is the range of combinations. Inclusion in the formulary should be based on cost-effectiveness, with leeway for individual decisions depending on patient preference and response.

> **Box 6.4** Indications for referral to a specialist (adapted from the British Hypertension Society guidelines[2])
>
> - Necessity for urgent treatment: blood pressure greater than 220/120 or impending complications (e.g. transient ischaemic attack, heart failure)
> - Suspected underlying cause (e.g. abnormal renal function)
> - Young age (<20 years or needing treatment before age 30 years)
> - Resistance to treatment
> - Multiple drug intolerance or contraindications
> - Special situations (e.g. hypertension in pregnancy)

Key points

- The minimum level to which blood pressure should be controlled is less than 150/90, with the optimal target being less than 140/85.
- For diabetics, the audit standard is less than 140/85, with an optimal target of less than 140/80.
- Up to 20% of patients with suspected mild hypertension prove to have normal blood pressures when they measure their blood pressures at home or when ambulatory blood pressure monitoring is used.
- Routine investigations should include a urine test for blood, protein and sugar, serum creatinine and electrolytes, serum total/HDL cholesterol, blood glucose and an ECG.
- Advise every patient on non-drug methods of lowering blood pressure.
- Tailor the drug to the patient.
- Use rational combinations of therapy.
- Refer to a specialist those patients with a blood pressure above 220/120 or with impending complications (e.g. transient ischaemic attack, heart failure), a suspected underlying cause, young age, resistance to drug treatment, multiple drug intolerance or contraindications, or special conditions (e.g. pregnancy).

Resources

The Blood Pressure Association, 60 Cranmer Terrace, London SW17 OQS. Tel. 020 8772 4994. Website: http://www.bpassoc.org.uk

References

1. Systolic Hypertension in the Elderly Programme Cooperative Research Group. Prevention of stroke by antihypertensive drug treatment in older persons with isolated systolic hypertension. JAMA 1991; 265:3255–3264.

2. Ramsay LE, Williams B, Johnston DG, et al. Guidelines for management of hypertension: report of the third working party of the British Hypertension Society 1999. J Hum Hypertens 1999; 13:569–592. Guidelines available at: http://www.hyp.ac.uk/bhs

3. Brookes M, Poulter NR. Improved hypertension management and control: results from the Health Survey for England 1998. Hypertension 2001; 38:827–832.

4. Prasad N, Isles C. Ambulatory blood pressure monitoring: a guide for general practitioners. BMJ 1996; 313:181–182.

5. Muscholl MW, Hense HW, Bröckel U, et al. Changes in left ventricular structure and function in patients with white coat hypertension: cross-sectional survey. BMJ 1998; 317:565–570.

6. Hayashi T, Tsumura K, Suematsu C, et al. Walking to work and the risk for hypertension in men: the Osaka health survey. Ann Intern Med 1999; 130:21–26.

7. Muller JE. Circadian variation in cardiovascular events. Am J Hypertens 1999; 1:35S–42S.

8. Jones JK, Gorkin L, Lian JF, et al. Discontinuation of and changes in treatment after start of new courses of antihypertensive drugs: a study of a United Kingdom population. BMJ 1995; 311:293–295.

9. Dahlof B, Devereux RB, Kjeldsen SE, et al. Cardiovascular morbidity and mortality in the Losartan Intervention For Endpoint reduction in hypertension study (LIFE): a randomised control against atenolol. Lancet 2002; 359:995–1003.

10. Yeo KR, Yeo WW. Workload implications of implementing national guidelines for hypertension. Br J Cardiol 2002; 9:524–530.

7. Management of hyperlipidaemia

F Machado

THIS CHAPTER REVIEWS

- Which patients should be considered for hyperlipidaemia screening.
- Which patients require treatment under current guidelines.
- Which patients should be referred.
- Which patients should be screened.

Box 7.1 Secondary causes of hyperlipidaemia

Metabolic/endocrine
- Poorly controlled diabetes
- Hypothyroidism
- Obesity

Renal
- Chronic renal failure
- Nephrotic syndrome

Liver
- Biliary obstruction

Drug
- Alcohol excess
- Thiazides
- Corticosteroids
- Oestrogens
- Progestogens

The average cholesterol of the UK population is around 6.7, and follows a normal distribution. It could therefore be argued that a substantial proportion of the population stand to benefit from statin prescribing. However, cholesterol alone is a weak predictor of coronary risk, so it is important that prescribing is rational.

Guidelines have been published recently to help prioritize appropriate treatment for those individuals at highest risk of developing coronary heart disease (CHD).[1]

For patients with established CHD the evidence is clear: the results of large, well-controlled trials have demonstrated the benefits of cholesterol reduction by statins on total and cardiac mortality. However, the evidence is less impressive for patients without previous CHD.

Aetiology

In 40% of all patients with hyperlipidaemia there is a secondary cause,[2] and this should be sought (Box 7.1). Basic investigations are:

- urea electrolytes and creatinine
- liver function tests
- γ-glutamyltransferase
- glucose
- thyroid function tests
- urine for blood and protein.

Presentation and diagnosis

Some patients may have signs of abnormal lipid levels (Box 7.2 and Fig. 7.1). However, most patients with hyperlipidaemia are asymptomatic and are diagnosed as a result of strategic screening by members of the primary healthcare team.

Risk factors that indicate screening for hyperlipidaemia include:

- established CHD
- evidence of atherosclerosis (e.g. peripheral vascular disease)
- history of familial hyperlipidaemia

- strong family history of early-onset CHD (e.g. under age 40 years)
- combination of risk factors for CHD, diabetes, hypertension and smoking.

Box 7.2 Signs of hypercholesterolaemia and hypertriglyceridaemia

Signs of hypercholesterolaemia
- Xanthelasma
- Tendon xanthomas
- Tuberous xanthomas
- Corneal arcus
- Polyarthritis

Signs of hypertriglyceridaemia
- Eruptive xanthomas
- Pancreatitis
- Hepatomegaly
- Lipaemia retinalis

Universal screening at regular intervals of all patients, irrespective of risk, is not recommended as it is not a cost-effective way of reducing the incidence of CHD.[3]

An increasing number of patients are asking to have a cholesterol check. The most common trigger for this is a cardiovascular event affecting a relative or friend. It is important to respond to this request by asking the patient about other risk factors for CHD and to explain to the patient that cholesterol level on its own is a poor predictor of the likelihood of having a cardiovascular event.[3] The patient also needs to be aware of the potential harm of screening.

Types of cholesterol testing

Total cholesterol can be measured most accurately from a venous blood specimen.

A patient's cholesterol level varies throughout the day, so it is important to confirm the presence of a raised cholesterol on two specimens separated by at least 2 weeks.

A fasting lipid profile will also measure high-density lipoprotein (HDL) cholesterol, from which the low-density lipoprotein (LDL) cholesterol can be calculated.

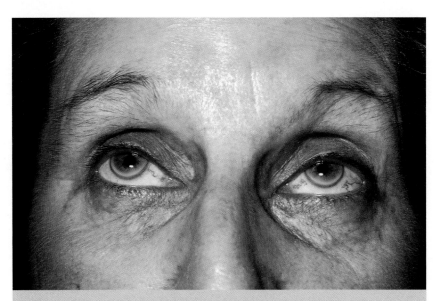

Figure 7.1 Subcutaneous cholesterol deposition on the medial aspect of the eyelids (xanthelasma). Courtesy of Professor GA Hitman. Reproduced with permission from Swash, *Hutchison's Clinical Methods*, 21st edn, Saunders, 2001.

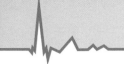

Box 7.3 Joint British recommendations on the prevention of CHD[1]

Secondary prevention: patients with CHD or other major atherosclerotic disease

- Lifestyle interventions regarding smoking, exercise and healthier food choices
- Rigorous control of blood pressure, lipids and glucose:
  - blood pressure <140 mmHg systolic and <85 mmHg diastolic
  - total cholesterol <5.0 mmol/l and LDL cholesterol <3.0 mmol/l
- Consider cardioprotective drug therapy:
  - aspirin, ACE inhibitors, beta blockers, statins
- Those who already have CHD and are at highest risk should have their risk factors modified. They will require rigorous control of blood pressure, cholesterol and glucose. Many will require treatment with a statin. Some argue that there is enough absolute benefit to justify statin therapy and cholesterol reduction in these patients, even if their cholesterol is already low

Primary prevention: patients without overt CHD or major atherosclerotic disease

- Three main groups should be identified and managed following a staged approac.

- Absolute CHD risk of ≥ 30% over 10 years, target and treat now:
  - blood pressure <140 mmHg systolic and <85 mmHg diastolic
  - total cholesterol <5.0 mmol/l and LDL cholesterol <3.0 mmol/l
  - diabetes optimally controlled and blood pressure reduced to <130 mmHg systolic and <80 mmHg diastolic
  - aspirin therapy if aged over 50 years and either hypertensive or male
- Absolute CHD risk of 15% over 10 years:
  - as resources allow, target progressively and treat as above
- Absolute CHD risk <15% over 10 years:
  - give appropriate lifestyle advice
  - drug treatment not required unless there is severe hypertension (>160/100) with target organ damage, diabetes with target organ damage, or familial hyperlipidaemia

To calculate an individual's cardiovascular risk using risk tables, such as the Joint British Societies Coronary Risk Prediction Chart,[1] the total and HDL fraction levels need to be known.

Management

All patients reviewed following a cholesterol assessment should be given lifestyle advice regarding:

- smoking
- weight loss, if indicated
- exercise
- moderate alcohol consumption
- other therapy, such as low-dose aspirin where appropriate
- advice about healthy dietary measures, including a move to a Mediterranean diet, which has been shown to have benefits on cardiovascular events, irrespective of cholesterol levels.

In addition, patients with diabetes and hypertension should be advised about the benefits of optimal management of blood glucose and blood pressure.

Patients should then have their cholesterol level interpreted with respect to their overall risk of developing CHD in the future.

Primary prevention

For primary prevention, there are a number of charts for assessing the patient's risk of a coronary event in the future. These can be used together with the recommendations of the joint committees on the management of patients at different risk. However, these charts have limitations and do not apply to:

- certain ethnic groups
- individuals with inherited dyslipidaemia
- patients with hypertension and target organ damage.

For details of secondary prevention, see Box 7.3.

Treatment options

All patients should be on a low-fat diet. Such diets are most effective in reducing cholesterol in patients who have had a myocardial infarction, who are possibly more motivated.

Patients should be assessed after 3 months to decide whether diet on its own is likely to reduce the cholesterol to acceptable levels. However, for many patients the main decision will be whether or not to prescribe a statin and, if so, which one.

Statins

There are now a number of statins, for some of which there is evidence from large, well-controlled trials to back their use in primary and secondary prevention of heart disease. There are substantial cost differences between statin preparations.

Statins appear to stabilize atherosclerotic plaques, and evidence suggests that it is not the absolute cholesterol level but the fact that the patient is on the trial dose of statin which is cardioprotective. This argument supports using the full trial doses of statins in all patients, rather than titrating dose to cholesterol response as has been done in the past.

Fibrates

Patients who do not respond to monotherapy with a statin may need additional treatment with a fibrate, but this increases the incidence of myositis and should be initiated and monitored in a hospital clinic.

Patients with predominantly raised triglyceride levels are often diabetic, and improvement of their control will reduce their triglyceride level.[4]

Patients should be encouraged to lose weight and moderate their alcohol intake. Those whose triglyceride level is persistently above 5 mmol/l should be treated with a fibrate, principally to reduce the chance of pancreatitis.

Recent discussion has focused on whether elderly patients (e.g. over 75 years old) should be managed in the same way.[5] Trials have largely focused on the under 75 population, but it can be argued that, if results are extrapolated, the elderly (whose absolute risks are higher than those of the young) have more to gain from statin therapy.

Referral criteria

Patients should be referred if:

- familial dyslipidaemia is suspected
- the patient does not respond to management with a single statin
- the patient experiences side-effects with statins.

Follow-up

Patients need to be seen regularly to check compliance with diet and treatment, and to identify possible side-effects of treatment.

It is important to reassess their risk factors and to measure blood pressure. It is wise to check for abnormal liver function at the same time. If the patient complains of muscle aches, creatinine kinase should be measured to identify myositis.

Patients who have abnormal liver function and myositis should discontinue treatment with statins and be referred to secondary care.

It is not clear whether regular repeat checking of cholesterol levels is of value, given that the absolute benefit from statin use may be dose related, although it does provide an opportunity to reinforce patient education about lifestyle.

Primary care groups

If national guidelines are implemented, the cost will be enormous. Previous estimates have suggested that, if the Standard Medical Advisory Committee guidelines on cholesterol prescribing were applied in just one health authority, this would account for 20% of the drug budget.[6]

This variation has implications for quality of care as well as cost-effectiveness. Clinical governance leads will need to work with GPs and their practice teams to implement national guidelines.

Practice team and resources

The practice team will need to have a clear vision of the importance of hyperlipidaemia. All members of the team should be alert to:

- identification of patients who should be screened
- identification of a patient's risk factors and their modification
- when patients should be considered for treatment
- monitoring of patients.

The coordinated care of preventive cardiovascular medicine may require extra resources for it to be successful in primary care.

Key points

- **40% of dyslipidaemia presenting in primary care has a secondary cause.**
- **The case for statin prescribing in the secondary prevention of CHD is clear.**

- The case in primary prevention is more controversial and would have huge cost implications for the NHS.

- Cholesterol levels alone are a weak predictor of coronary risk.

- Prescribing of statins for patients with high cholesterol but low risk should be avoided.

- Tables exist to allow GPs to assess overall risk, although they have limitations.

- Treatment of hyperlipidaemia should be approached from the angle of overall CHD risk management and not in isolation.

References

1. Wood D, Durrington P, Poulter N, et al (eds). Joint British recommendations on the prevention of coronary heart disease in clinical practice. Heart 1998; 80(suppl 2): S1–S29.

2. Feher D, Richmond W. Lipids and lipid disorders. London: Wolfe; 1995.

3. NHS Centre for Reviews and Dissemination. Cholesterol and coronary heart disease: screening and treatment. Effective Health Care 1998; 4(1).

4. Ballinger PM. The importance of hypertriglyceridaemia. Update 1999; 59:208–214.

5. Machado F. An age limit for statin therapy? Update 1999; 58:1050.

6. Freemantle N, Barbour R, Johnson R, et al. The use of statins: a case of misleading priorities? BMJ 1997; 315:826–827.

8. Acute management of myocardial infarction

AG Davies and C McLeod

THIS CHAPTER REVIEWS

- Acute management of myocardial infarction.
- GP thrombolysis.
- Prevalence of myocardial infarction.

Every year in the UK there are 500,000 cases of acute myocardial infarction. As most of these occur outside hospital, the prehospital phase of management is crucial. The advent of thrombolysis has made the early diagnosis of myocardial infarction paramount, but recent audit studies[1] have shown that the diagnosis and treatment of myocardial infarction leaves a good deal to be desired.

Diagnosis

The early diagnosis of myocardial infarction depends entirely on the electrocardiogram (ECG). Remember, however, that an initial normal ECG does not rule out a myocardial infarction

Early ECG changes after a myocardial infarction relate to convexly raised ST segments in a regional distribution (anterior, inferior, etc.) (Fig. 8.1) or the development of left bundle branch block. As ST segment changes are

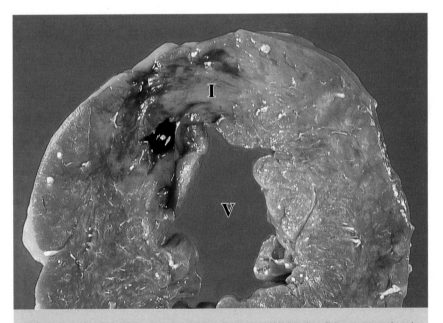

Figure 8.1 Rupture of myocardial infarct. The area of infarction (I) has ruptured and a track of blood runs from the ventricular chamber (V) to the epicardial surface. In this instance death was rapid after development of hemopericardium. Reproduced with permission from Stevens & Lowe, *Pathology*, Mosby, 2000.

effervescent, some authorities advocate giving thrombolysis in patients with any suspicious ECG change.[2]

GP thrombolysis has been proposed and trialled,[3] but GPs are reluctant to give thrombolysis because of the difficulty in interpreting ECG changes. This is not surprising, as most family doctors will see only two to three cases of myocardial infarction each year.

Immediate management

Aspirin, analgesia and thrombolysis

Once the GP is confident of the diagnosis the patient should be given:

- 300 mg of aspirin to chew (chewing facilitates absorption of the drug) – this reduces mortality by 23%

- glyceryl trinitrate by sublingual spray

- intravenous morphine or heroin for pain relief, together with an anti-emetic agent such as cyclizine.

Refer for urgent thrombolysis, to establish reperfusion. If thrombolysis is given within 6 hours of the onset of chest pain, mortality is reduced by 42%.[2] The earlier thrombolysis is given within the 6-hour window, the better is the chance of survival. In one study, treatment within 4 hours and at 13–24 hours reduced mortality by 50% and 35%, respectively.[4]

GP thrombolysis

The Grampian Region Early Anistreplase Trial (GREAT) study[3] demonstrated that it is feasible for GPs to give thrombolysis in the community. Their intervention before hospital admission allowed thrombolysis to be given, on average, 139 minutes sooner. The benefits were a 50% reduction in mortality, fewer cardiac events, smaller infarcts and better left ventricular function. The study concluded that where a delay of more than 30 minutes seems likely before a patient with suspected myocardial infarction reaches hospital, GPs should be encouraged to record ECGs and give thrombolysis, and be prepared to defibrillate.

Outside hospital the thrombolytic agents of choice are metalyse or tenecteplase, in a weight-dependent dose, given intravenously by bolus injection over 10 seconds. Avoid intramuscular or subcutaneous injections because of the risk of haemorrhage. Hydrocortisone should be available, as allergic reactions and anaphylactic shock have been reported. GPs who give thrombolysis must be prepared to monitor for arrhythmias and defibrillate if necessary.

Box 8.1 Indicators for and contraindications to GP thrombolysis

Indicators for GP thrombolysis are *all* of:
- a strong clinical suspicion of acute MI
- chest pain that is unrelieved by nitrates for 20 minutes to 12 hours
- an unequivocally abnormal ECG (i.e. ST elevation *or* left bundle branch left)

Contraindications to GP thrombolysis are:
- a normal ECG or no ECG
- a history of cardiovascular accident
- known intracranial pathology
- uncontrolled hypertension (>180/110)
- bleeding disorder
- anticoagulants
- surgery or major trauma within the last 10 days
- active gastrointestinal bleeding
- traumatic CPR (broken ribs)
- streptokinase or antistreplase within the last 5 days
- previous anaphylaxis with thrombolytic agents

The indicators for GP thrombolysis are listed in Box 8.1.

Key points

- **With the advent of easily administered thrombolysis, early diagnosis of myocardial infarction is paramount.**

- **An initial normal ECG does not rule out myocardial infarction.**

- **Treatment of acute myocardial infarction is with aspirin (300 mg to chew), glyceryl trinitrate and intravenous opiates (with an antiemetic), and early transfer to hospital.**

- **The earlier the patient is thrombolysed the better the prognosis.**

- **In some, mainly rural, areas GP thrombolysis is given before transfer to hospital.**

References

1. Birkhead JS. On behalf of the joint audit committee of the British Cardiac Society and a cardiology committee of the Royal College of Physicians of London. Time

delays in provision of thrombolytic treatment in six district hospitals. BMJ 1992; 305:445–448.

2. ISIS-2. Collaborative Group. Randomized trial of intravenous streptokinase, oral aspirin, both or neither among 17,187 cases of suspected acute myocardial infarction: ISIS-2. Lancet 1988; 2:349–360.

3. GREAT Group. Feasibility, safety and efficacy of domiciliary thrombolysis by general practitioners: Grampian Region Early Anistreplase Trial. BMJ 1992; 305:548–553.

4. Drug Therapeut Bull 1989; 27:81–82.

9. Atrial fibrillation

P O'Kane and G Jackson

THIS CHAPTER REVIEWS

- The prevalence of atrial fibrillation.
- The management of atrial fibrillation in primary care.
- Which patients are suitable for cardioversion.
- Which patients are at highest risk of embolic disease.
- Which patients should be offered anticoagulation.
- Follow-up of patients with atrial fibrillation.

Prevalence

Atrial fibrillation (AF), the complete absence of coordinated atrial systole, is a common arrhythmia. Its incidence in people over 22 years of age is 2% overall.[1] Its prevalence rises to 8.8% among people aged 80–89 years.[2]

AF is an important cause of embolic phenomena, such as cerebrovascular accident, which affects about 1.5% of people aged 50–59 years and up to 30% of those aged 80–89 years.[2] It is also associated with a 1.5- to 1.9-fold mortality risk.[3] As the population ages, the incidence of AF will increase.

Although AF is responsible for most arrhythmia-related hospital admissions, only one-third of community cases ever present to hospital. Most are managed in primary care.[4]

Presentation

AF is usually symptomatic. A rapid ventricular rate or irregularity may lead to chest pain, dyspnoea, fatigue or dizziness, which often occur during physical exertion when vagal tone is inhibited. Syncope can also occur.

Loss of atrial systole, even without a rapid ventricular rhythm, may severely compromise cardiac output. Cardiac failure can be precipitated if there is co-existing left ventricular dysfunction.

AF may also present with features of embolic phenomena, such as a transient ischaemic attack.

Classification

AF is traditionally classified as acute or chronic.

Acute atrial fibrillation

This implies a spontaneous resolution or successful cardioversion within 48 hours.

There are several acute causes of AF (Box 9.1), producing a dysrhythmia that is usually, although not necessarily, reversible within 48 hours. Significant underlying cardiac pathology (Box 9.2) is present in 70% of patients with AF. Patients without cardiac disease are described as having lone AF.

Chronic atrial fibrillation

This continues beyond 48 hours, and intervention is needed to re-establish sinus rhythm.[5] Chronic AF can be subdivided into paroxysmal, persistent and permanent forms.

Box 9.1 Acute causes of atrial fibrillation

- Acute alcohol or caffeine intake
- Acute myocardial infarction
- Acute pericarditis
- Acute myocarditis
- Pulmonary embolism
- Pneumonia
- Hyperthyroidism
- Electrocution
- After cardiac surgery (coronary artery bypass graft, mitral valvotomy and replacement)

The clinical impact of paroxysms increases with their severity and frequency. They are described as *persistent* when they occur continuously. *Permanent* AF implies resistance to previous cardioversion and an inability to return to sinus rhythm. The primary requirement in these patients is control of the ventricular rate, whereas the goal in paroxysmal or persistent cases is restoration and maintenance of sinus rhythm.[5]

Box 9.2 Cardiovascular causes of atrial fibrillation

- Valvular heart disease (mostly mitral valve disease)
- Obstructive coronary artery disease (may be without angina)
- Hypertension, particularly with left ventricular hypertrophy
- Cardiomyopathy
- Congenital heart disease (atrial septal defect)
- Constrictive pericarditis

These classification terms are not universally applied, and in practice it is often difficult to establish the pattern of AF. It is often more helpful to consider AF in relation to the underlying cause.

Action in primary care

Step 1: confirm diagnosis and seek cause

Clinically suspected AF should be confirmed by a resting or ambulatory electrocardiogram (ECG) (Figs 9.1 and 9.2). An ambulatory ECG may also define the temporal pattern.

The cause may be obvious from the history and examination, but it may be more difficult to exclude occult cardiac disease, which often requires referral or admission to the cardiology unit. It is essential to exclude hyperthyroidism in all newly diagnosed cases of AF.

Step 2: control ventricular rate

The next step is control of the ventricular rate to reduce symptoms. Indeed, this may be the only management

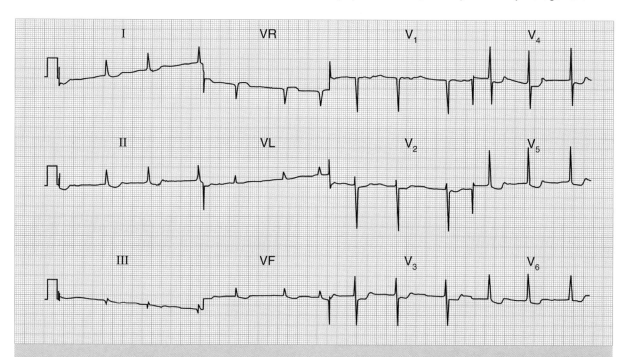

Figure 9.1 This ECG was recorded from a 60-year-old woman with rheumatic heart disease. She had been in heart failure, but this had been treated and she was no longer breathless. Atrial fibrillation with a ventricular rate of 60-65 beats/min. The downward-sloping ST segments (the 'reverse tick') indicate that digoxin has been given. Reproduced with permission from Hampton, *150 ECG Problems*, 2nd edn, Churchill Livingstone, 2003.

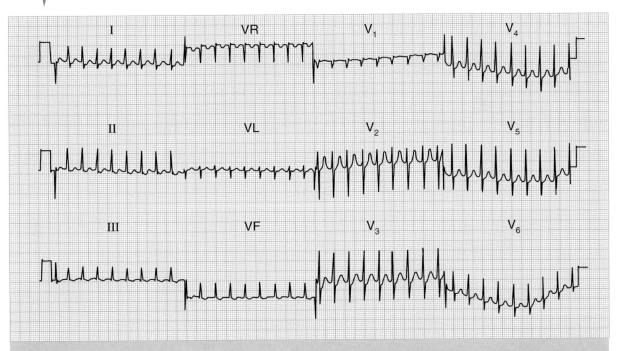

Figure 9.2 This ECG was recorded from a 26-year-old woman who had been admitted to the A&E department with palpitations. Reproduced with permission from Hampton, *150 ECG Problems*, 2nd edn, Churchill Livingstone, 2003.

required if the AF reverts spontaneously. The ventricular rate should be maintained at 60–80 beats/min resting and 90–115 beats/min during exercise. This will improve ventricular function. However, the risk of thromboembolism will probably remain the same.

Treatments for controlling the ventricular rate include digoxin, beta blockers, amiodarone and rate-limiting calcium channel antagonists such as diltiazem and verapamil.

Digoxin, perhaps the oldest and most widely used agent in AF, enhances vagal automaticity at the atrioventricular node, thus slowing the resting heart rate. However, this benefit is lost during exercise. Mild exertion often induces symptoms, even with a therapeutic serum digoxin level.

The positive inotropic effect of digoxin makes it useful in AF with associated poor left ventricular function. Regular monitoring of digoxin is of limited value because sensitivity to the drug is less predictable in cardiac disease. There is usually toxicity at levels of 1.5–3.0 mg/l.

Impaired renal function and hypokalaemia can increase serum digoxin concentration, so both should be monitored, particularly in the elderly and in patients taking potassium-losing diuretics.

Beta blockers, verapamil and diltiazem are increasingly used for ventricular rate control and are more effective than digoxin during exercise. Beta blockers reduce mortality after myocardial infarction. The main drawback is the negative inotropic effect, inducing pathological bradycardia and precipitating complete heart block, particularly with concomitant sick sinus syndrome.

Amiodarone can be effective for controlling ventricular rate, but should not be the first-line therapy because it produces serious adverse effects with long-term use.

Referral

AF can often be managed in primary care, for instance permanent AF requiring simple ventricular rate control. However, several groups of patients do require referral to the cardiology department for further investigation.

Immediate admission

Patients presenting with symptomatic AF with a rapid ventricular rate (>120 beats/min) will usually require immediate admission for stabilization and monitoring so

Table 9.1 Predisposing factors for stroke in atrial fibrillation

Clinical risks	Echocardiographic factors
Previous embolic or cerebrovascular event	Significant valve disease
Obstructive coronary artery disease	Left atrial thrombus
Congestive cardiac failure	Left ventricular dysfunction
Hypertension	Left atrial size >50 mm
Diabetes mellitus	Left atrial mechanical dysfunction

that the cause can be found. This is particularly important when there is co-existing left ventricular dysfunction, which often precipitates overt cardiac failure.

Patients who present with embolic phenomena should also be considered for hospital admission or urgent outpatient assessment.

Referral for investigation for cardiac disease

An ECG may identify previous myocardial infarction or left ventricular hypertrophy secondary to hypertension.

An exercise tolerance test is helpful if obstructive coronary artery disease is suspected, particularly in men aged over 50 years.

Transthoracic echocardiography is particularly important when there is a clinical suggestion of valvular disease or for assessing thromboembolic risk. It can be used to confirm left ventricular hypertrophy and to determine left atrial size, presence of thrombus, ventricular size and left ventricular ejection fraction.

A large left atrium, whether inducing or arising from AF, may contribute to the formation of atrial thrombi. The thromboembolic risk is increased further by the presence of left ventricular dysfunction.

Cardioversion

Spontaneous cardioversion occurs in nearly half the patients with paroxysmal or recent-onset AF. All newly diagnosed cases of AF should be considered for cardioversion. The decision to cardiovert is based on the likely benefit and the potential adverse outcome.

Restoration of sinus rhythm may relieve symptoms, improve exercise tolerance and avoid the need for medication.[5] Until recently, it was also thought to reduce the risk of thromboembolic disease.

However, several trials comparing the strategy of rhythm versus rate control have now been completed. The largest, with 4060 patients, showed that rate control was at least as good as rhythm control at reducing mortality. Importantly, sinus rhythm did not protect from stroke: 7.1% of the rhythm group and 5.5% of the rate group suffered an ischaemic stroke, but only 37% and 69%, respectively, were in AF at the time of the event.[6]

AF rapidly induces atrial remodelling, which reduces the chance of maintaining sinus rhythm. Thus, it is imperative to consider cardioversion at an early stage.

Pharmacological cardioversion is generally effective only for AF of recent onset. External electrical cardioversion under anaesthetic is the preferred method, having a success rate of 65–90%.[5]

Long-term anticoagulation

Non-rheumatic AF carries a 5.6-fold increase in embolic risk, rising to 17.6-fold when associated with rheumatic valve disease.[1] Embolic risk is higher at the onset of AF, within the first year, with frequent paroxysms and soon after cardioversion to sinus rhythm.[5] Factors that predispose to stroke are listed in Table 9.1.

Cardiovascular disease and advancing age in the presence of other risk factors increase stroke risk (Box 9.3). Thus a patient aged over 75 years with frequent paroxysms of AF and structural cardiac disease has a relatively high risk of a thromboembolic event.[7] Lone AF carries a low risk of stroke, but this risk increases with age.[8,9]

Risk versus benefit: warfarin or aspirin

Major trials have demonstrated an average relative risk reduction of embolism of 68% in patients with AF using warfarin with an international normalized ratio (INR) of

1.5–4.5.[8] More haemorrhagic events were associated with warfarin, particularly in the presence of uncontrolled hypertension and INRs greater than 3.0. The European Society of Cardiology recommends individual risk–benefit assessment, with introduction of warfarin to achieve an INR of 2.0–3.0 in patients who warrant anticoagulation.[5]

Aspirin, alone or in combination with low-dose warfarin (INR 1.5), has been shown to be less effective in stroke reduction among high-risk patients.[9] Aspirin, which is more convenient and theoretically safer than warfarin, is best reserved for medium- or low-risk patients with AF. The optimum daily dose is not clear (the various studies used 75–325 mg). We currently recommend 75 mg/day.

A major lesson from the AFFIRM trial is that patients who have had an episode of AF and exhibit other stroke risk factors should probably continue on warfarin even if they appear to be in sinus rhythm.[6] The future of stroke prevention in AF may be with a new oral direct thrombin inhibitor, ximelagatran, which has been compared against warfarin in a randomized, open-label trial and shown to be as effective with less overall bleeding. The additional benefit is that this agent does not require frequent monitoring.[10]

Follow-up

Follow-up of patients who have permanent AF involves monitoring the ventricular rate based on symptoms as well as clinical examination. Increasing dyspnoea on exertion

---

Box 9.3 Risk of stroke in atrial fibrillation

High risk (12% annually)
- Previous embolic or cerebrovascular event
- Significant valve disease
- Significant left ventricular dysfunction
- Left atrial thrombus
- Age >75 years with other clinical risks or echocardiographic signs

Moderate risk (8% annually)
- Age 65–74 years
- Age <65 years with other clinical risks or echocardiographic signs

Low risk (1% annually)
- Age <65 years with no other clinical risks or echocardiographic signs

---

may suggest poor rate control during exercise and prompt a change of medication.

The risk–benefit ratio of anticoagulation can be addressed regularly, particularly in the light of any new neurological symptoms, and the INR should be kept at a therapeutic level.

Preventing recurrence

Patients who have had successful cardioversion or those with paroxysmal AF should be followed up to make sure that they remain free from dysrhythmias. Maintaining sinus rhythm after cardioversion with antiarrhythmic therapy, especially amiodarone, should be considered when AF is likely to recur. Recurrence is likely when patients have long arrhythmia histories, large left atria, co-existent left ventricular dysfunction and associated mitral valve disease. Initiating the drug before cardioversion may reduce early recurrence.

Management of relapse

Patients who have successfully cardioverted AF may relapse despite treatment with antiarrhythmic therapy. In these situations the choice is between a further attempt at cardioversion or to accept the rhythm as permanent and aim therapy at ventricular rate control, and perhaps anticoagulation. If amiodarone is used to facilitate cardioversion, it should be switched to Digoxin with additional β-blocker to avoid long-term side-effects. Cardioversion may be considered again if symptoms are troublesome.

In difficult cases where AF proves resistant to rhythm control or symptoms persist despite adequate rate control, interventional strategies, such as permanent pacing or ablation techniques targeting the pulmonary vein, can be used.

Evidence-based treatment: problems with warfarin therapy

Reasons for the poor prescribing of warfarin in AF patients at high thromboembolic risk may include concern over cerebral haemorrhage, the problems associated with initiating therapy in elderly housebound patients and the inconvenience of safely monitoring anticoagulation. Patients' unwillingness to take warfarin may contribute.

An audit and qualitative study of 13,239 patients in general practice identified 132 cases of AF, with 100 at ▸

high risk of thromboembolism based on the established criteria.[11] Of this group, 28% were either too unwell or did not consent to an interview to discuss anticoagulation and 16% were on warfarin for an alternative reason. Approximately one-third of the remaining AF patients not already on warfarin but eligible for anticoagulation declined therapy after interviews detailing stroke risk and consequences.

There is as yet no single guideline available for managing patients with AF. However, the European task force has attempted to address this problem, and has produced a set of useful algorithms covering the main issues.[5]

Key points

- When a patient presents with AF it is essential to control ventricular rate, investigate for underlying cardiac disease then consider prompt cardioversion.

- An assessment of the risk of thromboembolic disease should follow.

- Those who remain in permanent AF despite intervention should have their ventricular rate controlled with digoxin, and perhaps beta blockers if required.

- Warfarin therapy should be discussed with patients in permanent AF at high stroke risk and also be considered in paroxysmal AF in the presence of other risk factors.

References

1. Kannel WB, Abbott RD, Savage DD, et al. Epidemiologic features of chronic AF. The Framingham Study. N Engl J Med 1982; 306:1018–1022.

2. Wolf PA, Abbott RD, Kannel WB. AF is an independent risk factor for stroke. The Framingham Study. Stroke 1991; 22:983–988.

3. Benjamin EJ, Wolf PA, D'Agostino RB, et al. Impact of AF on the risk of death. The Framingham heart study. Circulation 1998; 98:946–952.

4. Lip GYH, Golding DJ, Nazir M, et al. A survey of AF in general practice: the West Birmingham AF project. Br J Gen Pract 1997; 47:285–289.

5. Levy S, Breithardt R, Campbell WF, et al on behalf of the Working Group on Arrhythmias of the European Society of Cardiology. AF: current knowledge and recommendations for management. Eur Heart J 1998; 19:1294–1320.

6. Wyse DG, Waldo AL, DiMarco JP, et al. A comparison of rate control and rhythm control in patients with atrial fibrillation (AFFIRM). N Engl J Med 2002; 347:1825–1833.

7. Lip GYH. Does paroxysmal AF confer a paroxysmal thromboembolic risk? Lancet 1997; 349:1565–1566.

8. Lip GYH. Clinical implications of the stroke prevention in AF III trial: a clinician's perspective. Cardiac Electrophysiol Rev 1998; 2:49–51.

8. AF Investigators. Risk factors for stroke and efficacy of antithrombotic therapy in AF. Analysis of pooled data from five randomized controlled trials. Arch Intern Med 1994; 154:1449–1457.

9. Howitt A, Armstrong D. Implementing evidence based medicine in general practice: audit and qualitative study of antithrombotic treatment for AF. BMJ 1999; 318:1324–1327.

10. Halperin JL. The third Stroke Prophylaxis Using an Oral Thrombin Inhibitor in Atrial Fibrillation (SPORTIF III) trial. American College of Cardiology Annual Scientific Sessions, Chicago, IL, 2 April 2003.

10. Management of heart failure

A Bodner

THIS CHAPTER REVIEWS

- Diagnosis and definitions of heart failure.
- Treatment of heart failure in primary care.
- When to refer patients.

Pathology

The term 'heart failure' describes a clinical process rather than a disease. It means the heart is no longer able to pump blood around the body efficiently, and thus organs and muscles no longer receive the oxygen they require to function properly. The result is physical deterioration (Fig. 10.1). ▸

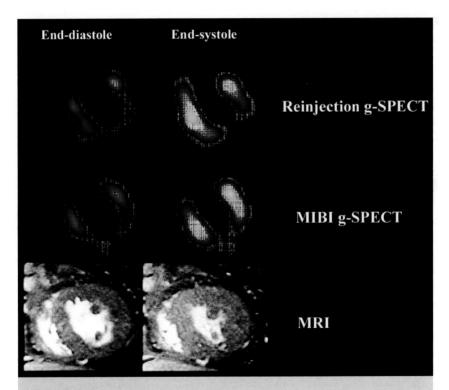

Figure 10.1 Typical left-ventricular end-diastolic (left) and end-systolic (right) short-axis g-SPECT and MRI images in a patient with old myocardial infarction. Regional wall motion and thickening were impaired in the anteroseptal and inferolateral regions. Reproduced with permission from Tadamura, Kudoh, Motooka et al, *Journal of the American College of Cardiology* 1999; 33(4):991–997.

In acute heart failure, left ventricular function is reduced suddenly with a resultant rise in end-diastolic pressure. Because forward pump action fails, a back pressure builds up in the pulmonary circulation, leading to pulmonary oedema.

The process is less dramatic in chronic heart failure, and involves not only cardiac pump failure but also several non-cardiac systems and organs, such as the lungs, liver and kidneys. The complex of congestive organ failure and autonomic and hormonal dysfunction causes chemical imbalance and clinical fluid retention.

Definition

Essential features are symptoms of heart failure (dyspnoea, ankle swelling). with objective evidence of cardiac dysfunction at rest.[1]

New York Heart Association classification of heart failure

- Class 1: no limitation; ordinary physical exercise does not cause fatigue, dyspnoea or palpitations. These patients would have to have objective evidence of cardiac dysfunction and a past history of treated symptoms in order to fulfil the basic definition.
- Class 2: slight limitation of physical activity; ordinary activity results in fatigue, dyspnoea, palpitation or angina; the patient is comfortable at rest.
- Class 3: marked limitation of physical activity; comfortable at rest, but less than ordinary activity results in symptoms.
- Class 4: unable to carry out any physical activity without discomfort; symptoms are present at rest.

Diagnosis

The diagnosis of heart failure is based on both history and clinical findings. Although the problem may present dramatically, it can also be covert, particularly in the elderly, whose functions may deteriorate gradually and whose symptoms may be confused with other medical conditions.

The principal symptoms of acute heart failure are:

- breathlessness
- fluid retention
- a rapid, weak pulse
- cold, clammy skin.

Examination may reveal low blood pressure and a raised jugular venous pulse. Gallop rhythm is an indication of

cardiac strain, while lung crepitations and peripheral oedema indicate acute fluid retention.

In chronic heart failure, sustained dyspnoea, abnormal fatigue and weight loss usually occur. The last two are common and are easily confused with respiratory, renal or malignant disease.

Examination usually reveals dependent oedema, hepatomegaly and ankle swelling. Muscle wasting often occurs. Cardiac signs of a displaced apex beat and a third heart sound suggest cardiac strain and possible poor left ventricular function.[2]

Breathlessness

At first, patients may be breathless only on exertion, but later the symptom also appears at rest. There may be breathlessness on lying down (orthopnoea) and the patient may wake up with breathlessness during the night (paroxysmal nocturnal dyspnoea).

There may be an apparent underlying cause in acute heart failure, such as coronary insufficiency. The patient may sit upright while trying to relieve the dyspnoea, and may cough up pink frothy sputum caused by blood-tinged congested alveolar exudate.

Chronic heart failure may be more difficult to diagnose, and breathlessness can occur in the absence of other causes and may be clinically silent.

It is important to be aware of pre-existing clinical conditions, such as pulmonary disease, long-standing hypertension, anaemia and conditions caused by chronic alcohol misuse, all of which can impair ventricular function.

Investigations

- A resting electrocardiogram (ECG) can be performed in the surgery to help to establish the presence of cardiac ischaemia, left ventricular hypertrophy or arrhythmia.
- Open access to an exercise ECG is useful to determine the degree of effort intolerance and to uncover covert ischaemia.
- Serum urea and electrolytes tests can rule out renal disorder before starting therapy.
- A full blood count, thyroid function and tests for cardiac enzymes may exclude anaemia, thyroid disease and myocardial infarction.
- Radiology may reveal pulmonary oedema, which appears as upper-lobe congestion and an enlarged cardiac size, and help to exclude diagnoses such as pneumonia, pneumothorax or malignancy.

- Echocardiography can confirm the presence of cardiac valvular dysfunction and also help to distinguish global impaired left ventricular function, as in ischaemic heart disease.

Management

Acute heart failure

Acute heart failure is a medical emergency warranting immediate referral to hospital. Oxygen and an intravenous diuretic, such as frusemide, can be administered in the practice while awaiting the ambulance.

Chronic heart failure

Management of chronic heart failure is lifelong. General management includes adjustments to lifestyle and occupation because of the limited cardiac reserve. Patients should stop smoking and restrict their alcohol intake, as both can impair cardiac function. Counselling about obesity, diet and salt intake and exercise are important. Rest should be advised only in acute heart failure or exacerbations of chronic heart failure.[1]

The patient's anxieties will need to be explored, including issues such as employment, driving and sexual intercourse. Regular vaccination against pneumococcal disease and influenza is advisable. There are several options for drug therapy, and these are described below.[3]

Diuretics

Treatment of mild heart failure can start with a mild-acting thiazide diuretic, which will counteract fluid overload. Loop diuretics such as frusemide (Frusol) are indicated for moderate failure, and combination diuretics such as co-amilofruse (Fru-Co) are used for severe or resistant symptoms.

The aldosterone antagonist spironolactone (Aldactone), used in combination with a loop diuretic, is a useful adjunct.

ACE inhibitors

ACE inhibitors are the mainstay of treatment, reducing mortality in heart failure and improving the prognosis and quality of life. All patients with left ventricular dysfunction should be taking an ACE inhibitor.[1,4,5]

Beta blockers

These are used in consultation with a specialist.

Digoxin

Digoxin should be used in patients with associated atrial fibrillation.

Aspirin

Aspirin is used for secondary prevention of coronary and cerebrovascular events. There is no evidence of its efficacy in heart failure.

Anticoagulation

There is no evidence of efficacy of anticoagulation, except in atrial fibrillation, where patients with heart failure are in a high-risk group for embolic disease.

Surgery (selected patients)

- Revascularization
- pacemakers
- heart transplantation.

Referral

Patients with heart failure should be referred when:

- the heart failure is not responding to medical treatment and seems to be worsening
- there is a need for further interventional investigation or treatment, such as coronary arteriography or cardiac valve surgery
- the diagnosis is unclear and possibly confused by co-existing conditions such as chronic airways disease or acute anxiety
- the patient and GP have concerns about home management.

Follow-up

The practice can take a multidisciplinary approach to follow-up. The practice nurse or health visitor can check drug compliance and social circumstances, while the GP will need to assess cardiac function.

Prevention

The prevalence of heart failure will increase with growing longevity. Prevention of the condition relies on lifelong pre-emptive control of risk factors. This needs to start early in life. Controlling blood pressure, moderating alcohol intake and stopping smoking will reduce the risk of cardiac morbidity and heart failure in the long term.[4]

Key points

- **Essential features are symptoms of heart failure (dyspnoea, ankle swelling) with objective evidence of cardiac dysfunction at rest.**

- Presentation can be covert in the elderly, in whom symptoms may be confused with other medical conditions.
- Symptoms of chronic heart failure are easily confused with respiratory, renal or malignant disease.
- Diuretics are used to counteract fluid overload.
- ACE inhibitors reduce mortality and improve the prognosis and quality of life.
- Beta blockers are also indicated (with care).
- Digoxin should be used in patients with associated atrial fibrillation.
- Anticoagulation shows no efficacy, except in atrial fibrillation, where patients with heart failure are in a high risk group for embolic disease.
- Controlling blood pressure, moderating alcohol intake and stopping smoking will reduce the risk of cardiac morbidity and heart failure in the long term.

References

1. The Task Force of the Working Party on Heart Failure of the European Society of Cardiology. Guidelines for the diagnosis of heart failure. Eur Heart J 1995; 16:741–751.

2. Coats A. Investigation and medical treatment of heart failure. Medicine 1998; 25:116–211.

3. The Task Force of the Working Party on Heart Failure of the European Society of Cardiology. The treatment of heart failure. Eur Heart J 1997; 18:736–753.

4. Department of Health. National Service Framework. Coronary heart disease. Emerging findings. London: HMSO; 1998.

5. SOLVD trial. Effect of enalapril on survival in patients with reduced left ventricular ejection fractions and congestive heart failure. N Engl J Med 1991; 325:293–302.

11. Managing transient ischaemic attacks

F Machado

THIS CHAPTER REVIEWS

- The presentation and urgency of transient ischaemic attack (TIA).
- The investigation and management of TIA.
- The identification of patients for surgical referral after TIA.
- The outlook after TIA.

A transient ischaemic attack (TIA) should be managed as a medical emergency. It indicates a high risk of permanent vascular injury to the brain (Fig. 11.1), and prompt assessment and treatment are essential to reduce the risk of stroke.

Relatively simple investigations can be used to identify patients whose risk can be reduced by drugs and/or surgery.

Presentation

Patients present either during a TIA or after the symptoms have resolved. The wide range of presenting features reflect the different areas of the brain that may be affected by the vascular obstruction.

The classical carotid artery territory TIA is easy to identify, and is often recognized by the patient. Vertebrobasilar TIAs are more difficult to diagnose, and if a patient presents with a temporary change in neuropsychiatric function, the possibility of a vascular event is often not considered.

Risk factors include hypertension, diabetes, coronary heart disease, hyperlipidaemia, smoking and a family history of vascular problems. A drug history is also necessary when evaluating the patient.

Examination

A full neurological examination should be performed to look for residual deficits. GPs performing an examination of the cardiovascular system should pay particular attention to:

- pulse rate, regularity and volume
- blood pressure
- heart murmurs
- carotid bruits
- peripheral vascular disease.

A carotid bruit in a patient with a TIA of carotid distribution supports the hypothesis that there is an embolism from the carotid artery. However, it is impossible to judge the degree of stenosis from auscultation alone. Sometimes no bruit is heard, even if there is a severe stenosis.

Investigations

Investigations by the GP

- Full blood count.
- Erythrocyte sedimentation rate.
- Urea and electrolytes.
- Glucose.
- Fasting lipids
- ECG.
- 24-hour or 7-day ECG if the patient reports palpitations.
- Thrombophilia and connective disease screen for young patients with TIAs.

Further investigations

Patients who have had carotid artery territory TIAs should undergo carotid artery Doppler studies to assess any stenosis of the carotid arteries. Many GPs do not have open access to Doppler studies, so patients have to be seen by a hospital consultant.

The patient may also require an echocardiogram, particularly if there is a heart murmur or atrial fibrillation. Again, open access to echocardiography varies between districts.

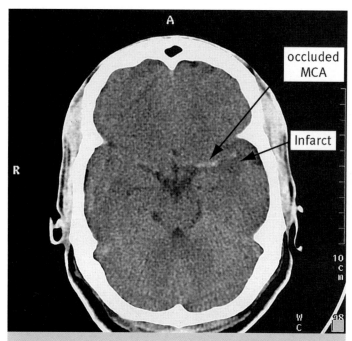

Figure 11.1 CT scan. Early cerebral infarction. There is occlusion of the left middle cerebral artery due to embolism from traumatic dissection of the wall of the left carotid artery, causing infarction in the left middle cerebral artery territory (MCA). Reproduced with permission from Swash, *Hutchison's Clinical Methods*, Saunders, 2001.

Management

Management of TIA includes educating patients about the risk of stroke and using therapeutic interventions.

Patient education

People who have had a TIA are often very anxious about having a stroke in the future. It is important to reassure patients that they have recovered from this acute episode. Nevertheless, they often need to modify their lifestyle to reduce the risk of stroke. The patient needs to understand that a TIA may indicate 'hardening of the arteries', not only to the brain but also to other vital organs such as the heart.

When discussing these events with patients it is best to avoid the term 'mini-stroke', as this may suggest that little harm is likely to result in the future. Indeed, patients need to be educated about the causes and treatment options for such 'brain attacks'.

Several major lifestyle changes may be needed, for example:

- smoking cessation
- weight loss
- increased exercise
- salt restriction
- alcohol restriction, particularly in hypertensive patients
- low-fat diet for patients with hypercholesterolaemia.

The importance of good control of hypertension should be stressed. Patients need to understand the target levels of treatment and the importance of regular monitoring.

Diabetics must be aware that good glycaemic control is essential.

Information leaflets, for example those produced by the Stroke Association, can be used to reinforce advice given in the surgery.

Therapeutic interventions

Any patient who presents with symptoms suggesting a TIA should be treated with either antiplatelet drugs (Box 11.1) or anticoagulation therapy. (See Ch. 9.)

Box 11.1 Antiplatelet treatments

- Aspirin (dispersible) 75 mg once daily
- Dipyridamole 200 mg modified-release capsules twice daily
- Dipyridamole + aspirin one capsule (dipyridamole 200 mg, aspirin 25 mg) twice daily
- Clopidogrel

Aspirin

Aspirin is the cheapest option. Indeed, until recently it was considered the best way of reducing morbidity and mortality after a TIA or stroke. However, the European Stroke Prevention Study has shown that, although low-dose aspirin and dipyridamole are equally effective, their efficacy is doubled when the two drugs are combined.[1] The combination is more expensive than aspirin alone, but because it prevents more strokes, it reduces overall costs in the long term. In fact, a study in New Zealand has concluded that there is no overall financial difference between aspirin and the dipyridamole and aspirin combination when both direct and indirect costs are considered.[2]

If the patient is intolerant of aspirin, dipyridamole can be used alone. Clopidogrel is another option.

Warfarin

Patients with atrial fibrillation should be considered for anticoagulation with warfarin.[3] A cause for the arrhythmia should be sought as it may be amenable to treatment (e.g. thyrotoxicosis and cardioversion should be considered, particularly if the arrhythmia is of recent onset). (See Ch. 9.)

Aspirin is an alternative for patients with non-rheumatic atrial fibrillation who do not want to take warfarin, or in whom the treatment would be difficult to manage. However, the patient should be aware that aspirin is only about half as effective as warfarin for the prevention of embolic stroke.

Antihypertensive agents

A TIA indicates end-organ damage, so any uncontrolled hypertension needs to be addressed. Recent trials have demonstrated that rigorous control of hypertension reduces the incidence of stroke, especially in diabetic patients.[4,5] Target blood pressure levels are 140/85 in non-diabetic patients and 135/80 in diabetic patients.

Of course, lower blood pressure targets often require the use of multiple agents, increasing the potential for side-effects and making the treatment more costly.

Patients who are normotensive at diagnosis must have regular reassessment of blood pressure.

Statins

Patients with a cerebrovascular cause for TIAs are at high risk of ischaemic heart disease. Their cholesterol target is ≤5 mmol/l, using a statin if diet alone is not effective.

Pravastatin is indicated to reduce the incidence of stroke in patients with ischaemic heart disease.[6]

Surgical referral

Endarterectomy halves the risk of stroke in patients with a carotid territory TIA and stenosis of >70%. These benefits outweigh the potential morbidity and mortality of the procedure.[7] Careful counselling is needed before the operation, and this is best provided by the surgical team.

Referral criteria in TIA

The need for referral depends on the GP's confidence that the patient has had a TIA, and on the availability of open-access Doppler and echocardiography studies.

Hospital referral is definitely needed when:

- there is doubt about the diagnosis
- further investigations are required
- a young patient has an unexplained TIA
- a patient has a carotid bruit and a TIA (refer to a surgeon with an interest in carotid endarterectomy).

The patient can be referred to a physician with a special interest in cerebrovascular disease, a cardiologist, a vascular surgeon or a neurosurgeon. A multidisciplinary clinic is ideal.

It is important that the patient is seen quickly, although sadly the current system is filled with delays. Delay may result in the patient having a further TIA or a stroke.

Follow-up

Patients must be followed up carefully to make sure their risk factors are managed optimally. GPs and practice and district nurses all need to identify patients who have had a TIA and to check their risk factors on a regular basis.

A TIA is also a very stressful experience, and patients may become depressed or anxious as a result. Primary ▶

healthcare teams can offer support and treatment where indicated.

The Stroke Association provides very useful contacts and support for patients and their carers who have suffered a TIA or stroke. Local groups operate in most areas. Such support organizations empower patients to discover what treatments and benefits should be available to them and to ask for them.

Practice and primary care trust issues

All team members need to be aware that TIAs warrant prompt treatment. In fact symptoms suggesting a TIA or stroke must be managed with the same urgency as chest pain. The practice should consider developing a protocol for the management of patients with TIAs, including:

- recognition of symptoms by all members of the primary healthcare team
- emphasis on the need for urgent assessment by a doctor
- a flow chart to follow for taking the history, examination and investigations
- a practice formulary
- awareness of standards for control of blood pressure and cholesterol levels, and of the need for good glucose control in diabetics.

Extra resources may be needed to meet increased prescribing costs for antiplatelet agents, statins and antihypertensive agents.

Structured care may require a dedicated clinic for patients at risk of stroke.

Key points

- TIA must be managed with the same urgency as chest pain.
- Risk factors include hypertension, diabetes, coronary heart disease, hyperlipidaemia, smoking and a family history of vascular problems.
- Patients who have had a carotid artery territory TIA should undergo carotid artery Doppler studies of both carotid arteries.
- Endarterectomy halves the risk of stroke in patients with a carotid territory TIA and a stenosis of >70%.

- Good control of hypertension and good glycaemic control are essential.
- Target blood pressure levels are 140/85 in non-diabetic patients and 135/80 (soon to be 120/75) in diabetic patients. The target cholesterol level is ≤5 mmol/l.
- Patients should be treated with antiplatelet drugs or anticoagulation therapy.
- Low-dose aspirin and dipyridamole are equally effective, but their efficacy is doubled when both drugs are combined. Clopidogrel is another option.
- Patients with atrial fibrillation should be considered for anticoagulation with warfarin: aspirin is only about half as effective as warfarin for preventing of embolic stroke.
- The Stroke Association provides very useful contacts and support for patients and their carers who have suffered a TIA or stroke.

Resources

The Stroke Association, Stroke House, Whitecross Street, London EC1Y 8JJ. Tel. 020 72 566 0300. Website: http://www.stroke.org.uk

References

1. Diener HC, Cunha L, Forbes C, et al. European Stroke Prevention Study. 2. Dipyridamole and acetylsalicylic acid in the secondary prevention of stroke. J Neurol Sci 1996; 143:1–13.

2. Scott G, Scott HM. Application of the findings of the European Stroke Prevention Study 2 (ESPS-2) to a New Zealand ischaemic stroke cost analysis. Pharmacoeconomics 1997; 12:667–674.

3. EAFT (European Atrial Fibrillation Trial) Study Group. Secondary prevention in non-rheumatic atrial fibrillation after transient ischaemic attack or minor stroke. Lancet 1993; 342:1255–1262.

4. Hansson L, Zanchetti A, Carruthers SG, et al. Effects of intensive blood pressure lowering and low-dose aspirin in patients with hypertension: principal results of the Hypertension Optimal Treatment (HOT) randomised trial. Lancet 1998; 351:1755–1762.

5. UK Prospective Diabetes Study Group. Tight blood pressure control and risk of macrovascular and microvascular complications in type 2 diabetes: BMJ 1998; 317:703–713.

6. Phehn JF, Davis BR, Sacks FM, et al. Reduction of stroke incidence after myocardial infarction with pravastatin: the Cholesterol and Recurrent Events (CARE) study. Circulation 1999; 99:216–223.

7. NASCET Collaborators. Beneficial effect of carotid endarterectomy in symptomatic patients with high-grade carotid stenosis. N Engl J Med 1991; 325:445–453.

12. Management of stroke in primary care

E Warren

THIS CHAPTER REVIEWS

- The social, psychological and financial implications of stroke.
- Planning secondary and tertiary stroke prevention strategies.
- The psychological needs of patients and carers.
- The management of post-stroke symptoms.
- Working with other agencies in patient management.
- Post-stroke patient surveillance.

Prevalence

Each year in the UK there are 110,000 first strokes, 30,000 recurrent strokes and 60,000 deaths from stroke.[1] An average GP will have four new strokes a year to deal with, as well as 12–15 patients with a past history of stroke.[2] Some 24% of severely disabled people in the community are stroke patients.[3]

Stroke care consumes around 5% of all NHS resources.[4] The Government's document *Saving Lives: Our Healthier Nation* has set a target to reduce deaths from stroke and coronary heart disease (CHD) in people under 75 years of age by a fifth before 2010 with the aim of saving 200,000 lives.[5] Stroke care has also been highlighted in the recently published National Service Framework for Older People.

Prognosis

The outlook following stroke is not very good. Patients and their carers are entitled to accurate information, however distressing this may be. Creating unrealistic expectations causes more problems in the long run. Changes to the lives of patients and their carers following a stroke are profound.

Successful management demands continuing surveillance of the patient for post-stroke physical effects, and an active watch for depression in both patients and carers. Primary care has a crucial role in post-stroke patient management and this is not always recognized by GPs.[6]

Death

Four out of five patients survive a stroke.[4] However, 10 years later the sufferer has only a 50% chance of still being alive: 15% will suffer a subsequent fatal stroke, while 40% will die of a myocardial infarction.[7] Stroke is only one manifestation of vascular disease.

Disability

Less than half of all stroke patients end up being fully independent.[8] Four out of five stroke patients live in the community, with 25% being entirely dependent on a carer, and a further 30% needing help with daily living tasks.

After 6 months, 50–80% of patients are able to walk independently, but only 22% can walk at their previous speed.[9]

Around a quarter of all stroke sufferers become depressed,[10] roughly twice the level in the normal elderly population (15%), and about the same as for other elderly people with a chronic debilitating illness. The extent of the cerebral damage does not correlate well with the risk of depression.

Recurrence

There is a 13% chance of recurrence in the first year following a stroke, and a 5% risk per year thereafter.[2]

Secondary prevention

Preventive measures are aimed at reducing overall atherosclerotic risk. Patients at the greatest risk have the most to gain. The Royal College of Physicians has published clinical guidelines on the management of stroke and its aftermath, providing a detailed review of worthwhile secondary prevention measures.[11]

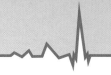

Box 12.1 Lifestyle advice after stroke

- Smoking advice, supplemented where appropriate by aids to cessation
- Dietary targets include:
  - achieving normal weight
  - reducing saturated fats
  - reducing salt intake to under 5 g/day
  - increasing fruit and vegetable intake to five portions a day
- Exercise for 20 minutes a day (where possible)
- Limit alcohol intake: 21 units a week for men and 14 units for women

---

Lifestyle advice (Box 12.1) should be offered to all stroke patients.[12]

Statins

Cholesterol should be reduced to <5.0 mmol/l using a statin if necessary.[13] (Cholesterol reduction may not reduce the chance of a further stroke, but will reduce cardiovascular risk.[14])

Antihypertensive agents

Hypertension should be brought under control gradually if it persists for more than a month following a stroke.[11]

Both diastolic and systolic blood pressure have a post-stroke linear relationship with the risk of a further stroke. Each 5 mmHg lowering of diastolic pressure is associated with a 34% decreased risk, and each 10 mmHg lowering of systolic pressure is associated with a 28% decreased risk.[15] This is the same percentage benefit as provided by a reduction in blood pressure in primary stroke prevention, but since individuals who have already had a stroke are at much greater risk of having another, the actual benefit is much greater.

The target blood pressure for secondary stroke prevention should be less than 130/80 in diabetics and less than 140/85 in non-diabetics.[16] It does not seem to matter which method is used to reduce blood pressure. However, evidence is gathering that angiotensin converting enzyme (ACE) inhibitors may confer an extra protective effect against stroke and heart attack.[15]

It has yet to be demonstrated that treating hypertension in the very old has conclusive benefits, but there is clear advantage to be gained from treating patients up to 80 years of age.[17]

Antiplatelet drugs

Following ischaemic stroke, the risk of future vascular events can be reduced by about a quarter by treatment with aspirin. Non-fatal myocardial infarctions are reduced by a third, and vascular deaths by one-sixth.[18] An initial dose of 300 mg followed by a daily dose of 75 mg is advised. The benefit is only seen following ischaemic stroke. In cases of haemorrhagic stroke, aspirin should not be used.[16] Benefit has been demonstrated from continuing aspirin for up to 2 years. The benefit probably remains continuous, and so indefinite use of aspirin is recommended.[18]

Modified-release dipyridamole 200 mg twice daily and the thienopyridines (e.g. clopidogrel) are about as effective as aspirin in secondary prevention, but are more expensive and have an additive effect when used with aspirin. They should be considered in patients allergic to aspirin or in those who suffer a vascular event while already taking aspirin.[14]

Anticoagulation with warfarin, keeping the international normalized ratio (INR) between 2 and 3, is recommended after an ischaemic stroke in patients with atrial fibrillation.[16] However, treatment should not commence within 14 days of the stroke, and then only if brain imaging has excluded haemorrhage.[11]

Recovery

Hospital admission following stroke often lasts 2–3 weeks during which time there should be intensive rehabilitative effort. It is important to plan properly so that community support structures can take over care on discharge.[11]

Stroke recovery has four distinct phases: crisis, treatment, realization and adjustment. Hospitals tend to concentrate on the first two and may lead patients and carers to believe that this is the only form of treatment available. Despondency results when it becomes evident that a degree of disability will persist.

Intrinsic recovery, the return of neurological function, occurs only over the first 3 months.

Functional recovery, the ability to do things, occurs through a combination of intrinsic recovery and adaptation, and may take up to a year, with just 5–10% of total improvement occurring in the latter 6 months. Further improvement after 12 months is very unlikely.[9] Despite this, one study found that 65% of spouses were still expecting full recovery 16 months after the stroke.[8]

There is a need for realistic information and explanation so that other ways of minimizing disability can be considered at an early stage. The Royal College of Physicians guidelines recommend that stroke patients who still have a residual disability at 6 months should be assessed for a period of further targeted rehabilitation.[11]

The GP's role

An early assessment should be made after discharge, and community services mobilized. Secondary preventive strategies should be implemented. GPs also have a role providing access to other services.

One study found that a third of stroke patients still had not seen their GP 3 months after discharge, 27% had received no inpatient physiotherapy and 67% no outpatient physiotherapy.[20]

Discussion of prognosis is appropriate. Advice on resuming normal activities can be useful, especially in relation to sexual activity: only a third of patients return to their previous levels of sexual activity after a stroke.[9]

Driving is not advised for a month after a stroke[21] and the DVLA will need to be informed. If the patient is left with epilepsy, substantial motor or visual loss or significant sensory inattention, then he or she should not drive. If there is doubt about driving ability, the DVLA can arrange an independent medical examination and a formal driving test.

Advice on this and other matters will be much needed by the patient and carers. Excellent literature is available from the Stroke Association.

Symptom control

Depression is common among stroke patients and responds to antidepressants in standard doses. It should be distinguished from emotionalism, which also frequently accompanies a stroke. The patient may become weepy and distressed for no obvious reason, to their embarrassment and the distress of their carers. Emotionalism may show some response to antidepressants.[10] In general, emotionalism is best seen as a type of illness behaviour, and care must be taken by carers and professionals that the behaviour is not inadvertently reinforced.

Most stroke patients have other age-related pathology, so when considering medication it is usually wise to begin with a small dose.

Post-stroke pain

Muscle pains

Spastic muscles are prone to spasm. Pain, in particular shoulder pain, may be present. Muscle and even bone injuries may occur, and pressure areas need regular review. Pain may respond to simple analgesia such as paracetamol or ibuprofen 400 mg (if there are no contraindications).

Thalamic syndrome

Central post-stroke pain (thalamic syndrome) affects 2–6% of stroke victims and is more common in younger patients. The onset of symptoms is typically several weeks or months after the stroke. An area of burning pain is felt, often associated with autonomic instability and allodynia (pain following non-painful stimuli). There is invariably an area of sensory loss to pinprick testing which extends beyond the bounds of the pain.[22] The pain is central in origin and results from the damaged cerebrum. Standard analgesics, however powerful, often do not work. Nortriptyline and amitriptyline in standard antidepressant doses may help. Clinical response takes 4–6 weeks.

Other symptoms

The patient or carer may not volunteer the fact that insomnia or incontinence are problems unless the GP enquires.

Leg swelling and contractures in the affected limbs will be visible on clinical examination. Pressure sores and fractures are more common in stroke patients.

Falls are more common following a stroke because of impaired balance-maintaining senses (proprioception, sight, vestibular function).[23] In addition, because of the age of the average stroke patient, there will probably be some pre-existing impairment of the other balance systems.

Supporting patient and carer

Most of the care of stroke patients is done by informal carers in the community. The majority are spouses, who are often elderly themselves. Some 14% of carers will give up work to care for the stroke patient. Around 12% of stroke carers are depressed. This figure rises to 40% in the case of spouses.[8] The patient's partner is thus more likely to be depressed than the patient.

Financial advice is often needed. Some benefits are particularly relevant to stroke patients, such as the Attendance Allowance or, for those under 65 years of age, the Disability Living Allowance.

The local Social Services department may be able to assist with respite admissions and day-care facilities giving the carer a well-earned rest.

The Stroke Association, other voluntary bodies and many hospital stroke units provide Stroke Clubs for the support of patient and carer, but these facilities are not well publicized.

Key points

- **The care of stroke patients could be improved.**
- **Stroke and cardiovascular disease are intimately linked and post-stroke care also includes overall reduction of vascular risk.**
- **The incidence of clinical depression in carers is high, particularly in spouses.**
- **The contribution of informal carers is significant.**
- **Most stroke patients have physical and psychological symptoms in addition to the stroke itself. Such symptoms should be actively sought and alleviated where possible.**
- **Many stroke patients have financial problems.**

Resources

The Stroke Association, Stroke House, Whitecross Street, London EC1Y 8JJ. Tel. 0207 490 2686. Website: http://www.stroke.org.uk

References

1. Bath PMW, Lees KR. ABC of arterial and venous disease. Acute stroke. BMJ 2000; 320:920–923.

2. Dennis M, Warlow C. Strategy for stroke. BMJ 1991; 303:636–638.

3. Greveson G, James O. Improving long-term outcome after stroke – the views of carers. Health Trend 1991; 23:161–162.

4. Sandercock PA, Lindley RI. Management of acute stroke. Prescribers' J 1993; 33:196–205.

5. Fowler G. Stroke: the general practice perspective. Geriatric Med 1999; 29:30–31.

6. Forster A, Young J. Stroke rehabilitation: can we do better? BMJ 1992; 305:1446–1447.

7. Marshall J. Why patients at risk of stroke should take aspirin. Monitor Weekly 1994; 7:43–44.

8. Cassidy TP, Gray CS. Stroke and the carer. Br J Gen Pract 1991; 41:267–268.

9. Hewer RL. Stroke-induced disability. Update 1994; 48:375–385.

10. House A. Depression after stroke. BMJ 1987; 294:76–78.

11. Royal College of Physicians. CEEU Projects: Stroke. National clinical guidelines. London: Royal College of Physicians;1999.

12. Action for Stroke Group. Preventing further events – a stroke management checklist. London: Action for Stroke Group; 2001.

13. British Cardiac Society, British Hyperlipidaemia Association, British Hypertension Society, British Diabetic Association. Joint British recommendations on prevention of coronary heart disease in clinical practice: summary. BMJ 2000; 320:705–708.

14. Gubitz G, Sandercock P. Prevention of ischaemic stroke. BMJ 2000; 321:1455–1459.

15. Rodgers A, MacMahon S, Gamble G, et al. Blood pressure and risk of stroke in patients with cerebrovascular disease. BMJ 1996; 313:147.

16. Lees KR, Bath PMW, Naylor AR. ABC of arterial and venous disease. Secondary prevention of transient ischaemic attack and stroke. BMJ 2000; 320:991–994.

17. Ramsay LE, Williams B, Johnston GD, et al. British Hypertension Society guidelines for hypertension management 1999: summary. BMJ 1999; 319:630–635.

18. Underwood MJ, More RS. The aspirin papers. BMJ 1994; 308:71–72.

20. Crowe S. Stroke prevention: more than just monitoring BP. Monitor Weekly 1993; 6:41–42.

21. The Stroke Association. Driving after a stroke or TIA. London: The Stroke Association; 1994.

22. Bowsher D. Central post-stroke pain and its treatment. London: The Stroke Association; 1994.

23. Overstall PW. Falls after strokes. BMJ 1995; 311:74–75.

13. Prevention of coronary heart disease

F Machado and J Coope

THIS CHAPTER REVIEWS

- Current thinking on primary and secondary prevention of coronary heart disease (CHD).
- The problems associated with implementing best practice.

The prevention of CHD is one of the most important tasks for general practice. CHD remains the principal cause of death in developed countries and, more significantly, 20% of these deaths occur below the age of retirement and a further 20% curtail normal life expectancy.[1] Many risk factors are now known, some of which are causal and reversible. These include smoking, hypotension, diabetes, obesity and hypercholesterolaemia.

Secondary prevention of CHD

In the UK 2–3 million people have established CHD. Half of all deaths from CHD occur in people who are known to have CHD, and reducing the mortality in this group of patients would have a major impact on overall mortality from the disease.

A number of interventions have been shown to be effective in the secondary prevention of CHD, particularly in the post-myocardial infarction (MI) patient.

Stopping smoking

About a third of patients will stop smoking after an infarct,[2] but all should be encouraged to do so because there is a 50% reduction in mortality over 2 years in patients who stop smoking following MI compared with those who continue to smoke.[3]

Aspirin therapy

Aspirin has been shown to reduce death, reinfarction and non-fatal cardiovascular accident by 12%, 31% and 42%, respectively, when given shortly after infarct.

The Antiplatelet Trialist Collaboration concluded that antiplatelet therapy prev.1LDL) cholesterol.[11] A recent report, the Joint British Recommendations on the Prevention of CHD in Clinical Practice, has advised that total cholesterol should be <5 mmol/l and LDL cholesterol <3 mmol/l.[12]

Control of hypertension

Blood pressure should be rigorously controlled in patients with CHD. Levels of <140 mmHg systolic and <85 mmHg diastolic are advised by the Joint British Recommendations on the Prevention of CHD in Clinical Practice.[12]

Hormone replacement therapy

Hormone replacement therapy (HRT) reduces both total cholesterol and LDL cholesterol, but is not as effective as simvastatin.[13] However, a randomized controlled trial of oestrogen and medroxyprogesterone acetate in postmenopausal women with established CHD did not demonstrate a reduction in the overall rate of CHD events during a follow-up period of 4 years, and recent research from the USA suggests a slight increase in MI in women taking HRT. The HRT group had an increased rate of thromboembolic and gall-bladder disease.[14] The results of the UK WISDOM trial are still awaited.

Cardiac rehabilitation and exercise

A combination of exercise and psychological and educational interventions is the most effective form of cardiac rehabilitation.[15] Exercise improves physical aspects of recovery at no additional risk, but a sole intervention is not sufficient to reduce risk factors for morbidity or mortality.

Many patients who might benefit do not receive cardiac rehabilitation, particularly the elderly, women and certain ethnic groups. However, an overview of 22 randomized controlled trials of cardiac rehabilitation programmes ▶

demonstrated a reduction in cardiac mortality and total mortality of 22% and 20%, respectively.[16]

Primary prevention

Until recently, a number of multiple intervention trials provided the main focus for primary prevention of CHD. These interventions included:

- smoking cessation
- exercise
- dietary advice
- weight control
- antihypertensive drugs
- cholesterol-lowering drugs.

A systematic review of randomized controlled trials of multiple risk factor interventions in primary care showed that small changes in risk factors for CHD had no significant effects on CHD mortality or total mortality.[17] In patients with hypertension and in other risk groups, risk-factor interventions have some beneficial effects.

The efficacy of lipid-lowering therapy in primary prevention has been shown conclusively.[18,19] Guidelines for cholesterol screening and treatment have been produced by a variety of organizations. It is important to remember that cholesterol is one of several risk factors that make up an individual's absolute risk of CHD.

The first step in primary prevention must be to calculate the individual patient's absolute risk of a CHD event. This is often presented as an annual percentage. The Sheffield Risk Tables,[20] probably the best known in the UK, identify individuals with an annual risk of >3%. However, they have been criticized for underestimating the risk as they do not take into account an individual's family history or ethnic background.

A joint report from the British Cardiac Society, the British Hyperlipidaemia Association, the British Hypertension Society and the British Diabetic Association recommends a staged approach to individuals based on their risk (Fig. 13.1).[12] Top priority for prevention is given to patients with CHD or other major atherosclerotic disease. Recommendations are lifestyle interventions, rigorous control of blood pressure, lipids and glucose, and cardioprotective drug therapy in selected patients.

For primary prevention it recommends risk stratification with identification of high-risk groups. Those with an absolute CHD risk of 30% over 10 years are targeted for aggressive treatment of hypertension, diabetes and cholesterol, and

aspirin therapy if aged >50 years and hypertensive or male or both.

As resources allow, those with a 15% risk over 10 years are targeted progressively and treated as above, but those with lower risk should only be targeted if they fall in particular groups likely to regress swiftly to higher risk strata (i.e. severe hypertension (systolic >160 mmHg and/or diastolic >100 mmHg), associated target organ damage, diabetes with associated target organ damage, or familial hyperlipidaemia).

Implementing prevention in primary care

There are nine key questions for the GP in CHD prevention:

- Has a fasting lipoprotein level been recorded? If the patient has an LDL level >3.5 mmol/l, has he or she received dietary advice? If he or she has persistent hyperlipidaemia, has he or she been prescribed an effective dose of a statin?
- Do we know whether the patient smokes? If the patient is smoking, has he or she been given advice on stopping?
- Is the patient obese? Has he or she been given dietary advice?
- Has the patient's blood pressure been reviewed recently? If he or she is receiving antihypertensive therapy, is he or she achieving his or her target?
- Has the patient been given advice on exercise and a healthy diet?
- Is the patient taking low-dose aspirin?
- If the patient has a history of MI in the past 3 years, is he or she taking a beta blocker?
- If the patient has symptoms of left ventricular failure, is he or she taking an ACE inhibitor or an angiotensin II blocker?
- If the patient has atrial fibrillation, have anticoagulants been considered?

A major concern about implementing prevention of CHD is the cost, especially that of statins. In response to the Standing Medical Advisory Committee's guidelines on the use of statins,[21] a group from Warwickshire Health Authority estimated that approximately 17,000 people aged 35–69 years would be taking a statin, accounting for about 20% of the drug budget.[22]

Preventive coronary care in general practice has been shown to be haphazard.[23] This reinforces the findings of

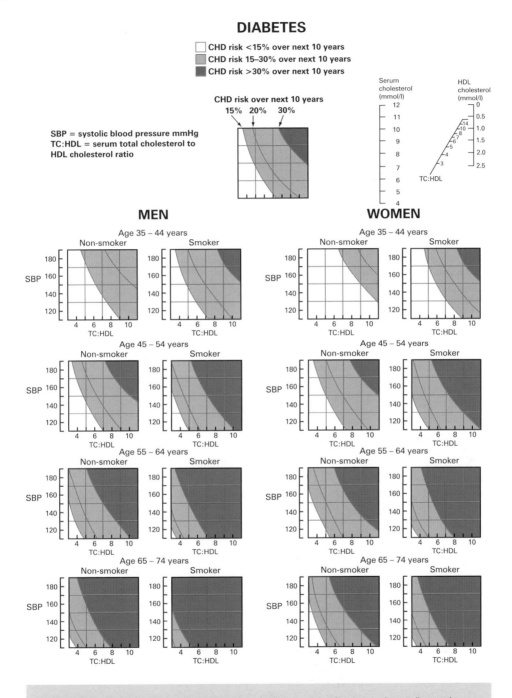

Figure 13.1 Joint British recommendations on the prevention of coronary heart disease in clinical practice. Reproduced with permission from Wood, Durrington, Poulter et al (eds), *Heart*, 1998; 80(suppl 2):S1–S29.

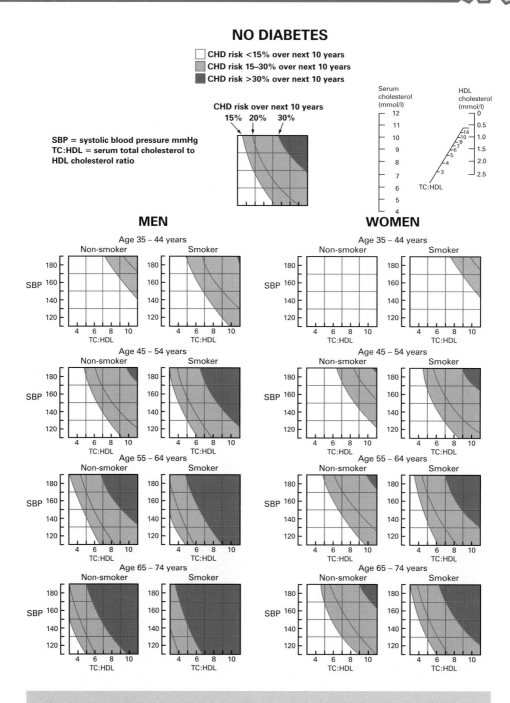

Figure 13.1 Joint British recommendations on the prevention of coronary heart disease in clinical practice (contd).

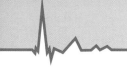

the British Cardiac Society's ASPIRE study in secondary care.[24] Risk-factor recording was incomplete, with smoking history and blood pressure the most commonly recorded and history of hyperlipidaemia and cholesterol levels the least well recorded. However, the biggest barrier for implementing evidenced-based practice may be convincing patients that they need to take part in life-long prevention.

Patients' enthusiasm about improving their health may be reduced if they experience side-effects from medication and do not have the motivation to continue that a closely controlled trial provides. GPs deal with individuals and we must recognize that observations of effectiveness on groups of patients do not guarantee benefit to the individual patient. The way we present data to our patients may affect their perception of the benefits.[25]

Key points

- In the UK, 2–3 million people have established CHD.
- A secondary prevention strategy may include: advice to stop smoking, aspirin therapy, treatment with beta blockers, ACE inhibitors, controlling blood pressure, lowering cholesterol with a statin and a programme of cardiac rehabilitation.
- To identify patients who will benefit from primary prevention, the coronary risk of the individual should be calculated.
- Cholesterol levels alone are a poor predictor of who will develop CHD.
- Implementing a prevention programme will require extra resources.
- The biggest barrier to implementing evidenced-based practice may be convincing patients that they need to take part in life-long prevention.

References

1. Mortality statistics: cause, 1995. Series DH2; 22. London: The Stationery Office; 1997.
2. Burt A, Thomley P, Illingworth D, et al. Stopping smoking after myocardial infarction. Lancet 1974; i:304–306.
3. Wilhelmsson C, Vedin JA, Elmfeldt D, et al. Smoking and myocardial infarction. Lancet 1975; 1:415–420.
4. Antiplatelet Trialist Collaboration. Collaborative overview of randomised controlled trials of antiplatelet therapy. I. Prevention of death, myocardial infarction and stroke, by prolonged antiplatelet therapy in various categories of patients. BMJ 1994; 308:81–106.
5. Yusuf S, Peto R, Lewis J, et al. Beta blockade during and after myocardial infarction: an overview of the randomised trials. Prog Cardiovasc Dis 1985; 27:335–371.
6. Mehta RH, Eagle KA. Secondary prevention in acute myocardial infarction. BMJ 1998; 316:838–842.
7. Ebrahim S, Davey Smith G. Health promotion in older people for the prevention of coronary heart disease and stroke. London: Health Education Authority; 1996.
8. Scandinavian Simvastatin Survival Study Group. Randomized controlled trial of cholesterol lowering in 4444 patients with coronary heart disease: the Scandinavian Simvastatin Survival Study (4S). Lancet 1994; 344:1383–1389.
9. Sacks F, Pfeffer M, Moye L, et al. The effect of pravastatin on coronary events after myocardial infarction in patients with average cholesterol levels. N Engl J Med 1996; 335:1001–1009.
10. The Lipid Study Group. Prevention of cardiovascular events and death with pravastatin in patients with coronary heart disease and a broad range of initial cholesterol levels. The Long-Term Intervention with Pravastatin in Ischaemic Disease (LIPID). N Engl J Med 1998; 339:1349–1357.
11. Rosengren A. Cholesterol: how low is low enough? BMJ 1998; 317:425–426.
12. Wood D, Durrington P, Poulter N, et al (eds). Joint British recommendations on the prevention of coronary heart disease in clinical practice. Heart 1998; 80(suppl 2):S1–S29.
13. Sbarouni E, Kyriakides ZS, Kremastinos DT. The effect of hormone replacement therapy alone and in combination with simvastatin on plasma lipids of hypercholesterolemic postmenopausal women with coronary artery disease. J Am Coll Cardiol 1998; 32:1244–1250.
14. Hully S, Grady D, Bush T, et al. Randomized trial of estrogen plus progestin for secondary prevention of coronary heart disease in postmenopausal women. Heart and Estrogen/progestin Replacement Study (HERS) Research Group. JAMA 1998; 280:605–613.
15. NHS Centre for Reviews and Dissemination. Cardiac rehabilitation. Effective Health Care 1998; 4:1–12.

16. O'Connor GT, Buring JE, Yusuf S, et al. An overview of randomised trials of rehabilitation with exercise after myocardial infarction. Circulation 1989; 80234–244.

17. Ebrahim S, Davey Smith G. Systematic review of randomised controlled trials of multiple risk factor interventions for preventing coronary heart disease. BMJ 1997; 314:112–117.

18. Shepperd J, Cobbe S, Ford E, et al. Prevention of coronary heart disease with pravastatin in men with hypercholesterolaemia. N Engl J Med 1995; 333:1301–1307.

19. Downs JR, Clearfield M, Weis S, et al. Primary prevention of acute coronary events with lovastatin in men and women with average cholesterol levels: results of AFCAPS/TexCAPS. Air Force/Texas Coronary Atherosclerosis Prevention Study. JAMA 1998; 279:1615–1622.

20. Management of hyperlipidaemia. Drug Therapeut Bull 1996; 34:89–93.

21. Standing Medical Advisory Committee. The use of statins. London: Department of Health; 1997.

22. Freemantle N, Barbour R, Johnson R, et al. The use of statins: a case of misleading priorities? BMJ 1997; 315:826–827.

23. Campbell NC, Thain J, George Deans H, et al. Secondary prevention in coronary heart disease: baseline survey of provision in general practice. BMJ 1998; 316:1430–1434.

24. ASPIRE Steering Group. A British Cardiac Society survey of the potential for the secondary prevention of coronary heart disease: ASPIRE (action on secondary prevention through intervention to reduce events). Heart 1996; 75:334–342.

25. Pringle M. Preventing ischaemic heart disease in one general practice: from one patient, through clinical audit, needs assessment, and commissioning into quality improvement. BMJ 1998; 317:1120–1123.

UROLOGY

14. Benign prostatic hypertrophy

THIS CHAPTER REVIEWS

- How to assess disease severity.
- How to investigate benign prostatic hypertrophy (BPH).
- When to treat BPH.
- Which treatments are best.
- When to refer a patient.

Prevalence

Benign prostatic hypertrophy (BPH) is a common, benign growth of the prostate arising periureterically and leading to obstructive and irritative urinary symptoms.

It is common with increasing age: at the age of 55 years around 25% of men have a decreased urinary stream; by the age of 75 years the percentage rises to 50–80%. Over 20% of men need a medical or surgical intervention for the condition by the age of 75 years.

The only racial difference in prevalence is in Japanese men, who have a lower prevalence.

Risk factors

Age and normal androgen hormone status are the risk factors. BPH is not seen in 20-year-old men or those castrated before puberty.

Family history predisposes to early difficulty, with autosomal-dominant inheritance. Around 50% of men requiring a transurethral resection of the prostate (TURP) under 60 years of age have fathers who are also affected by BPH.[1]

Aetiology

Prostatic hyperplasia increases urethral resistance, leading to compensatory changes in bladder detrusor function. This, together with age-related changes in both the bladder and the nervous system, causes symptoms of lower urinary tract irritation, as well as obstruction.

Presentation

Prostatism involves prostate enlargement, bladder outflow obstruction and lower urinary tract irritative symptoms (Box 14.1). Men with predominantly obstructive symptoms are more likely to experience acute retention.

Symptoms may interrupt normal activities or sleep, create anxiety or create a perception of reduced general health. The degree of distress can be very different for patients with the same symptom scores on objective assessment.

The size of the prostate does not correlate with symptom severity or degree of obstruction.

Diagnosis

Medical history

A detailed medical history should focus on the urinary tract, previous surgical procedures, general health issues and the patient's fitness for surgical procedures.

Physical examination

The general examination should pay attention to fitness, blood pressure and signs of renal insufficiency. The abdominal examination should include palpating the kidneys and bladder, which is palpable post-micturition if there is at least 150 ml of residual urine.

Digital rectal examination is essential to assess the size and normality of the prostate gland, although prostate size does not correlate with symptom severity.

Neurological examination may need to be considered if neurological bladder problems are suspected.

Investigations

Investigations include urinalysis, serum creatinine and serum prostate specific antigen (PSA).

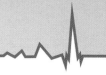

Obstructive symptoms

- Decreased force of stream
- Hesitancy
- Post-void dribbling
- Sensation of incomplete emptying
- Overflow incontinence
- Inability to voluntarily arrest stream
- Urinary retention

Irritative symptoms

- Frequency
- Nocturia
- Urgency
- Urge incontinence

Other symptoms

- Gross haematuria
- Clinically apparent bladder distension
- Prostatic enlargement (the normal size is about the size of a horse chestnut)
- Symptoms of renal failure

Complications of BPH

- Prostatitis
- Haematuria
- Urinary retention – the risk is probably around 1% per year (often with evidence of a precipitating event)
- Obstructive uropathy and chronic renal failure
- Bladder stones

Urinalysis

If urinalysis indicates a urinary tract infection or haematuria, a non-BPH cause of the symptoms is likely, and should be investigated before treating for BPH.

Serum creatinine

Serum creatinine should exclude renal insufficiency caused by obstructive uropathy. Up to 10% of patients with prostatism may have renal insufficiency.

Serum prostate specific antigen

Of men with BPH 11–33% have occult prostatic cancer. Prostate cancer can also cause prostatism.[1-3] In most men

with a 10-year or greater life expectancy, the knowledge of concomitant prostate cancer will alter management of the BPH. (Conversely, early detection of small, low-grade prostate cancer in an 80-year-old man may not be beneficial.)

PSA and digital rectal examination together increase the detection rate of prostate cancer compared with rectal examination alone. Therefore, measurement of the serum PSA should be performed in patients in whom identification of cancer would alter BPH management. A prostate has not been fully assessed without a serum PSA measurement.

There is overlap between serum PSA values in BPH and in clinically localized prostate cancer – 28% of men with proven BPH have a serum PSA >4.0 ng/ml. Men with a PSA in the range 4–10 ng/ml and a non-suspicious rectal examination have a 25% risk of prostate cancer.

PSA is significantly raised in prostatitis, prostatic infarction and after urinary tract instrumentation and prostatic biopsy, but rectal examination does not significantly raise it.

Imaging

Ultrasound of the upper urinary tract is indicated if there is:

- raised serum creatinine
- haematuria
- urinary tract infection
- a history of urolithiasis
- a history of urinary tract surgery.

Additional tests

Transrectal ultrasound can be useful to estimate prostate size or where malignancy is suspected.

Urethrocystoscopy is recommended for men with prostatism with a history of haematuria, urethral stricture (or risk factors such as urethritis or urethral injury), bladder cancer or previous lower urinary tract surgery.

Uroflowmetry and other pressure flow studies may be helpful in determining treatment choice.

Symptom assessment

The International Prostate Symptom Score (IPSS) (Box 14.2) is a scoring instrument for baseline assessment of symptom severity which is used in prostate assessment clinics. Symptoms are classified as mild, moderate or severe depending on symptoms score.[2] Pragmatically, GPs tailor a shortened version for convenience in the 10-minute consultation.

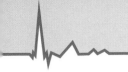

Ask the patient:

- How many times do you typically get up to urinate from the time you go to bed until the time you get up?

Score: 0 for none, 1 for 1, 2 for 2, 3 for 3, 4 for 4, 5 for 5 or more

Then for the following questions score: 0 for not at all, 1 for less than 1 time in 5, 2 for less than half the time, 3 for about half the time, 4 for more than half the time, 5 for almost always

- How often have you had a sensation of not emptying your bladder completely after you have finished urinating?
- How often have you had to urinate again less than 2 hours after you finished urinating?
- How often have you found that you stopped and started again several times when you urinate?
- How often have you found it difficult to postpone urination?
- How often have you had a weak urinary stream?
- How often have you had to push or strain to begin urination?

Total score: 0–7 = mild, 8–19 = moderate, 20–35 = severe

Referral

Patients should be referred if:

- the diagnosis of BPH is in question
- complications of BPH are suspected
- the patient has severe or intolerable symptoms
- there are indications for surgery (see below)
- PSA is raised
- there are suspicious findings on rectal examination.

Treatment options

Treatment options are medical, surgical or watchful waiting. With appropriate management, more than 70% of patients improve or stabilize.

Medical therapies investigated for BPH include alpha blockers, androgen suppression, aromatase inhibitors and plant extracts, but only the first two are of proven benefit. If successful, therapy will be lifelong. Medical therapy should not be offered to patients with absolute indications for surgical intervention.

Watchful waiting

Without absolute indications for surgery, delaying treatment will not have irreversible consequences, so watchful waiting may be the patient's choice. Dietary changes, such as avoiding caffeine, may help, as may avoiding cold and allergy remedies, and other medications, such as anticholinergics, which can exacerbate symptoms.

Alpha blockers

BPH is caused in part by bladder outlet obstruction mediated by the smooth muscle of the prostate: contraction is mediated by α-1A receptors.

Prazosin (Hypovase) was one of the first α-1 antagonists; the longer acting terazosin (Hytrin BPH) and doxazosin (Cardura) were then developed as once-daily alternatives. Titration up to the therapeutic dose may be necessary. Tamsulosin (Flomax MR) is α-1 subtype A specific, which reduces the side-effect of orthostatic hypertension.

The main contraindication to terazosin and doxazosin is a history of orthostatic hypotension. Terazosin should not be co-administered with verapamil. Tamsulosin does not affect blood pressure, so titration is not required.

Maximum clinical response is observed within 2 weeks and is dose dependent. There is no advantage to the lowest effective dose, so titrate to full doses, which are tolerated by 90% of patients.

Some 30% of males with BPH also have hypertension. α-1 Blockers can be administered to hypertensive patients who are controlled on medication, and on achieving a BPH response the other antihypertensive may be withdrawn. The use of α-1 blockers in normotensive patients does not appear to significantly lower their mean blood pressure.

Androgen suppression

The development of the prostate is dependent on dihydrotestosterone (DHT). Testosterone is converted to DHT by 5-α-reductase. Reducing prostate volume may decrease bladder outlet obstruction resulting from BPH. 5-α-Reductase inhibitors attempt to shrink the whole prostate to reduce symptoms caused by the periurethral prostate.

Finasteride (Proscar) is the only drug to achieve androgen suppression with acceptable tolerance in BPH, and is recommended for patients with large prostates who do not respond to α-1 blockers. Finasteride reduces prostate volume by approximately 20% within 6 months. However, overall improvements in symptom score are modest. It has been assumed that patients with large prostates are likely ▶

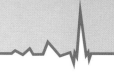

to achieve the greatest benefit, but there is a lack of clear evidence.[1]

Side-effects of finasteride can include impotence and decreased ejaculatory volume. It should not be given to patients whose partners are trying to conceive or who are pregnant as it can affect the foetus.

On average, finasteride reduces mean serum PSA levels by approximately 50%, but its effect on individual patients' serum PSA levels is variable.

Surgery

Transurethral resection of the prostate

Transurethral resection of the prostate (TURP) is now the gold standard for surgical management of BPH. TURP successfully relieves symptoms in 70–95% of patients, and 75–95% patients are satisfied with the result more than 5 years after surgery. The outcome is best for men who were most bothered by their symptoms. The incidence of short-term complications and need for re-treatment after surgery is low.

Most common early complications are failure to void, bleeding and clot retention.[1]

Indications for TURP are:[1]

- moderate to severe symptoms, which interfere with quality of life
- acute or refractory urinary retention
- recurrent infection
- recurrent haematuria
- serious complications of BPH
- bladder stones
- renal insufficiency
- large bladder diverticula
- a high residual urine volume is sometimes considered an indication

Medical treatments may be appropriate while awaiting surgical treatment.

Transurethral incision of the prostate

Transurethral incision of the prostate is almost as effective as TURP, but is reserved for patients in whom only a small volume of tissue needs to be resected.[1]

Open prostatectomy

Open prostatectomy, which has a significantly higher level of morbidity, is usually reserved for patients with very large prostates.[1,2]

Balloon dilatation of the prostate

Balloon dilatation of the prostate is less effective than surgery, but has fewer complications. It is useful in patients with smaller prostates.[1,2]

Newer alternatives to TURP

Clinical trials of ultrasound treatment using thermal tissue ablation are still in progress. It is well tolerated and does not harm the rectum. The median lobes are not treated. Patients need to lie still, and intravenous sedation is needed.[1,3]

YAG laser therapy has been used to treat bladder and prostate cancer and BPH. It is established, durable, effective and safe.[3]

Urethral stents, as temporary or permanent solutions for obstruction, are relatively new, and there have been good results in patients too ill for other procedures.[3]

Follow-up

In the UK, there is no clear consensus about monitoring and follow-up, and regular testing for PSA is not currently recommended, although it is available on request. Follow-up should aim to monitor symptom recurrence and suspicious features.

In the USA, the prostate score is assessed biannually,[4] and PSA and rectal examination are done annually. Regular urodynamic studies are also recommended.

Key points

- **Assessment of prostatism is incomplete without a PSA measurement.**
- **Occult malignancy co-exists with BPH in 11–33% of patients.**
- **Prostate size correlates poorly with symptoms.**
- **International symptom scores are a useful way of monitoring treatment response.**
- **Minimally invasive surgical techniques are likely to become more popular.**
- **TURP is very safe, with a high patient satisfaction rate.**
- **As the most common indication for treatment is to improve quality of life, patients should direct treatment choice unless there are absolute indications for surgery.**

References

1. McConnell JD. Benign prostatic hyperplasia. In: Walsh PC, Retik AB, Vaughan ED, et al (eds). Campbell's urology, 2nd edn. Philadelphia: WB Saunders; 1998, p 1429–1449. Available at: http://www.mdconsult.com

2. Jennings C. Benign prostatic hyperplasia. In: Dambro MR (ed). Griffith's 5-minute clinical consult. Baltimore: Lippincott Williams and Wilkins; 1999, p 868.

3. Abrams P, Wein A. Recent advances: urology. BMJ 2000; 321:1393–1396.

4. Thompson I, Carroll P, Coley C, et al. Prostate specific antigen: best practice policy. Available at: http://www.cancernetwork.com/journals/oncology/o0002e.htm

15. Prostate cancer

M Selby

THIS CHAPTER REVIEWS

- How prostate cancer presents.
- The usefulness of screening.
- The importance of staging and Gleason grading.
- The treatments currently in use.
- The evidence that the treatments help.

Prevalence

Prostate cancer is the most common non-dermatological malignancy worldwide. It accounts for 70% of all male cancers, and is identified microscopically in 30–50% of men at post mortem. The disease kills 19 men per 100,000 per year in the UK. Only lung cancer has a higher mortality.

There is no conclusive evidence yet about the benefits of treatment, even when the cancer is confined to the prostate, although most urologists advocate a radical approach.

Presentation

Adenocarcinoma accounts for 99% of cases of prostate cancer. There is a broad spectrum of aggression, ranging from low-grade and slow-growing tumours (patients have a good chance of dying of something unrelated) to highly malignant tumours that swiftly breach the capsule and metastasize, leading to painful and distressing terminal illness.

Benign prostatic hyperplasia (BPH) commonly co-exists: 11–33% of men with BPH have occult malignancy.

Most cancers are silent until advanced, and patients commonly present with symptoms of bony metastasis, thrombosis, hypercalcaemia and cord compression, although periurethral disease may cause earlier symptoms typical of prostatism. In advanced disease, there may be marrow suppression, renal failure and lower body oedema.

Risk factors

Asian men, who have genetically low levels of α-1-reductase, are at lowest risk. African men have the highest incidence, with higher-grade tumours and poorer survival. This may relate to higher testosterone levels.

Family history increases risk. An affected first-degree relative increases the chance of clinical disease two- to three-fold. The risk is four-fold if two first-degree relatives are affected.

There is no proven increase in prostate cancer after vasectomy.

Age is an important risk factor. Men under the age of 40 years have a 1 in 10,000 risk of invasive prostate cancer. The risk increases to 1 in 103 at the age of 40–59 years, and 1 in 8 at the age of 60–79 years. A 50-year-old man with a life expectancy of 25 years has:

- a 42% risk of prostate cancer
- a 10–15% risk of clinically evident prostate cancer
- a 3% risk of fatal prostate cancer.

Referral

Always refer a patient with suspected prostate cancer if the man has a life expectancy of more than 10 years, if he is symptomatic or if his prostate-specific antigen (PSA) level is >10 ng/ml.

Non-referral is an option for frail patients if life expectancy is less than 10 years, there are no symptoms, the PSA is <10 ng/ml and there are strong contraindications to a transurethral biopsy.

Prognosis (and likelihood of unpleasantly symptomatic disease) depends on tumour grade, which cannot be determined without biopsy.

If diagnosis may alter management, the patient should be referred. The differential diagnoses are BPH, urinary infection, prostatitis and prostatic stones.

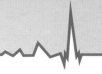

Investigation

Investigation by the GP

The GP may decide to arrange midstream urine tests (dipstick and microscopy) for infection and haematuria, and serum creatinine to evaluate renal function.

Radiographs may be appropriate if there is bone pain and tenderness. Prostatic lesions are typically sclerotic, and are commonly found in the vertebrae, ribs, long bones and pelvis.

If the history or examination (Box 15.1) raises suspicion of prostatic disease the GP will wish to consider testing PSA levels. This test is controversial, due to the high level of false-positive results it generates. The effectiveness of PSA as a screening tool is discussed in Chapter 16.

The PSA test is more likely to pick up slow-growing tumours, which have a low probability of causing illness, as tumours spend a much longer period with PSA in the slightly elevated range. Rapidly growing highly malignant tumours probably progress from normal to highly elevated PSA levels in a very short period, but will also generally become clinically obvious in this time (Boxes 15.2 and 15.3).

Investigation by the urologist: free PSA

If the PSA level is 4–10 ng/ml and the rectal examination is normal there is a 25% chance of carcinoma being present. If there are reasons not to do a biopsy, further tests may aid the decision.

Free PSA measures the percentage of unbound to total PSA. A low percentage of free PSA suggests malignancy. A high free PSA suggests benign disease or low-grade

---

Box 15.1 History and examination in suspected prostate cancer

Features in the history that suggest prostate cancer

- Prostatism (obstructive or irritative symptoms)
- Impotence (due to neurovascular bundle involvement)
- Pain on ejaculation
- Haematospermia due to seminal vesicle involvement
- Reduced volume of ejaculate due to obstruction of the ejaculatory duct
- Perineal pain
- General malaise (advanced prostate disease can cause intractable nausea)
- History of bone pain and tenderness, typically worse on movement, and there may be tender areas
- Pathological fracture
- Unexplained phlebitis or deep vein thrombosis
- Family history
- Symptoms of hypercalcaemia (constipation, dehydration, confusion, low mood)
- 'Gone off feet' – consider cord compression

Examinations for prostate cancer

- Abdominal examination for palpable bladder or kidneys
- Digital rectal examination – this is normal in 10% of symptomatic prostate cancer; look for an area of firmness or induration, loss of the median sulcus or irregular enlargement
- Examination of other painful areas
- Examination for vertebral tenderness and sensory loss if the patient has back pain

---

Box 15.2 The PSA test: sensitivity and specificity

- With a cut-off of 4 ng/ml, the sensitivity of PSA for prostatic cancer is 46%, the specificity is 91% and the positive predictive value is 32% (compared with 21% for rectal examination alone)
- PSA picks up 75% of organ-confined cancers, compared with 56% detected by rectal examination alone
- A man with a PSA of 4–10 ng/ml and a normal rectal examination has a 25% chance of prostate cancer, but this is most likely to be of low grade
- Levels above 10 ng/ml are highly suggestive of cancer
- PSA is normal in 20% of cases of prostatic cancer
- PSA is mildly raised in 30–50% of men with BPH – there is overlap between prostate cancer and BPH in the range 4–10 ng/ml
- Some laboratories increase the cut-off level with age, but this is not yet backed by guidelines or evidence

---

Box 15.3 What alters the PSA level?

- Digital rectal examination raises PSA by about 0.4 ng/ml
- Finasteride lowers PSA variably, on average by 50%
- Transrectal biopsy and transurethral resection of the prostate elevate PSA for 2–3 weeks
- Prostatitis and prostatic infarction raise PSA to high levels

malignancy. When PSA is 4–10 ng/ml and rectal examination is normal:

- a free PSA >25% lowers the risk of cancer from 25% to 8%
- a free PSA <10% raises the risk from 25% to 56%, and the disease is more likely to be aggressive.

The PSA density (the PSA level divided by the prostate volume as determined by ultrasound) is sometimes helpful. A density >0.15 is an indication for biopsy.

Transrectal ultrasound is used to detect or assess the extent of disease and to guide needle biopsy. It misses about half of lesions smaller than 1 cm. Transrectal biopsy usually involves six fine-needle aspirations. The procedure is painful, but is often performed in outpatients. There is a small risk of retrograde ejaculation.

Computed tomography and bone scans are usually reserved for patients with confirmed disease.

Treatment

Treatment depends on the patient's age, general health and life expectancy, the staging and grade of tumour and patient choice.

Treatment by Gleason grade

The Gleason grade of the tumour (Box 15.4) has enormous prognostic significance, but few if any large randomized controlled trials of treatments have used Gleason grading to compare treatments.

Treatment by stage

Most trials have looked at tumour stage, and staging is either clinical stage (Box 15.5) or by the TNM system (Box 15.6 and Fig. 15.1). In practice most organ-confined cancers are of low Gleason grade.

Box 15.4 Gleason grading

This is a histological scoring system. Various features are assigned scores of 1–5 which are then added to give total tumour score
- Score 1–5: prognosis generally good
- Score 6–10: prognosis intermediate to poor
- Score >10: anaplastic lesions, with very poor prognosis

Radical treatments (prostatectomy and pharmacological or surgical androgen deprivation) are widely used for disease confined to the prostate gland, in the hope of cure. There is little evidence for benefit of aggressive treatment in early (usually low grade) disease. However, the randomized controlled trials of treatments for early disease largely predate the availability of PSA testing.

Box 15.5 Clinical tumour staging

- Stage A: confined to prostate, impalpable
- Stage B: confined to prostate, palpable nodule
- Stage C: local extension
- Stage D: regional lymph nodes or distant spread

Box 15.6 TNM staging

- T0: clinically unsuspected
- T1: clinically unapparent
- T2: confined within prostate
- T3: outside capsule or extension into vesicle
- T4: fixed to other tissue
- N0: no evidence of nodal involvement
- N1: regional node involvement
- M0: no evidence of distant metastases
- M1: evidence of distant metastases

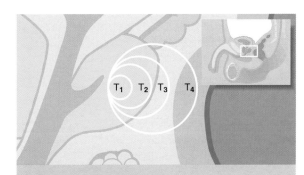

Figure 15.1 Prostatic cancer: TNM tumour grades on palpation. Note that palpation is more accurate when performed under general anaesthesia. Reproduced with permission from Burkitt & Quick, *Essential Surgery*, 3rd edn, Churchill Livingstone, 2001.

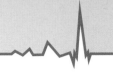

Such treatments carry a very high morbidity. However, most urologists believe that radical treatment of early disease offers patients the best chance. As a result, there are unlikely to be trials comparing radical treatment with no treatment in early aggressive disease.

The prognosis for aggressive tumours, which usually present after breaching the capsule, remains extremely poor. Hormonal treatments can be effective in advanced disease, while radiotherapy has a role in palliation. Androgen blockers, such as flutamide, are widely used when PSA rises, but there is little evidence as yet for benefit.

Treatment options

Watch and wait

A watch-and-wait approach, used alone, may be as good as any other treatment in clinically localized disease. However, it is appropriate only if the patient is fully informed and agrees to this course of action.

Surgery

Radical prostatectomy (removal of the prostate, capsule, seminal vesicles, vas, pelvic fascia and some lymph nodes) can be performed retropubically or perineally. It can result in urinary difficulties, and a few men become incontinent.

Mortality is 1.5–5% and is age-related. All men have retrograde ejaculation after the operation. Ability to achieve and sustain an erection is always lost, but up to 70% of patients regain this within a year (the chances are better in men under the age of 50 years).

There is a small risk of urinary incontinence and of faecal incontinence. The risk of major cardiopulmonary complications within 30 days of surgery can be as high as 8% among those aged over 65 years.

Cryotherapy has not yet been fully evaluated.

Radiotherapy

External beam radiation is a long-established treatment for prostate cancer. Sixty percent of men develop rectal and bladder symptoms during treatment, and 12% develop chronic cystitis. Other complications are proctitis, urethral stricture and chronic diarrhoea. Sexual function is preserved in three-quarters of men but falls off with time.

Brachytherapy

Brachytherapy (implantation of radioactive seeds into the prostate) has raised high hopes. The aim is to target the

prostate with minimal damage to surrounding tissue (the deposition of radiation energy decreases as a square function of the distance from the source). Bladder toxicity can be substantial, with 14% of patients having severe symptoms at 2 years.

Androgen deprivation

Orchidectomy is the most effective method of androgen deprivation. It is often used, particularly in the USA, with radical prostatectomy in localized disease. Side-effects include hot flushes and loss of libido as testosterone levels fall, which young patients tolerate poorly. Gout, hyperglycaemia, osteoporosis and gynaecomastia are also common.

Gonadotrophin releasing hormone (GnRH) analogues such as goserelin are the mainstay of androgen deprivation treatment for non-localized disease, and may be used as an adjunct to prostatectomy for localized disease. Treatment is lifelong.

Androgen receptor blockers, such as flutamide (Drogenil) and bicalutamide (Casodex), are used for 2–3 weeks to cover the androgen flare when GnRH analogues are initiated, otherwise there is a risk of boosting disease and causing obstruction or cord compression. There is no clear evidence that continued use confers greater benefit, and these drugs are not always well tolerated. However, they are in widespread use as an adjunct treatment when PSA levels rise.

The *steroidal androgen blockers*, such as cyproterone and medroxyprogesterone, are second-line treatments. Diethylstilbestrol is occasionally used for the same reason. Adrenal enzyme synthesis inhibitors, such as ketoconazole, are sometimes used.

The benefits of 5-α-reductase inhibitors, such as finasteride, are unproven.

Asymptomatic men do not tolerate androgen ablation well, leading to investigation of treatment cycling in ongoing trials.

Other therapies

Chemotherapy for prostate cancer has not yet been established, but studies now suggest that the disease may not be as resistant to chemotherapy as was once thought. The future may also see the development of immune therapy, using retroviruses to deliver cytokines directly to tumour cells.

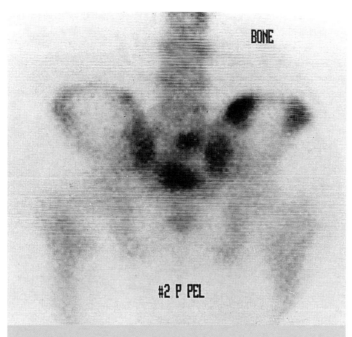

BONE

#2 P PEL

Figure 15.2 A bone scan showing multiple hot spots caused by metastatic carcinoma of the prostate. Reproduced with permission from Henry & Thompson, *Clinical Surgery*, Saunders, 2001 (courtesy of Gordon Williams).

Follow-up

Patients with known prostate cancer should undergo review every 3–6 months, with rectal examination and PSA testing. Bone scans (Fig. 15.2) and x-rays are indicated if PSA rises or symptoms develop.

Key points

- Prostate cancer is usually silent until it reaches an advanced stage.
- 25% of men with a PSA of 4–10 ng/ml and a normal rectal examination have prostate cancer.
- Patients with suspected prostate cancer and a life expectancy of >10 years should always be referred.
- Few large randomized controlled trials of treatments have used Gleason grading to compare treatment outcomes.
- Most urologists believe that radical treatment of early disease offers patients the best chance. The prognosis for aggressive tumours, which usually present after breaching the capsule, is poor.
- The challenge is to find a reliable method of detecting early cancer, particularly aggressive disease, while it is still confined to the prostate.
- Hormonal treatments can be effective in advanced disease, while radiotherapy has a role in palliation.

Resources

British Medical Journal: Clinical Evidence, issue 4, December 2000. Available at: http://www.clinicalevidence.org

Iversen P, Madsen PO, Corle DK. Radical prostatectomy versus expectant treatment for early carcinoma of the prostate: 23 year follow-up of a prospective randomized study. Scand J Urol Nephrol 1995; 172:65–72.

MEDLINE. Available at: http://194.200.197.82

Middleton RG, Thompson TM, Austenfeld MS, et al. Prostate cancer: clinical guidelines panel summary report on the management of clinically localised prostate cancer. J Urol 1995: 154:2144–2148.

Prostate Cancer Clinical Trialists Collaborative Group. Maximum androgen blockade in advanced cancer: an overview of 22 randomised trials with 3283 deaths in 5710 patients. Lancet 1995; 346:265–269.

US guidelines on prostate screening give guidelines for PSA screening asymptomatic men >50 years old and makes it clear that neither of the two large urology associations support this. Available at: http://www.guidelines.gov/index.asp

Wilt TJ, Brawer MK. The prostate cancer intervention versus observation trial. Oncology 1997: 11:1133–1139.

16. Prostate cancer screening and prognosis

M Selby

THIS CHAPTER REVIEWS

- The suitability of screening tests for prostate cancer.
- How the situation in the UK compares with that in the USA.
- The usefulness of prostate specific antigen testing.
- The prognosis.
- The effect of treatment on prognosis.

Prevalence

Prostate cancer is common. It kills 19 men per 100,000 per year in the UK, yet most patients with low-grade disease have a good prognosis, apparently regardless of whatever the doctor does.

As most urologists believe, despite a lack of evidence, that early disease should be treated radically, should screening be available, at least for men with symptoms possibly indicating prostatic disease? The USA has had a full screening programme since 1992, but there is little evidence that this has had any effect on overall mortality so far, despite the increased use of radical treatments. However, it may be too early to draw conclusions.

Which treatments give the best prognosis?

The understanding of the prognosis of prostate cancer is poor. More trials are needed, looking at the Gleason score (histopathological grade), before firm conclusions may be reached. Urologists believe radical treatment offers a chance of cure. So do most patients. However, there is no clear evidence that any one treatment is more effective than any other for asymptomatic men whose cancer has been picked up by a raised prostate-specific antigen (PSA) level alone.

Prognosis without treatment

Prognosis varies with tumour stage and Gleason classification. The 5-year survival by tumour grade is:

- well differentiated tumours: 98%
- moderately differentiated tumours: 92%
- poorly differentiated tumours: 29%.

In clinically localized cancer with a Gleason score less than 6, 70% of men are free from symptom progression at 5 years and 40% at 10 years. Once metastatic disease has developed, the median time to death is 5 years.

Gleason grading

Different histological patterns are assigned scores of 1–5, which are then added to give total tumour score:

- score 1–5: prognosis generally good
- score 6–10: prognosis intermediate to poor
- score >10: anaplastic lesions, with very poor prognosis.

On average, the time between a raised PSA level and clinical detection by rectal examination or from symptoms is 8–10 years. Thus men with palpable tumours or symptoms have already survived 8–10 years compared with those picked up early by PSA measurement. However, in those with aggressive disease there is a much shorter gap between a raised PSA level and tumour spread.

Disease confined to the prostate: prognosis with treatment

Low-grade disease carries a good prognosis, whatever the doctor does. Where the tumour is grade 1 on the Gleason scale, the 10-year survival is 94% after prostatectomy, 90% after radiotherapy, and 93% after conservative management. There are no similar figures available for higher grade disease.

Survival rates after prostatectomy for localized disease are 97% at 5 years and 85% at 10 years. This is perhaps ▶

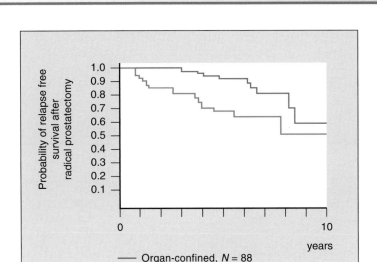

Figure 16.1 Capsular penetration by prostate cancer cells correlates with risk of tumour recurrence after radical prostatectomy. Data supplied by Dr DF Paulson. Reproduced with permission from Kirby, *Prostate Cancer*, Mosby, 1996.

unsurprising, since most of these tumours will be of a low Gleason grade.

Existing evidence suggests that watchful waiting may be as good as most treatments for localized asymptomatic prostate cancer, although one trial suggests that hormone treatment alone adds 5 years to life. However, most specialists feel that combined radical prostatectomy with radiotherapy and possibly surgical or medical androgen deprivation offers the best chance of curing localized disease. Results from the Mayo Clinic in the USA suggest that aggressive treatment can delay metastases.

There is no positive evidence for brachytherapy, cryosurgery or radiotherapy. One trial suggests that prostatectomy is better than brachytherapy when the Gleason score is greater than 6.

Most urologists add androgen blockade to androgen deprivation when the PSA level eventually rises, although again the evidence of benefit is very limited.[1-3]

Locally advanced disease

Survival rates after radical treatment for locally advanced disease with capsular penetration (Fig. 16.1) are 68% at 5 years and 42% at 10 years. These figures fall to 15% and zero when there is high-grade histology as well as capsular penetration.

Several trials give conflicting results. Androgen deprivation therapy alone has been shown to improve survival and reduce major complications, yet one trial has found that orchidectomy gives no benefit.[1,3,4] Overall, the available evidence suggests that radical treatment improves survival for patients with locally advanced symptomatic disease.[4,5] This means simultaneous interventions with radical prostatectomy, orchidectomy, androgen deprivation and androgen blockade, but the side-effects are severe.

Overall, the picture is unclear, suggesting as is does that radical treatment is more of an advantage in locally advanced disease than in localized disease. Perhaps the group who are picked up while asymptomatic have lower grade disease on average.

Metastatic disease

There is some evidence that androgen deprivation treatment improves survival in metastatic disease, although no one method seems to be better than any other.[1,3]

Starting treatment early may reduce complications compared with waiting until the disease progresses, but it

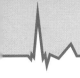

does not seem to affect mortality. Adding androgen blockers, such as flutamide and bicalutamide, does not appear to give any extra benefit.

Adding orchidectomy to these treatments does appear to increase survival in trials, but at a high cost in terms of adverse events.

Radiotherapy and strontium-89 both provide symptomatic relief from bone pain, but only strontium-89 reduces the number of new sites. Strontium-89 is a calcium displacing radionuclide given as an intravenous single-dose treatment and costs around £1000. It has an affinity for sclerotic tissue.

Chemotherapy may give palliative benefit, particularly for pain, but the evidence so far does not suggest that is prolongs survival.

Hormone-independent metastatic disease

Palliative chemotherapy, radiation and strontium-89 may relieve symptoms but do not improve survival.

Palliative care

The slow course of advanced disease means that many patients need palliative care for several months. A high proportion of adult hospice beds in the UK are occupied by men with prostate cancer.

Treatment with androgen deprivation and blockade is usually indefinite, or is continued at least until the patient can no longer take medication. Stopping treatment may worsen pain.

Bone pain

Bone pain is gnawing and becomes worse with movement. It responds best to targeted radiotherapy or the radionuclide strontium-89. Treatment with strontium is very expensive, but it is superior to external beam radiation.

Non-steroidal anti-inflammatory drugs are helpful. However, patients with advanced disease are frail and care must be taken with the choice of agent. Gastroprotective medication may be advisable.

Opiates provide partial relief of bone pain. Paracetamol may also be helpful.

Nausea

Nausea is common in prostate cancer and may be severe and intractable. Haloperidol delivered by syringe driver is often effective.

Pathological fractures

These require pinning. Stabilization produces pain relief, but the fractures will not heal. If surgical treatment is impossible, careful nursing and traction may suffice.

Hypercalcaemia

Hypercalcaemia is common and is a poor sign in prostate cancer. It is treated with rehydration and intravenous pamidronate titrated against corrected calcium levels and takes up to 3 days to work.

The speed of recurrence of hypercalcaemia is an indicator of deterioration. It is important to maintain a high index of suspicion for hypercalcaemia, as malaise, nausea and constipation may be present anyway.

Cord compression

This is suggested by 'going off feet', weakness, radicular pain, sphincter disturbance, sensory loss and central back pain with tenderness. The last symptom is absent in 10% of cases.

Emergency radiotherapy is the treatment of choice to prevent permanent paralysis. Every hour of delay reduces the chance of retrieval of function, and the patient is at risk of irreversible paralysis and loss of sphincter control.

Treatment with 16 mg oral dexamethasone or 120 mg oral prednisolone immediately reduces the swelling and buys time. Even so, radiotherapy should be given within 24 hours of onset.

Screening

Screening asymptomatic men

There is no clear evidence that detection and treatment of asymptomatic disease makes any difference to survival. The group picked up by PSA testing of asymptomatic men, those with early but relatively benign disease, do not appear to benefit from the treatments currently offered.

PSA testing also currently has a too high false-positive rate to be ideal.[6] As the prostate enlarges through life the chance of picking up mildly raised PSA and generating invasive testing becomes high in the older age group. PSA would pick up aggressive disease, but as this spreads rapidly an extremely short inter-testing interval would be necessary in order to have any chance of detecting the disease at a treatable stage.

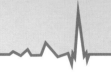

Screening symptomatic men

Measuring PSA in men with prostate symptoms is common, although whether this constitutes screening is a moot point. One could argue that it is screening, as although they do have symptoms they are not necessarily symptoms of prostate cancer, they are just an at-risk group.

Nevertheless, again, where PSA testing detects aggressive disease it tends to detect it too late. A large number of men with benign prostatic hypertrophy will test in the range 4–10 ng/ml and require biopsy, and most men with aggressive disease will test higher because by the time they are symptomatic their disease has spread. In other words, the group of greatest interest, those with aggressive but early disease, present too late.

Wilson's screening criteria state that there must be an interval in which effective intervention is possible. PSA testing does not pick up the right men at the right stage. PSA thus fails the essential criteria of a screening tool, in that it is unlikely to pick up the disease while it is still in a phase that is amenable to treatment and in which treatment would bring clear benefit. The PSA test is not specific enough to rule out benign prostatic disease and, without very frequent repeat testing, it is in effect not sensitive enough to pick up early aggressive disease.

Nevertheless, it is an essential tool in evaluating the symptomatic prostate in order to inform the patient about the cause of symptoms, likely progression and treatment options.

US policy

There has been widespread PSA screening of asymptomatic men in the USA since 1992, with increased rates of radical treatment.[6] All men over 50 years old are offered an annual PSA test and rectal examination. Screening begins at the age of 40 years for African-American men and patients with a positive family history. Biopsy is indicated if the PSA level is >4 ng/ml or increases by more than 0.75 ng/ml per year.

The annual death rate has declined from 19 per 100,000 to 18 per 100,000 men. However, the greatest declines have been in areas with the lowest screening uptake and lowest uses of radical treatment, and countries with low rates of PSA testing do not have higher death rates.

The US cancer screening trial is currently evaluating the policy in a study of 74,000 men.

UK policy

Screening of symptomatic patients for prostatic carcinoma is felt to be inappropriate because men with early but aggressive disease are less likely to be symptomatic, and symptoms are more likely to be due to benign prostatic hyperplasia. This point of view is understandable, but is arguably illogical, for the following reasons:

- Urological opinion is that tumours confined to the prostate should be offered radical treatment.
- The argument is that patients with aggressive disease often present late. By the time symptoms appear or the PSA level rises the disease has often breached the capsule. However, there is some evidence suggesting that treatment may be of benefit in locally advanced disease.

It can be argued that assessment of the symptomatic prostate is incomplete without a PSA test. Most guidelines do not yet suggest it, but it is hard to find a urologist who does not check the PSA level of all patients referred with prostatism.

Current research

The prostate cancer prevention trial is a double-blind multicentre randomized controlled trial looking at whether finasteride prevents prostate cancer in 18,000 men over the age of 55 years. Half will receive finasteride daily for 7 years, and half will receive placebo.

Key points

- **The PSA level is not highly sensitive or specific for early disease.**
- **Aggressive tumours are usually not localized at presentation.**
- **Combined rectal examination and PSA test is more sensitive than either used alone.**
- **In a man with a normal rectal examination and a PSA level in the range 4–10, the chance of cancer is 25%.**
- **There is insufficient evidence to be certain whether radical treatments are beneficial in early disease, whatever the histological grade or the tumour.**
- **There is evidence to support some hormonal therapies in late disease.**
- **Despite a lack of evidence as yet, most urologists believe that radical treatment offers hope of cure in early localized disease.**

Resources

US guidelines on prostate screening. Available at: http://www.guidelines.gov/index.asp

References

1. Prostate Cancer Clinical Trialists Collaborative Group. Maximum androgen blockade in advanced cancer: an overview of 22 randomised trials with 3283 deaths in 5710 patients. Lancet 1995; 346:265–269.

2. Middleton RG, Thompson TM, Austenfeld MS, et al. Prostate cancer: clinical guidelines panel summary report on the management of clinically localised prostate cancer. J Urol 1995; 154:2144–2148.

3. British Medical Journal: Clinical Evidence, issue 4, December 2000. Available at: http://www.clinicalevidence.org

4. Wilt TJ, Brawer MK. The prostate cancer intervention versus observation trial. Oncology 1997; 11: 1133–1139.

5. Iversen P, Madsen PO, Corle DK. Radical prostatectomy versus expectant treatment for early carcinoma of the prostate: 23 year follow-up of a prospective randomized study. Scand J Urol Nephrol 1995; 172:65–72.

6. MEDLINE. Available at: http://194.200.197.82

17. Haematuria and proteinuria

M Selby

THIS CHAPTER REVIEWS

- The role of the GP in detecting haematuria and proteinuria.
- The investigation and treatment of haematuria to exclude serious underlying conditions.
- The presentation and management of proteinuria.

Haematuria and proteinuria, together or separately, are common findings in general practice. Most GPs regard a significant amount of blood or protein in the urine as an indication for referral to exclude serious kidney disease or renal tract malignancy. However, microscopic haematuria and proteinuria are both commonly detected in well patients.

Haematuria

The prevalence of haematuria in general practice is quoted as 1–14%. The blood may originate from the kidney (glomerular) or the collecting system (non-glomerular). The likely causes are outlined in Box 17.1.

A 'normal' limit for microscopic haematuria is not agreed. Recommendations vary between 2 and 5 erythrocytes/high power field.

All definite haematuria, whether gross or microscopic, requires investigation to exclude serious underlying conditions.[1,2] It should also be re-evaluated once or twice, with testing repeated twice at intervals of 6 months if the initial follow-up is negative. Occult cancer will show within a year.[1,3]

The chance of detecting a nephrological or urological condition varies with age. In men and women aged over 50 years, pathological explanations are found in up to 80% of cases of haematuria, and further investigations uncover life-threatening conditions in 12–34%.[4] The risk is lower in younger patients and in women.

All children with haematuria should be referred.

Anticoagulants are more likely to provoke haematuria from pre-existing lesions than to cause it de novo, so patients on anticoagulants should also be investigated.

Microscopic haematuria has also been linked to the use of aspirin. The balance of opinion is that this is not normal in aspirin users, and indicates acute tubular nephrotoxicity.[5]

It is important to remember that blood is not the only substance which can colour urine red (Box 17.2).

Investigations

If white cells are present, urinary culture is mandatory and cytological examination of urine is recommended.

If urinalysis does not explain the findings, the kidneys and bladder should be examined by ultrasound, which is as sensitive as intravenous urography and more cost-effective.[6] A plain film radiograph of the abdomen should also be obtained, mainly to rule out urinary calculi.

If no explanation is found, the patient should be referred for cystoscopy. If this is negative, Coulter counter analysis of the excreted erythrocytes may be carried out to determine whether the haematuria is glomerular or non-glomerular in origin. Dysmorphic erythrocytes, especially if associated with substantial proteinuria, suggest a glomerular origin. Further studies may then include renal biopsy. If the haematuria is not glomerular, then intravenous urography may be needed. If a definite diagnosis cannot be made, investigations should be repeated whenever gross haematuria occurs or after 4–6 months.

Most GPs adopt a pragmatic approach to well patients, with dipstick haematuria only. This involves:

- excluding infection by microscopy and culture
- excluding contamination due to menstruation
- repeating the test and investigating or referring if haematuria persists or if there are other worrying features.

Confirmed infection should be treated and then followed up with further urinalysis, because renal tract abnormality increases the risk of infection.

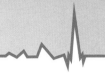

Box 17.1 Causes of haematuria

Haematological
- Sickle cell disease
- Coagulation disorders
- Anticoagulant therapy

Infection
- Glomerulonephritis
- Tuberculosis
- Cystitis
- Prostatitis
- Urethritis
- Tropical infections (e.g. schistosomiasis, yellow fever, blackwater fever)

Inflammation
- Henoch–Schönlein purpura
- Immunoglobulin A nephropathy
- Goodpasture's syndrome
- Arteritis
- Post-irradiation

Structural
- Calculi (renal, bladder, ureteric)
- Simple cysts
- Polycystic renal disease
- Congenital vascular anomalies

Surgery
- Invasive procedures to the prostate or bladder

Toxins
- Sulphonamides
- Cyclophosphamide
- Non-steroidal anti-inflammatory drugs
- Phenols
- Turpentine

Trauma
- Kidney trauma due to a catheter or foreign body
- Prolonged severe exercise
- Rapid emptying of an overdistended bladder (e.g. after catheterization for acute retention)

Tumour
- Hypernephroma
- Wilms' tumour
- Carcinoma of the bladder, prostate or urethra

Other
- Genital bleeding, including child abuse
- Menstruation
- Factitious, including Munchausen's disease by proxy

Box 17.2 Causes of red or dark urine

- Haematuria
- Haemoglobinuria (dipstick positive, but no red cells on microscopy)
- Myoglobinuria
- Food, such as beetroot
- Drugs, such as rifampicin and senna
- Porphyria (urine darkens on standing)
- Obstructive biliary disease

Macroscopic haematuria usually requires early referral, with urine cytology. Recurrent gross haematuria in patients with benign prostatic disease is usually considered an indication for surgery, so referral is needed.

Common causes
Non-glomerular causes
In a study of 1000 patients[1] the common causes of non-glomerular haematuria were:
- inflammatory conditions of the urethra and prostate (usually trigonitis) (37%)
- benign prostatic hyperplasia (16%)
- cystitis (7%)
- transitional carcinoma of the bladder (6%)
- stones in the renal pelvis or ureter (3%)
- altogether, 8% had some form of cancer.

In a screening study of men aged over 50 years, pathological conditions were found in 31 of 44 patients who had haematuria. One-third of the 44 had either cancer of the urinary tract or other conditions requiring immediate treatment.[4]

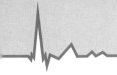
Glomerular causes

The most common cause of glomerular haematuria is immunoglobulin A nephropathy (characterized by recurrent episodes of gross haematuria in association with respiratory infection and seen in young patients), followed by the other glomerulonephritides. Glomerulonephritis presents in many different ways, and an accurate diagnosis cannot be made clinically.[7] Early referral for assessment and renal biopsy is essential so that treatable conditions can be detected. Early treatment is more likely to preserve or improve renal function.

Underlying glomerulonephritis is considered to be the cause of end-stage renal failure in about a quarter of patients accepted onto dialysis programmes.[7] Most other renal cases are due to vascular malformations, simple cysts or stones and thin basement membrane disease (Box 17.3).[8] The latter (also called benign familial haematuria) involves thinning of the glomerular basement membrane and a mild glomerulonephritis.[9] It is suggested by a lifelong history of haematuria, minimal proteinuria and normal renal function.

Proteinuria

Presentation

Patients with proteinuria are unlikely to notice any alteration in their urine, although it may be more frothy. Thus proteinuria in healthy patients is commonly picked up on routine dipstick testing.

Proteinuria may indicate primary renal disease, although a degree of proteinuria is seen in urinary tract infection and viral illnesses. The causes of significant proteinuria are listed in Box 17.4.

Minor albuminuria may occur transiently after exercise, during fever or in heart failure, but rarely rises to the nephrotic range (Table 17.1). Tests should be repeated if such a cause is suspected.

Orthostatic proteinuria is urinary leakage of protein in well patients that is absent in the morning sample but appears through the day. It appears to be benign.

Nephritic and nephrotic syndromes

Nephritic syndrome is the abrupt onset of haematuria, proteinuria (usually moderate), reduced renal function and salt and water retention, causing oedema and hypertension. *Nephrotic syndrome* is heavy proteinuria (>3.5 g/24 h) associated with hypoproteinaemia, distinct oedema and, often, hypercholesterolaemia.

Box 17.3 Features suggesting a renal cause of haematuria

- Hypertension
- Altered renal function tests
- Proteinuria
- Known previous renal problems
- Renal mass
- Glomerular red cells in urine

Common causes include various types of glomerulonephritis and systemic disease, such as diabetes and systemic lupus erythematosus. These may lead to renal failure, venous thromboembolism, hypercholesterolaemia and infection, although the incidence of severe complications is low.

Mild haematuria and low-level proteinuria (<2 g/day) in the absence of renal impairment or hypertension are associated with a good long-term prognosis. Management includes treating the cause and supporting fluid regimens.

Investigation and management

If a patient has persistent proteinuria on dipstick testing, it may be useful to quantify protein excretion with a 24-hour collection. Normal urinary excretion of protein is <150 mg/day, and if 24-hour collection shows total excretion in the normal range there is no need for further action.

Alternatively, the protein/creatinine ratio could be checked, which makes allowance for the variable dilution and is easier for the patient.[10]

Proteinuria of <2 g/24 h may be due to failure of tubular reabsorption, as some low molecular weight protein is filtered at the glomerulus and reabsorbed by tubular cells. However, greater degrees of albuminuria are almost always due to glomerular disease.

Patients with higher levels of proteinuria or other renal symptoms, such as hypertension or oedema, should be referred for investigation, as should any children with proteinuria. The urgency of the referral depends on the degree of proteinuria and the patient's clinical condition. Depending on the age of the patient it may be appropriate to ask for urine protein electrophoresis to look for abnormal proteins.

Nephrotic levels of protein excretion require urgent referral for investigation and management of fluid balance. While

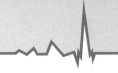

awaiting this, the GP should exclude congestive heart failure and malignant hypertension.

In many types of renal disease, the degree of proteinuria is proportional to the risk of progressive loss of renal function. Treatments such as angiotensin-converting enzyme inhibitors that reduce the risk of progression also reduce proteinuria.

Key points

- Dipstick haematuria and proteinuria are most likely to be caused by infection, stones or contamination; however, they may indicate serious disease and should be followed up.
- Occult malignancy producing microscopic haematuria will become clinically apparent within a year.

Box 17.4 Causes of proteinuria

Renal
- Primary renal disease (e.g. glomerulonephritis, renal vein thrombosis)

Systemic
- Malignant hypertension
- Congestive heart failure
- Diabetes
- Amyloidosis
- Sarcoidosis
- Sickle cell disease
- AIDS-related nephropathy

Malignancy
- Multiple myeloma (Bence Jones proteins are present in around 30% of cases, but are not always detected by dipstick testing)
- Leukaemia
- Hodgkin's disease

Infection
- Pyelonephritis, especially when complicated by stones, obstructive uropathy or diabetes
- Cystitis

- Malaria
- Tuberculosis

Inflammation
- Systemic lupus erythematosus
- Rheumatoid arthritis
- Goodpasture's syndrome
- Radiation nephritis
- Wegener's granulomatosis

Tubular disease
- Cystinosis

Functional
- After heavy exercise
- Chronic catheterization (debris)
- Pregnancy
- Orthostatic proteinuria
- Benign proteinuria due to fever, heat or cold exposure

Toxins
- Heavy metals
- Drugs

Table 17.1 Protein levels and their significance

Excretion (g/24 h)	Protein/creatinine	Significance
<0.15	Not raised	Normal
0.3-0.5	Not raised	Dipstick tests positive
0.5-2.5	20-250	Source equivocal
>2.5	>300	Glomerular disease likely
>3.5	>400	Nephrotic range, definitely glomerular

- Urgency of referral depends on the degree of proteinuria and the patient's clinical condition.
- Proteinuria may indicate primary renal disease, although a degree of proteinuria is seen in urinary tract infection and viral illnesses.
- Have a low threshold for referral of children and the elderly, and refer where symptoms suggest renal disease.

References

1. Mariani AJ, Mariani MC, Macchioni C, et al. The significance of adult haematuria: 1000 haematuria evaluations including a risk–benefit and cost-effectiveness analysis. J Urol 1989; 141:350–355.

2. Savige J, Buzza M, Dagher H. Haematuria in asymptomatic individuals [editorial]. BMJ 2001; 322:942–943.

3. Schroder FH. Microscopic haematuria requires investigation [editorial]. BMJ 1994; 309:70–72.

4. Messing EM, Young TB, Hunt VB, et al. Urinary tract cancers found by home screening with haematuria dipstick in healthy men over 50 years of age. Cancer 1989; 64:2361–2367.

5. Faivre J-MR. Haematuria and aspirin [letter]. BMJ 2001; 22 June.

6. Corwin HL, Silverstein MD. The diagnosis of neoplasia in patients with asymptomatic microscopic haematuria: a decision analysis. J Urol 1988; 139:1002–1006.

7. Mason PD. Glomerulonephritis: diagnosis and treatment. BMJ 1994; 309:1557–1563.

8. Davison A, Cumming A, Swainson CP, et al. Diseases of the kidney and urinary system. In: Haslett C, Chilvers ER, Hunter JAA, et al (eds). Davidson's principles and practice of medicine. Edinburgh: Churchill Livingstone; 1999.

9. Kincaid-Smith P. Thin basement membrane disease. In: Massry SG, Glassock RJ (eds). Textbook of nephrology. Philadelphia: Lippincott.

10. Greene H (ed). Decision making in medicine. St Louis: Mosby; 1998.

18. Urinary tract infection in adults

THIS CHAPTER REVIEWS

- Which clinical examination is helpful in which circumstances.
- The advantages and disadvantages of a midstream sample urine test.
- The differential diagnosis for dysuria and frequency and how this guides management.
- The rational use of antibiotics in dysuria and frequency.
- Which patients need further investigation.

Prevalence

One in five women will have an episode of dysuria and frequency in a given year,[1] and half of women will have one at some time in their lives.[2] Episodes are more common in the sexually active aged 20–50 years, the pregnant, the elderly and those with diabetes.[2] Only half of episodes present to a doctor,[3] but dysuria and frequency accounts for up to 3% of all GP consultations[2] and 6% of consultations among women aged 15–44 years.[3]

Only half of those who present with this set of symptoms have a urinary tract infection. Most infection, including recurrent infection, is ascending via the urethra. It is much less common in men (only a fifth of that in women) due to their longer urethras.[4] It is rare in younger men, but becomes more common in the sixth decade and beyond. This increase with age is attributable to lower urinary tract irritation caused by prostatic enlargement.[5]

Asymptomatic bacteriuria

Asymptomatic bacteriuria can be found in 2% of women aged 20–50 years, in 10% of women aged 65–70 years[6] and up to 50% of those who live in an institution.[5] In the non-pregnant it appears to cause no harm.[6] Up to 20% of institutionalized elderly men are also affected.[5]

In pregnant women, the prevalence of asymptomatic bacteriuria is as high as 7%.[6] Nearly a third of these progress to pyelonephritis, and there is an increased risk of mid-trimester miscarriage, premature labour and intrauterine growth retardation.[2] All pregnant women should routinely have a urine culture at the first antenatal appointment. If bacteriuria is present it should be treated and followed up with repeated cultures throughout the pregnancy.[2]

Diagnosis

Most women who present to their GP with symptoms of lower urinary tract infection (UTI) will be issued with a prescription and will get better. However, some will not get better, especially those in whom the diagnosis of UTI is incorrect. Only half of women presenting with dysuria and frequency have a demonstrable UTI. Conversely, half of non-pregnant women with proven bacteriuria will be better within 3 days without drug treatment.[2]

The symptoms of UTI are listed in Box 18.1. Loin pain may suggest an upper UTI, and abdominal palpation can be helpful. However loin pain is found in lower UTI one-third of the time, and upper UTI is not associated with loin pain up to one-third of the time. Clinical examination in women is unlikely to be fruitful. Some specialists suggest vaginal examination, but this is not supported unless vaginal pathology is suspected.[2,7]

In men, UTI is more likely to be the result of renal tract abnormality. Examination of the abdomen (for loin pain and ▶

Box 18.1 Symptoms of urinary tract infection

Lower UTI	Upper UTI
• Dysuria	• Fever
• Urinary frequency	• Malaise
• Urgency	• Nausea
• Nocturia	• Loin pain

palpable bladder), testes, epididymis and prostate may be appropriate.[4]

Use and abuse of the MSSU

A midstream sample of urine (MSSU) is one collected after the first 10 ml or so of urine have been discarded. A lower UTI exists when bacteria are actively multiplying in the bladder.[8] Significant bacteriuria is deemed to exist when 100,000 or more bacteria per millilitre can be seen in an MSSU (the Kass criterion, developed in 1956).[5] A single positive MSSU indicates an 80% probability that bacteria are replicating in the bladder.

The risk of contamination is minimized when the woman holds the labia apart while collecting the specimen. The specimen should be cultured within 2 hours, or 24 hours if stored at 4°C. The addition of 1.8% boric acid to the MSSU stops organisms multiplying and white cells lysing, so that the specimen stays usable for several days at room temperature. Culture takes at least 48 hours, but microscopy can be reported immediately.

Although in widespread use, the Kass criterion is not beyond criticism. Bacterial counts are lowered by dilution. Unusual organisms, or ones that are difficult to culture, may be a significant finding at levels below 100,000 bacteria/ml.[5] In men, contamination of an MSSU is less likely, so that lower bacterial counts may well be significant (i.e. 1000 bacteria/ml).[4,6]

Following a positive MSSU, a repeat should be done after treatment, to confirm cure.

In suspected UTI a quick result can be obtained by dipstick testing. If dipstick testing for either nitrite or leucocytes (or both) is positive, the patient should be treated as having a UTI.[2] The presence of nitrites has a positive predictive value of nearly 90% that an MSSU will be positive, and an absence of nitrites has a nearly 80% negative predictive value. The corresponding figures for leucocyte dipstick tests are 60% and 90%.

Managing dysuria and frequency

In half of women who present with dysuria and frequency it is not possible to find a UTI. This may be because of the deficiencies of dipstick and MSSU testing, or because no infection is present. The differential diagnosis for dysuria and frequency is given in Box 18.2. If a UTI cannot be found, and no other cause for the symptoms can be discovered, the symptoms are unexplained and a diagnosis of urethral syndrome can be made.

Box 18.2 Differential diagnosis of dysuria and frequency

Women

- UTI
- Urethral syndrome
- Atrophic vaginitis
- Vaginal infection, including *Chlamydia*
- Urolithiasis
- Trauma ('honeymoon cystitis')
- Pelvic inflammatory disease
- Interstitial cystitis
- Urethritis (gonococcal, non-gonococcal, trichomonal)

Men

- UTI
- Urethritis (sexually transmitted disease)
- Urolithiasis
- Prostatitis

Simple or complicated UTI?

UTI should be considered as having two distinct forms: simple or complicated.[2] Simple UTI is dysuria and frequency in women aged 20–50 years with lower UTI symptoms only, who are not pregnant or diabetic and who do not have recurrent symptoms (four or more episodes a year) or a known renal tract abnormality. All other UTIs are considered to be complicated.

Symptomatic measures, such as a hot water bottle, may help in all cases of UTI. Pain and fever can be helped by analgesics, such as paracetamol 1 g four times daily. Altering the pH of the urine by adding bicarbonate of soda to drinks may relieve symptoms.[2] Patients are normally recommended to drink lots of fluid, but the value of this is disputed.[2]

Management of simple UTI

If the dipstick urine test is positive, the patient should be prescribed a 3-day course of trimethoprim 200 mg twice daily. Most infections respond clinically. Longer courses are no more effective.[9] Trimethoprim does not affect the efficacy of the combined oral contraceptive pill.[10] Cephalosporins have a similar range of activity, but are

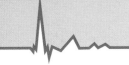

more expensive and more likely to disrupt gut flora. Nitrofurantoin is also effective and does not disrupt gut flora; however, it may cause nausea. If the dipstick urine test is negative, look for alternative causes of the symptoms.

Management of complicated UTI

An MSSU should be taken, and a 7-day course of antibiotic treatment begun while waiting for the result.[2]

In pregnancy, use of cephalosporins and nitrofurantoin appears to be safe, but trimethoprim is not safe in the first trimester. Follow-up with repeated MSSUs is needed for the duration of the pregnancy.

In men, 70% of those with a proven UTI will have a renal tract abnormality,[7] most commonly bladder outflow obstruction in elderly men. They should be referred to a urologist.[4] The organisms responsible are the same in men as in women, as is the choice of suitable antibiotics.[2] If symptoms are caused by prostatitis, the patient should take a 30-day course of antibiotics.[4]

The combination of diabetes, renal tract abnormality, infection and stones is particularly dangerous and can lead to destructive pyelonephritis.

In elderly women, the typical symptoms of UTI may be absent, or only elicited by specific questioning. Organisms may be unusual, and so treatment is best informed by an MSSU.

Upper UTI (pyelonephritis)

Patients with symptoms of an upper UTI who are well enough to remain at home should be treated with a quinolone or co-amoxiclav for 14 days. Fever and loin pain are commonly present in lower UTI and can be absent in upper UTI. A patient who is severely unwell because of a UTI should be admitted to hospital for intravenous treatment. Other patients should be investigated for an underlying cause, including stones and urinary tract abnormality (e.g. obstruction).

Recurrent UTI

Four or more episodes of dysuria and frequency in a year, at least one of which has produced a positive MSSU, defines recurrent UTI. Self-help measures may be effective. Patients with a recurrent simple UTI should be referred to hospital for radiological investigation of the renal tract.[9] Cranberry juice is often recommended, but there is limited evidence that it prevents or treats UTI.[11] Lifestyle

---

Box 18.3 Self-help in recurrent UTI[12]

- Wear cotton underwear
- Wipe front to back after micturition/defaecation
- Drink plenty, but limit caffeine and alcohol
- Void regularly, and ensure the bladder is empty ('double micturition')

---

modifications that can help in recurrent UTI are listed in Box 18.3

Honeymoon cystitis/urethritis

If the renal tract is normal, recurrence may be the result of sexual activity. Gel can be used if lubrication is a problem. Emptying the bladder and a perineal wash down (front to back) after intercourse may help. A single dose of trimethoprim 200 mg after coitus can prevent an attack.

Atrophic vaginitis can cause dysuria, and also predisposes to UTI. Topical oestrogen cream may help.

In the absence of any of the above, and after confirmation has been obtained that the renal tract is normal, prophylaxis against UTI may be considered through daily use of a small dose of antibiotic (e.g. trimethoprim 100 mg nightly).

Urethral syndrome

Women with frequency and dysuria and a negative MSSU are sometimes said to have urethral syndrome. The cause is not known, although lactobacilli or other organisms that are difficult to culture have been suggested as a possible cause.[13,14] Other suggestions are allergy to bath products, urethral congestion related to sexual intercourse and atrophic vaginitis. This has to be a diagnosis of exclusion.

Key points

- **The use of dipstick tests for nitrite and/or leucocyte makes the rational use of antibiotics in UTI more likely.**
- **The MSSU has limitations.**
- **A simple UTI needs only 3 days of antibiotics.**
- **There are many other causes, apart from a UTI, for dysuria and frequency.**
- **All patients with a complicated UTI need further investigation.**

References

1. Waters WE. Prevalence of symptoms of urinary tract infection in women. Br J Prev Soc Med 1969; 23:263–266.

2. Urinary tract infection. MeReC Bull 1995; 6:29–32.

3. Thomas M, Kyi M, Moorhead J. Cystitis and pyelitis: urinary tract infections in women. Matern Child Health 1990; 15:340–344.

4. Dhillon G. Urinary infections in men. Update 1998; 56:871–874.

5. Wilkie ME, Almond MK, Marsh FP. Diagnosis and management of urinary tract infection in adults. BMJ 1992; 305:1137–1141.

6. Brooks D. Management of cystitis. Update 2000; 60:492–499.

7. Shah J. Cystitis: treat quickly, and suggest hygiene precautions. Practitioner 1998; 242:698–702.

8. Brooks D. Acute dysuria and frequency in women. Update 1995; 51:269–274.

9. Managing urinary tract infections in women. Drug Therapeut Bull 1998; 36:30–32.

10. Miller DM, Helms SE, Brodell RT. A practical approach to antibiotic treatment in women taking oral contraceptives. J Am Acad Dermatol 1994; 30: 1008–1011.

11. Kontiokari T, Sundqvist K, Nuutinen M, et al. Randomised trial of cranberry–lingonberry juice and Lactobacillus GG drink for the prevention of urinary tract infections in women. BMJ 2001; 322:1571–1573.

12. Van Shaik S, Cranston D. Urinary tract infections in adults. Update 1996; 53:412–416.

13. Maskell R. Antibacterial agents and urinary tract infection: a paradox. Br J Gen Pract 1992; 42:138–139.

14. Brumfitt W, Hamilton-Miller JMT, Gillespie WA. The mysterious 'urethral syndrome'. BMJ 1991; 303:1–2.

19. Swellings in the groin and scrotum

JE Thistlethwaite

THIS CHAPTER REVIEWS

- Common and important causes of swelling or pain in the groin or scrotum.
- The investigation and management of enlarged inguinal nodes.
- The presentation and management of common conditions of the groin and scrotum.
- Testicular torsion.
- When to refer patients.
- When to refer urgently.

Box 19.1 Diagnosis: key questions

- Has the lump or swelling appeared suddenly?
- Is there any history of trauma?
- Is the patient otherwise well?
- Are there associated symptoms, such as malaise, pyrexia or dysuria?
- Is there any possibility of a sexually transmitted disease?
- What does the patient think the problem might be?

Box 19.2 Differential diagnosis of groin and scrotal swellings

- Enlarged lymph glands
- Abscess
- Inguinal hernia
- Femoral hernia
- Hydrocele
- Varicocele
- Maldescended testis
- Tumour
- Aneurysm
- Epididymitis
- Torsion
- Epididymal cysts

When a patient presents with a groin swelling, the GP needs to consider the patient's own ideas and fears, as well as the clues uncovered by the history and examination. For many patients, a recently discovered lump is cancer until proved otherwise. A lump or swelling in the groin, especially in the scrotum, can be particularly worrying to men who rarely see a doctor and are not used to being examined in such an intimate area.

Diagnosis

Although the exact location of a lump is apparent on examination, the patient can be asked to point to the swelling so the doctor knows what is meant by 'groin'.

A discrete lump needs to be differentiated from swelling. It is important to find out:

- when the lump or swelling first appeared
- if there is any pain associated with it
- whether it is getting bigger.

The patient should be asked if he or she has been feeling unwell in any way (Box 19.1). Enlarged lymph glands may be due to conditions such as infection or malignancy, and may be associated with non-specific symptoms of ill health, such as weight loss or pyrexia. Patients should also be asked about any recent change in bowel habit. A scrotal swelling may be the first symptom of Crohn's disease or carcinoma of the sigmoid colon.[1,2] There are several possible causes of a swelling in the groin (Box 19.2), and it is important to ask the patient what he or she thinks is wrong.

Examination

The physical examination should take place in a room with a couch and a good light. It is not good practice to ask a male patient to drop his trousers in the consulting room and attempt to examine him standing up. Both men and women should be given time to undress and should be given clear instructions about what clothes they need to remove.[3]

At this point the doctor needs to decide whether a chaperone is needed (Box 19.3). A male doctor examining a male patient may feel relatively comfortable, as may the patient. A male patient is likely to feel embarrassed if being examined by a female doctor.

When examining a patient's genitalia, whatever the sex, I always wear gloves. This helps to emphasize that the procedure is a medical examination. The patient should be asked to demonstrate where the swelling is. They may need to do this standing up, but then should be asked to lie down. Inspection is followed by palpation, starting with abdominal palpation to relax the patient, continuing with the groins and then the scrotum or perineum.

Examination may provide clues to the diagnosis. For example, an unobstructed inguinal hernia will often disappear when the patient lies down, and gives an impulse on coughing.

Hernia

If a hernia is suspected, the groin should be examined with the patient standing. A hernia is not reducible if it contains adherent omentum or, more seriously, if it is strangulated

---

Box 19.3 Examination: key questions[3]

- Do I need a chaperone?
- Have I explained why I need to examine the genitalia?
- Is the swelling painful?
- Are there other swollen glands?
- Is this an obstructed hernia?
- Is there a possibility of torsion?
- Is there a possibility of malignancy?

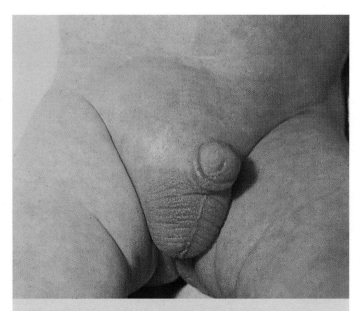

Figure 19.1 Irreducible inguinal hernia. This 14-month-old boy was known to have a reducible inguinal hernia, but after a bout of crying it became irreducible. With sedation and rest the hernia reduced spontaneously, but was repaired on the next available operating list. Reproduced with permission from Burkitt & Quick, *Essential Surgery*, 3rd edn, Churchill Livingstone, 2001.

(Fig. 19.1). A patient with a strangulated hernia needs immediate surgical admission.

The important signs are tenderness and absence of the cough impulse. If the hernia contains bowel, there may be symptoms and signs of intestinal obstruction.

Inguinal and femoral hernias can be distinguished by the fact that the former originate from above the inguinal ligament and the latter from below. Femoral hernias are uncommon in males, and even in females inguinal hernias are more common at all ages.

Whatever kind of hernia is present, the patient should be referred for treatment.

Maldescended testicle

A lump in the groin and an absent testicle strongly suggests a diagnosis of a maldescended testicle.

Enlarged glands

Enlarged glands in the groin are usually multiple and subcutaneous. Possible causes are (Box 19.4):

- If infection is suspected, examine the patient for the source. Possible sites are the genitalia, legs and feet.
- In Hodgkin's disease, the groin glands are rarely affected alone. Other glands may be smoothly and softly

enlarged, and abdominal palpation may reveal an enlarged spleen.

- Secondary spread of cancer, from the ovaries or bowel for example, may also result in palpable glands, but these tend to be hard and painful.
- Palpable lymph glands might be a sign of sexually transmitted disease, particularly HIV infection. Primary and secondary syphilis are rare nowadays. Acute attacks of genital herpes may cause painful enlargement of the inguinal glands, but there will also be genital ulceration. The persistent generalized lymphadenopathy of HIV infection commonly involves the inguinal glands.

Box 19.4 Causes of enlarged lymph glands

- Infection
- Lymphoma
- Lymphatic leukaemia
- AIDS
- Secondary malignancy
- Lymphogranuloma inguinale
- Tuberculosis
- Syphilis (now rare)

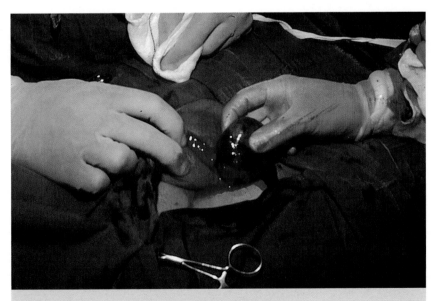

Figure 19.2 Black non-viable testis after testicular torsion.

Scrotal swelling

Swellings that extend into the scrotum may be due to a hydrocele, hernia, varicocele or trauma. Congenital hydroceles are seen most commonly in infants, although some remain undiagnosed until later in life. A hydrocele is translucent.

A hernia has a cough impulse and may be reduced into the abdomen. A varicocele is a swelling mainly in the scrotum, usually on the left side. A haematoma may follow a kick in the groin, and later there will be bruising.

Swellings in the scrotum may be due to acute epididymitis, malignant disease of the testicle or torsion. Many GPs worry about missing a torsion of the testis. Whereas most would suspect the diagnosis in young and adolescent boys who present with testicular pain and swelling, there may be doubts in older men.

Acute testicular bruising will also present with swelling and pain, but there will be a clear history. In young children with abdominal pain and scrotal bruising where injury is denied, physical abuse should be remembered. Injuries to the scrotum are often seen in physical and sexual abuse and the child may deny injury.

Acute testicular torsion

Sudden onset of pain, perhaps associated with vomiting, may be diagnostic. However, some boys present with a minor pain attack before complete torsion occurs. Presentation may be with abdominal pain and vomiting, and the scrotum should be examined in men and boys with unexplained abdominal pain (Fig. 19.2).

The peak incidence of the condition is between 14 and 16 years of age, but torsion accounts for nearly 90% of acutely presenting scrotal symptoms in the 13–21 year age group.[4] In 80% of cases the testes are salvaged if surgery is within 12 hours.

Investigations

Few investigations are helpful in the diagnostic or decision-making process, although a full blood count may help to identify the cause of swollen glands. The blood film may suggest lymphatic leukaemia or anaemia associated with lymphoma.

An ultrasound scan of the scrotum may aid the diagnosis of lumps. However, if torsion is suspected, investigation is not appropriate as prompt surgical assessment is necessary.[5]

If epididymitis is suspected, the patient should be asked to provide a urine sample.

When it comes to mumps infection, the GP has to decide whether to trust to clinical judgement or to send off a sample of blood.

Testicular carcinoma is the most common malignancy in young men, and the incidence has more than doubled in the past 25 years. There is an 80% cure rate for patients who are referred and evaluated without delay.[6] Many would say that a lump in the testicle of a young man should be regarded as cancer until proved otherwise.

There appears to be less awareness among young men about testicular cancer than in women about breast cancer.[7] There are arguments for and against advising and training men in self-examination.[1,8,9]

Management

Most causes of swelling require referral, either for a firm diagnosis or for treatment. An exception is infection causing enlarged glands. The infection can be treated appropriately and the glands checked later, although an inguinal abscess may need drainage.

Treatment can be prescribed if the doctor is confident that the patient has acute epididymitis. Antibiotics are not needed if there is no pyuria on urinalysis; analgesia and a scrotal support are sufficient.[10]

Where there is suspicion of sexually transmitted infection, the GP may consider referral to the genitourinary clinic.

If malignancy is likely, the doctor needs to decide what to tell the patient. This may depend on what the patient has already suspected. It is difficult to justify an urgent referral without alerting the patient to the possible diagnosis.

Key questions to ask regarding the management of the condition are listed in Box 19.5.

Referral

An elderly patient with an uncomplicated hernia may ask to be fitted with a truss. However, as elective surgery has a better outcome than emergency surgery, particularly for femoral hernia, all elderly patients should be considered for early referral.[11]

Some GPs are happy to drain hydroceles in the surgery.

These treatment options need to be explored with the patient. Some people are afraid of hospitals, and their expectations of treatment are based on this fear. It may help to explain that modern surgery for hernia repair often involves day-case surgery.

References

1. Simoneaux SF, Ball TI, Atkinson GO. Scrotal swelling: unusual first presentation of Crohn's disease. Pediatr Radiol 1995; 25:375–376.

2. Bryan NP, Jackson A, Raffery AT. Carcinoma of the sigmoid colon presenting as a scrotal swelling. Postgrad Med J 1997; 73:47–48.

3. Royal College of Obstetricians and Gynaecologists. Intimate examinations. Report of a working party. London: RCOG Press, 1997.

4. Thomas DFM. Testicular torsion – how not to miss it. Trends Urol Gynaecol Sex Health 1998; 3:39–42.

5. Fisher R, Walker J. The acute paediatric scrotum. Br J Hosp Med 1994; 51:290–292.

6. O'Callaghan A, Mead GM. Testicular cancer. Postgrad Med J 1997; 73:481–486.

7. Katz RC, Meyers K, Walls J. Cancer awareness and self examination practices in young men and women. J Behav Med 1995; 18:377–384.

8. Peate I. Testicular cancer: the importance of effective health education. Br J Nursing 1997; 6:311–16.

9. Bueton SA. Testicular cancer: to screen or not to screen? J Med Screening 1996; 3:3–6.

10. Lau P, Anderson PA, Giacomanfonio JM, et al. Acute epididymitis in boys: are antibiotics indicated? Br J Urol 1997; 79:797–800.

11. Clamary VL. Femoral hernia: intestinal obstruction is an unrecognised source of morbidity and mortality. Br J Surg 1993; 80:230–232.

Box 19.5 Management: key questions

- Am I sure of the diagnosis?
- Does this patient need to be admitted now?
- How long will the patient have to wait before being seen in outpatients?
- Should I organize an ultrasound scan while the patient is waiting to be seen?
- Do all hernias need referral?
- At what age can I be sure that this is not a torsion?
- What should I tell the patient?

Key points

- There are many different causes for swelling in the groin and scrotum.

- A good history and examination are important to exclude serious pathology.

- The doctor needs to consider the patient's own ideas and worries, particularly in relation to cancer.

- A lump in the testicle of a young man should be regarded as cancer until proven otherwise.

- There may be a possibility of sexually transmitted disease.

20. Progressive renal disease

K Baboolal

THIS CHAPTER REVIEWS

- Management approaches to slow deterioration of renal function.
- The management of comorbid contributory conditions.
- The management of end-stage renal disease.
- The prevention and treatment of complications.
- When to refer patients.
- When renal replacement is appropriate.

Box 20.1 Key elements in the management of renal disease

Detection of renal injury
- Urinalysis
- Serum creatinine and urea
- Blood pressure
- Referral to a renal specialist

Prevention of progressive renal injury
- Blood pressure control
- Diabetes control

Detection and treatment of comorbid risk factors
- Cardiovascular disease
- Anaemia
- Renal bone disease
- Preparation for renal replacement therapy

Box 20.2 The aims of treatment

- To slow down deterioration in renal function and delay the need for renal replacement therapy
- To prevent and treat comorbid complications
- To anticipate and plan renal replacement therapy

Presentation

Renal disease is characterized by a reduction in glomerular filtration rate, proteinuria and hypertension. Whatever the underlying cause, renal function can progressively deteriorate to end-stage renal failure.

A management programme (Box 20.1) should treat not only the underlying cause of renal injury but also prevent or slow down the progressive decline in renal function (Box 20.2). The rate at which renal function declines is variable. Male patients who present with uraemia, poorly controlled hypertension and heavy proteinuria (>3 g/24 h) tend to have a more rapid decline in renal function.

Hypertension and proteinuria are important determinants of the rate at which renal function declines, and therefore treatments have been designed to slow down the rate of decline in renal function by reducing blood pressure and proteinuria.

Management of renal disease and comorbid risk factors

Blood pressure reduction

Large randomized trials of patients with both diabetic and non-diabetic renal disease have demonstrated that a

reduction in blood pressure slows down the rate of decline in renal function.[1-4] Ideally, the systolic blood pressure should be below 140 mmHg and the diastolic pressure below 90 mmHg. Hypertension not only accelerates loss of renal function in patients with renal impairment, but also contributes to cardiovascular mortality.[5,6]

103

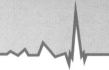

ACE inhibitors

Recent studies suggest that the rate of decline in renal function is slower with angiotensin converting enzyme (ACE) inhibitors than with other antihypertensive agents.[1,2] The beneficial effect may be attributable to mechanisms other than the antihypertensive effect of these agents, such as their effectiveness in reducing proteinuria.

Care should be taken when using ACE inhibitors in patients with renal failure as their use may lead to dangerous levels of hyperkalaemia, especially when used with other potassium retaining drugs. In addition, ACE inhibitors can cause a decline in blood pressure and glomerular filtration rate in volume-depleted patients. Renal function and serum potassium should be checked after their introduction in any patient, but especially in those with renal dysfunction.

Protein restriction

Protein restriction was recommended in the past. However, trials have shown that protein restriction has no beneficial effect in delaying the onset of end-stage renal failure.[7] In addition, other studies have shown that patients who were poorly nourished at the start of renal replacement therapy were at increased risk of morbidity and mortality. This approach has since been abandoned.

Diabetic control

In patients with diabetic renal disease the development of overt diabetic nephropathy (proteinuria >500 mg/24 h, impaired glomerular filtration rate and hypertension) is preceded by the development of microalbuminuria. The progression of microalbuminuria (incipient nephropathy) to overt diabetic nephropathy can be prevented by tight diabetes control.[8] It is now established practice to aim for optimum glucose control and to reduce the blood pressure, preferably with an ACE inhibitor, to prevent diabetic renal disease or to slow its progression.

Cardiovascular disease

The existence of proteinuria identifies patients as having renal injury and is an important prognostic indicator of long-term renal function. Proteinuria is also a very strong independent risk factor for cardiovascular disease.[9] In addition, patients with renal disease often have multiple other risk factors for cardiovascular disease, including hypertension, hyperlipidaemia, anaemia, left ventricular hypertrophy and impaired glucose tolerance. It is therefore not surprising that patients, both before dialysis and those on renal replacement therapy, have a very high cardiovascular mortality.

The management of these patients is therefore aimed at correcting and modifying cardiovascular risk factors. Some studies suggest that modification will reduce mortality. The UKPDS Hypertension in Diabetes and Hypertension Optimal Treatment (HOT) studies[5,6] have demonstrated that cardiovascular mortality can be reduced by tight control of blood pressure in diabetic patients.

The British Hypertension Society guidelines now recommend a blood pressure level of <140/85 in hypertensive patients to reduce cardiovascular mortality. In diabetic patients with hypertension and proteinuria >1 g/24 h, the blood pressure should be <125/75.[10]

Cholesterol

The total and low density lipoprotein (LDL) cholesterol targets for primary coronary heart disease prevention in high-risk patients also apply to those with chronic renal disease.[11,12] Statin therapy can be used to treat patients with chronic renal failure. However, in renal transplant recipients, care should be taken when prescribing statins and cyclosporin, as this combination can result in rhabdomyolysis.

Anaemia

Anaemia contributes significantly to morbidity and mortality associated with uraemia, exacerbating symptoms such as tiredness and lethargy. It also exacerbates the symptoms of clinically apparent or silent ischaemic heart disease and left ventricular dysfunction. Anaemia is a major independent risk factor for cardiac morbidity in patients with renal failure.

Anaemia can be treated with an injection of recombinant human erythropoietin. In small studies the treatment of anaemia has been shown to reduce left ventricular hypertrophy, which is a major risk factor for cardiovascular mortality. The major adverse effect of erythropoeitin therapy is worsening hypertension.

Renal bone disease

Renal bone disease is a complication of renal failure and describes a number of bone disorders that can occur at the same time. These include bone disease as a consequence of secondary hyperparathyroidism and altered vitamin D metabolism.

Renal bone disease is caused by a loss of calcium, phosphate retention and reduced vitamin D synthesis by the diseased kidney. Altered bone metabolism occurs early in the progression of renal injury and is apparent when the glomerular filtration rate is less than 50 ml/min. The predominant lesion may vary within an individual and between individuals and is dependent on factors including the underlying renal disease, the degree of acidosis and type of renal replacement therapy.

Therapy aims to normalize serum phosphate. Calcium carbonates are used as phosphate binders, and dietary phosphate intake is restricted. In addition, synthetic vitamin D analogues are used to correct hypocalcaemia by increasing calcium reabsorption from the gut. Unfortunately, they also increase phosphate reabsorption from the gut, and thus should not be used until phosphate control has been achieved.

Renal replacement therapy

Therapies for patients with progressive renal failure are aimed at delaying the onset of renal replacement therapy. Eventually, however, renal replacement therapy becomes inevitable. At present, renal replacement therapy involves haemodialysis, chronic ambulatory peritoneal dialysis and transplantation, including living related and unrelated transplantation. During renal replacement therapy most patients will try all three options, sometimes more than once.

Patient education is essential in ensuring compliance and choosing the appropriate therapy to suit the individual and their way of life. Late referral is associated with a significant increase in morbidity and mortality in patients with uraemia.[13] It is therefore imperative that patients are referred early to renal units so that renal replacement therapy can be planned and potential donors identified.

Key points

- Renal disease is detected clinically as a reduction in glomerular filtration rate, proteinuria and hypertension.
- Treatments are designed to reduce hypertension and proteinuria. ACE inhibitors are especially useful.
- Protein restriction has no beneficial effect.
- Proteinuria is a predictor of prognosis in renal failure and a strong predictor of cardiovascular disease in diabetic and non-diabetic patients.
- Tight control of hypertension is especially important in diabetic patients.
- Correction of anaemia improves symptoms of

tiredness and lethargy. A major adverse effect is the worsening of hypertension.

- Renal bone disease may be treated with phosphate binders (calcium carbonate) and synthetic vitamin D analogues.
- Patient education is essential to ensuring compliance and choosing the appropriate therapy to suit the individual and their way of life.

References

1. Lewis EJ, Hunsicker LG, Bain RP, et al. The effect of angiotensin converting enzyme inhibition on diabetic nephropathy. N Engl J Med 1993; 329:1456–1462.

2. Maschio G, Alberti D, Janin G, et al. Effect of the angiotensin converting enzyme inhibitor benazapril on the progression of chronic renal insufficiency. N Engl J Med 1996; 334:939–945.

3. Bjork S, Nyberg G, Granerus G, et al. Beneficial effects of angiotensin converting enzyme inhibitors on renal function in patients with diabetic nephropathy. BMJ 1986; 293:471–474.

4. Bakris GL, Copley JB, Vicknair N, et al. Calcium channel blockers versus other antihypertensive therapies on the progression of NIDDM associated nephropathy. Kidney Int 1996; 50:1641–1650.

5. United Kingdom Prospective Diabetes Study Group. Tight blood pressure control and risk of macrovascular and microvascular complications in type 2 diabetes: UKPDS 38. BMJ 1998; 317:703–713.

6. Hansson L, Zanchetti A, Carruthers SG, et al. Effects of intensive blood pressure lowering and low dose aspirin in patients with hypertension: principal results of the Hypertension Optimal Treatment (HOT) randomised trial. Lancet 1998; 351:1755–1763.

7. Klahr S, Levey AS, Becj GJ. The effects of dietary protein restriction and blood pressure control on the progression of chronic renal disease. N Engl J Med 1994; 330:877–884.

8. DCCT Research Group. The effect of intensive treatment of diabetes on the development and progression of long term complications in IDDM. N Engl J Med 1999; 329:977–986.

9. Bulpitt CJ, Beevers DG, Butter A. The survival of treated hypertensive patients and their cause of death: a report from the Department of Health and Social Security hypertension care computing project. J Hypertens 1986; 4:93–99.

10. Ramsey LE, Williams B, Johnston G, et al. British Hypertension Society Guidelines for hypertension management 1999: summary. BMJ 1999; 319:630–635.

11. West of Scotland Coronary Prevention Group. Prevention of coronary heart disease with pravastatin in men with hypercholesterolaemia. N Engl J Med 1995; 335:1301–1307.

12. Scandinavian Simvastatin Survival Study Group. Randomised controlled trial of cholesterol lowering in 4444 patients with coronary heart disease: the Scandinavian Simvastatin Survival Study (4S). Lancet 1994; 344:1383–1389.

13. Dunn EJ, Burton CJ, Feest TG. The care of patients with diabetic nephropathy: audit, feedback, and improvement. Q J Med 1999; 92:443–449.

21. Urology: some common presentations

M Selby

THIS CHAPTER REVIEWS

- Common urological presentations and conditions.
- Likely diagnoses and recommended GP investigations.

Haematuria

Common causes

- Menstruation/other female genital tract blood loss.
- Prostatic enlargement (benign or malignant).
- Bacterial infection (bladder or renal, prostatitis).
- Calculus (renal, ureteric or bladder).
- Renal inflammation (e.g. glomerulonephritis).
- Post-streptococcal nephritis.
- Bladder inflammation (e.g. radiotherapy bladder damage).
- Henoch–Schönlein purpura (in children).
- Anticoagulant use (warfarin, streptokinase).
- Tumour (renal cell carcinoma, bladder cancer, prostatic cancer).
- Wilms' tumour (children).
- Trauma (to kidney, from catheter, from foreign body in urethra, prolonged exercise, rapid emptying of large bladder volume).
- Surgery (e.g. transurethral resection of the prostate, bladder tumour diathermy, cystoscopy).

Other causes (some rare in the UK)

- Coagulation disorders (haemophilia, iidiopathic thrombocytopenic purpura (ITP), sickle cell disease).
- Haemolytic uraemic syndrome (in children).
- Endometriosis of the bladder.
- Congenital (cysts, aneurysms).

- Renal vein thrombosis.
- Tuberculosis, tropical infection (bilharzias, malaria).
- Toxins, including non-steroidal anti-inflammatory drugs (NSAIDs), cyclophosphamide and some antibiotics.
- Immunoglobulin A nephropathy (in children).

Tests

- History and examination: abdomen, kidneys and temperature.
- Urine culture: if positive, treat and then repeat with another midstream urine sample.
- Urine culture: if negative, intravenous pyelogram (IVP) or renal ultrasound scan.
- Urea and electrolytes, creatinine, calcium and uric acid levels.
- Cystoscopy if haematuria is persistent and unexplained.

Referral criteria for outpatient department

- Persistent haematuria without infection.
- Child.

Refer urgently or admit:

- Mass, suspected calcium, large blood loss, renal trauma.
- Systemically unwell, suspected renal failure.

Enuresis

Primary enuresis

- Involuntary voiding day or night for >5 years.
- Usually a combination of a low bladder volume and failure to wake.
- 3% boys and 2% girls at age 10 years, 1% males at age 30 years.
- >75% have a family history.

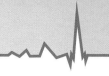

• 10% per year of those still affected remit spontaneously.

Investigations
• History: primary or secondary.
• Constant trickle: exclude congenital anomalies.
• Midstream urine test.
• Bursting test to assess the bladder volume.
• Review of drinking habits (often dry all day then thirst in evening).

Treatments
Treatments include:
• an explanation of bladder function
• bladder stretch exercises
• enuresis alarm systems (useful for patients aged >7 years, with support)
• desmopressin nasal spray or nocturnal tablet
• imipramine (rarely, not prescribed by the GP)
• star charts (with intensive support)
• referral to an enuresis clinic, if available
• contact with ERIC (the enuresis support centre).

Secondary enuresis
Likely causes are:
• infection
• diabetes
• psychological (e.g. anxiety, life change).

Urinary tract infection (UTI)

What is a UTI?
• A pure culture of $>10^5$ organisms/cm^3.
• In symptomatic patients a culture of 10^2 to 10^4 organisms/cm^3 may be significant.
• White cell count >200 cells/cm^3 may be significant.

What organisms are involved?
• 95% enterobacteriacaea.
• *Escherichia coli*.
• *Proteus* spp.
• *Pseudomonas* spp.
• *Enterococcus* spp.
• *Staphylococcus saprophyticus*.

• Consider *Chlamydia*, *Gonorrhoea* and *Trichomonas* if the culture is negative and there are symptoms and pus cells.

How do we get a UTI?
• Most cases: ascending infection.
• Babies <3 months old: most commonly blood borne.

Presentation
• Dysuria.
• Frequency.
• Urgency.
• Haematuria.
• Abdominal pain, tenderness.
• Temperature.
• Vomiting.
• Loin pain.
• Pyrexia of unknown origin, swinging fever.
• Offensive urine.

Investigation (adults)
For a single episode of a UTI:
• Urine dipstick test: this may show nitrites (which suggests *Proteus* spp.), leucocytes, blood or protein.
• Midstream urine test: repeated after treatment.
For repeated episodes of a UTI:
• Check the blood glucose level.
• Consider investigation for stones and urinary obstruction.

Upper versus lower UTI
• Loin pain and systemic malaise may indicate ascending infection.
• Consider an increased risk of upper UTI in diabetes and pregnancy, and in cases of known stones or known reflux.

Note: The combination of diabetes, stones and infection predisposes to pyelonephritis and renal damage.

Treatment of uncomplicated lower UTI
A lower UTI is uncomplicated if there is no co-existing pathology and the patient is an adult and not systemically unwell. Treatment is with a locally recommended antibiotic

(usually trimethoprim) for 3 days. Resistance to antibiotics is as follows:

- trimethoprim, in the community around 10%
- amoxicillin, 30% resistant
- ciprofloxacin, norfloxacin and ofloxacin, <1%.

Treatment of complicated UTI

Treatment is with an oral antibiotic for a minimum of 1 week. Consider admission if:

- there are rigors and loin pain (the patient needs an urgent intravenous urogram)
- the patient is systemically unwell, a diabetic or has known renal disease
- the patient is pregnant (if the patient is not admitted there should be early review, as there is a risk of preterm labour and a high risk of ascending infection).

Upper UTI: pyelonephritis

Symptoms:

- loin pain (not always)
- systemically unwell
- swinging fever
- nausea and vomiting.

Treat for a minimum of 1 week.

Consider admission for intravenous therapy if:

- the infection is not resolving
- the patient is systemically unwell
- there are complicating features (e.g. diabetes, stones, pregnancy).

UTI in children

Diagnosis

Diagnosis is as described above, but with the following additional symptoms. In babies:

- lethargy
- vomiting
- diarrhoea
- poor feeding
- febrile convulsion (>6/12 old)
- sepsis (poor perfusion and capillary refill, floppy or irritable)

- may show few signs other than pyrexia of unknown origin.

In children:

- vomiting and pyrexia of unknown origin
- dysuria
- abdominal or loin pain
- febrile convulsion
- secondary enuresis
- suprapubic tenderness, offensive urine, loin pain.

Note: All babies and children with unexplained fever should have urine dipped.

Admission

- Consider admission if the child is systemically unwell.
- Consider admission in babies under 3 months old, as Gram-negative infection is more likely.

Follow-up

- UTIs in young children require further investigation to exclude reflux and scarring.
- Antibiotic prophylaxis may be indicated (trimethoprim 1 mg/kg daily)
- Proven UTI in a child under 3 years old should usually be referred.
- Most renal scarring occurs well under the age of 2 years.
- Children of 3 years old or more should have an ultrasound scan and an abdominal plain film radiograph. A normal ultrasound scan at age 3 years or more makes subsequent reflux and scarring very unlikely.
- Children under 2 years of age will undergo a DMSA scan and a micturating cystogram. Follow-up in children aged 2–3 years is a grey area.
- Check a midstream urine sample if there is any pyrexial illness.

Child with known renal scarring

- Paediatric follow-up.
- Monitor growth and blood pressure.

Child with reflux

Surgical reimplantation of ureters may be indicated if disease is bilateral and severe. The majority improve with watchful waiting.

Urolithiasis

Aetiology

- Diabetes.
- Recurrent infection.
- Hypercalciuria (renal, tubular or hypercalcaemia).
- Raised uric acid.
- Chronic diarrhoea.
- Dehydration.
- Urine stasis (neuropathic bladder, bladder outflow obstruction).
- Diuretics.
- Chemotherapy.

Stone types

- Calcium oxalate and/or calcium phosphate: 70% of cases.
- Uric acid: 10% of cases.

Presentation

- Loin pain.
- Ureteric colic.
- Nausea and vomiting.
- Pain referred to genitalia.
- Ileus (occasionally).
- Recurrent UTI.
- Haematuria.
- Persistent pyuria.

Investigations

- Midstream urine test.
- Bloods: urate, calcium, phosphate, urea and electrolytes, creatinine.
- Abdominal x-ray and ultrasound scan of the renal tract.

Treatment

- Advise high fluid intake.
- For uric acid stones, give allopurinol.

Treatment options are:

- percutaneous nephroureterolithotomy
- ureteroscopy
- stent.

Referral

Indications for referral are:

- persistent pain, fever, nausea
- recurrent stones
- recurrent UTI
- a solitary kidney with obstructive stones
- proximal ureteric stones, especially those >1 cm.

Non-referral is an option for small uncomplicated ureteric or renal stones, if:

- they are not obstructing
- there are no complications in the patient's history
- the patient is not diabetic.

Prostatic hypertrophy: benign

Presentation

- Lower urinary tract irritation: frequency, urgency, dysuria, nocturia.
- Bladder outflow obstruction: hesitancy, poor stream, double voiding, terminal dribble, palpable bladder post-voiding, acute retention.
- Other: haematuria, recurrent UTI, stones.

Diagnosis in general practice

- On symptoms.
- Check the prostate specific antigen (PSA) level: it is elevated in 30–50% of cases.
- Urea and electrolytes, creatinine.
- Midstream urine to rule out infection.
- Digital rectal examination: smoothly enlarged prostate, preservation of median sulcus.
- Prostate size correlates poorly with symptoms.

Referral

Refer if:

- symptoms are intolerable
- the patient is not responding to treatment
- there is suspicion of malignancy (e.g. the PSA level is raised)
- there is macroscopic haematuria

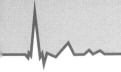

- there is recurrent UTI.

GP treatment options

- 70% improve with appropriate treatment.
- Avoid caffeine, cold and allergy remedies.
- Stop tricyclic antidepressants.
- Alpha blockers titrated to full dose.
- Finasteride (for 6 months for full effect).

Hospital investigations

- Transrectal ultrasound.
- Free PSA and PSA density if there is diagnostic uncertainty.
- Uroflowmetry.

Hospital treatments

- As GP treatment options, above.
- Transurethral resection of the prostate.
- Open prostatectomy (for very large prostates).
- Bladder neck incision.
- Bladder neck laser therapy, diathermy, coils and stents are under evaluation.

Prostatic malignancy

Presentation

- Often silent until late stage.
- Bone pain (especially hip, back, chest wall).
- Unexplained clot or phlebitis.
- Reduced ejaculate.
- Haematospermia.
- Impotence (neurovascular bundle involvement).
- Perineal pain.
- Symptoms of prostatism (see above).
- Hard or indurated gland on digital rectal examination.
- Late cases: anaemia, nausea, renal failure, lower body oedema, cord compression, hypercalcaemia.

Diagnosis

- Raised PSA level (>10 ng/ml is virtually diagnostic; 4–10 ng/ml is a grey area – see below).

- If no malignancy is seen on ultrasound, the percentage free PSA and the PSA density (= PSA/prostate volume) may help clarify the situation.
- Ultrasound guided biopsy (misses 50% of lesions <1 cm).

Management options

Watchful waiting is the GP's decision only if:

- the patient's life expectancy is <10 years and
- the patient is symptomatic and
- the patient is fully informed and
- investigation not desired.

Always refer if:

- the patient's life expectancy is >10 years
- the PSA level is >10 ng/ml
- the patient is symptomatic.

Treatment

- There is no clear evidence-based consensus on who should be treated.
- There is a lack of clear evidence for radical treatment, but most urologists believe it justified in early aggressive disease.
- Most trials evaluate treatment by tumour stage, but not by the Gleason grade, which is probably more significant in localized disease.
- There is some evidence of benefit with early zoladex.
- Tumours of a high Gleason grade caught before breaching the capsule are most likely to benefit from radical treatment.

Treatment options

- Hormonal: gonadotrophin analogues; these are poorly tolerated in young men.
- Androgen receptor blockers: these have no proven benefit other than to block tumour flare at the initiation of treatment with gonadotrophin analogues.
- Surgery: radical prostatectomy; this carries a high morbidity (chronic bladder problems, impotence, risk of faecal incontinence).
- Orchidectomy (total androgen deprivation).
- Brachytherapy: this carries a high incidence of bladder toxicity.
- External beam radiation to the gland and bony metastases.
- Strontium-89: a single treatment for bony metastases.   ▸

Screening controversy

- The PSA level in the range 4–10 ng/ml with a normal rectal examination has a poor positive predictive value due to overlap with benign prostatic hypertrophy..
- Investigation carries its own morbidity.

Imperfect testicular descent

Prevalence

This is common, occurring in 2–3% of babies and in 1.5% by the age of 3 months.

Diagnosis

- The imperfectly descended testicle may be located high, in the inguinal canal or in the abdomen.
- Distinguish from retractile testes, which can be brought down and do not need treatment. Review occasionally to make sure that the testis is not ascending to the inguinal canal (uncommon).

Treatment

Refer for investigation:

- ultrasound scan to locate the testis if it is not palpable
- hormone tests to prove that testicular tissue is present.

Problems

- There is a risk of infertility if the testis is not brought down by the age of 2 years.
- Rarely, torsion.
- There is a risk of malignancy, this being highest for an intra-abdominal testis left in situ after puberty.

Treatment

- Orchidopexy, at age 1–2 years, probably reduces the risk of cancer (uncertain).
- Unilateral abdominal testes are removed.
- Bilateral intra-abdominal testes need staged orchidopexy.

Torsion of the testis

Presentation

- Pain in the testis.
- Swelling of the testis.
- Pain in the abdomen.

- Nausea and vomiting, without urinary symptoms.
- Swollen testicle, which may be retracted.
- In the neonate, painless discoloured hemiscrotum (torsion in utero).

Referral

- Urgent, as there is a risk of irreversible testicular damage.
- 80% of testes can be salvaged if detorsion is carried out within 12 hours.
- Most urologists recommend bilateral orchidopexy.

Epidydimo-orchitis

Aetiology

The causes of epidydimo-orchitis are infection or trauma:

- in men aged >35 years with other urological disease, the cause is commonly Gram-negative rods
- in young men, the cause is usually *Neisseria gonorrhoea* and *Chlamydia*
- the condition is sometimes seen in young boys who have urinary reflux, usually due to *Escherichia coli*.

Presentation

- Pain in the scrotum.
- Scrotal erythema.
- Pain on ejaculation.
- Pain in the abdomen.
- Fever (sometimes).
- Rarely, tuberculous.

Diagnosis

- Tender epidydimis.
- Painful red scrotum.

Investigations

- Culture any discharge.
- Midstream urine test if there are urinary symptoms.

Treatment

- Boys: trimethoprim and other locally recommended treatment.

- Men aged >35 years: ciprofloxacin 500 mg twice daily for 10–14 days (septrin in the USA).
- Sexually active men: doxycycline 100 mg twice daily covers *Gonococcus* spp. and *Chlamydia*.
- Diabetics: risk of extensive scrotal infection and Fournier's gangrene.
- Department of genitourinary medicine: for contact tracing, where appropriate.

Balanitis

Balanitis is inflammation of the superficial tissues of the penile head.

Aetiology

- Poor hygiene.
- Trauma (e.g. zipper).
- Sexually transmitted infections.
- Allergy (e.g. to condoms).

Symptoms

- Itch and soreness.
- Dysuria.
- Discharge.
- Oedema.
- Rarely, ulcers.
- Rarely, urinary retention.

Treatment

- Antibiotic cream, applied liberally.
- Adults: retract and bathe the prepuce.
- Children: bathe frequently, do not force retraction (although balanitis often dissolves adhesions).
- Circumcision is not indicated unless the condition is recurrent.

Phimosis

The term 'phimosis' is sometimes used to mean a normal but non-retractable foreskin. No treatment is necessary:

- 8% of boys have non-etractile foreskin at 6 years of age and 1% at 16 years at age.

- If an adolescent is concerned, gentle gradual retraction using emollients or mild steroid creams can be tried to break down adhesions.
- Circumcision is not indicated.
- Ballooning of the prepuce with micturition is of no significance.

Non-retractable foreskin scarred by repeated attempts to retract it requires circumcision.

In balanitis xerotica obliterans (lichen sclerosis of the prepuce, with fixing of foreskin, dysuria, poor stream and bleeding), circumcision and metal dilatation are necessary.

Paraphimosis

Presentation

- An acute condition.
- The foreskin is tight and retracted and will not pull distally.
- The glans is oedematous and painful.

Treatment

- Prolonged gentle compression, with analgesia.
- Anaesthesia for emergency circumcision or dorsal slit is occasionally required.

Incontinence

Prevalence

- Affects 1–5% of men and 10–25% of women.
- Probably affects 50% of residents in nursing homes.

Transient incontinence

This is usually due to a UTI or constipation. Treat the underlying cause.

Urge incontinence

- Involuntary urine loss; large volume loss with a strong urge to void.
- Usually there are involuntary detrusor contractions ('detrusor instability', or 'detrusor hyperreflexia' in patients with neurological impairment).

Treatments

- Bladder training is helpful for urgency.
- Bladder relaxants (e.g. tolterodine, oestrogen).

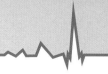

Stress incontinence

This is involuntary urine loss with increased intra-abdominal pressure. It is usually due to:

- displacement of the bladder neck (e.g. prolapse)
- failed incontinence surgery
- prostatectomy
- radiation
- cord lesions.

Treatment
- Pelvic floor exercises.
- Surgery (anterior repair, Manchester repair, sling, hysterectomy).

Overflow incontinence

This is overflow of an overdistended bladder due to:

- drugs
- faecal impaction
- a neurogenic bladder (e.g. diabetes, cord injury, vitamin B_{12} deficiency)
- a bladder outflow obstruction (e.g. prostatism, urethral stenosis).

Treatment
- Treat obstructing lesions.
- Bladder washouts if there is an indwelling catheter.

Sensory urgency incontinence

This is decreased bladder compliance and increased irritability due to:

- radiation therapy
- interstitial cystitis
- meningomyelocoele
- pelvic surgery
- renal reflux may complicate the condition.

Treatment
- Bladder training and bladder relaxants (anticholinergics, muscle relaxants, tricyclic antidepressants).

Sphincteric incontinence

This is urethral hypermobility due to pelvic floor weakness. Sphincter malfunction is due to, for example, previous major abdominopelvic surgery or ageing.

Investigations
- Full examination, including balance and neurology, and examination of the vaginal wall for prolapse.
- Midstream urine test: urea and electrolytes and creatinine; exclude diabetes.

Treatment
Treatment is by various specialist surgical procedures (e.g. urethral bulking agents, artificial sphincters). Surgery less likely to succeed if:

- the patient is elderly
- prior surgery has failed
- there is radiation damage or detrusor instability
- the patient is postmenopausal.

Carcinoma of the kidney: child

- Wilms' tumour (nephroblastoma).
- 80% of cases occur at age <5 years; the condition is rare after 10 years of age.
- Rare association with aniridia.
- Presents as a mass in a well child.
- Poor appetite or poor weight gain, occasionally.
- Abdominal pain and pallor from haemorrhage into the tumour.
- Haematuria and hypertension are uncommon.
- 5% of tumours are bilateral.
- 15% of tumours are metastatic at presentation.
- Refer urgently.

Treatment
- Nephrectomy (all children).
- Chemotherapy (all children).
- Radiotherapy in advanced disease.
- Prognosis is good: 80% cure (60% of metastatic cases).
- Relapse carries poor prognosis.

Carcinoma of the kidney: adult

- Hypernephroma (clear cell carcinoma, Grawitz tumour) in >90% of cases.
- Transitional cell carcinoma of the renal pelvis in 8% of cases.
- Other forms are rare (e.g. sarcomas).

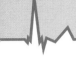

Presentation

- Classic triad (haematuria, mass, flank pain): 5–10% of cases.
- Haematuria: 50–60% of cases.
- Raised erythrocyte sedimentation rate: 50–60% of cases.
- Mass: 25–50% of cases.
- Anaemia: 30% of cases.
- Flank pain: 40% of cases.
- Hypertension: 30% of cases.
- Weight loss: 30% of cases.
- Fever: 10% of cases.
- Hepatic dysfunction: 10–15% of cases.
- Hypercalcaemia: 5% of cases.
- Erythrocytosis: 5% of cases.
- Variocoele: 3% of cases.

Aetiology

- There are hereditary forms.
- Exposure to lead, cadmium, asbestos, petroleum products, phenacetin or diuretics increases risk.

Treatment

- Refer all cases urgently.
- Surgical nephrectomy is only effective management for stages 1 to some stage 3 tumours.
- Invasion is down the renal vein, with most going to the lung, bone or nodes.
- The response rate to chemotherapy is only 5%.
- Angioinfarction is used for palliation.
- Radiotherapy is used for palliation.
- The response rate to immunotherapy (interleukin-2) is about 25%.

Prognosis

- Stage 1 (not through the capsule): 80–100% survival.
- Stage 2 (still within fascia): 70–80% survival.
- Nodal or distal involvement: 10–25% survival.

Acute renal failure

Aetiology

- Pre-renal: hypoperfusion, heart failure, cirrhosis, sepsis, extension of aneurysm to renal arteries.

- Post-renal: outlet obstruction (prostate enlargement, stones, tumour, renal vein occlusion).
- Intrinsic: glomerulonephritis, nephrotic syndrome, acute tubular necrosis, drugs and toxins, contrast media.

Presentation

- Oedema.
- Pallor.
- Oliguria (not always).
- Altered consciousness, seizure.
- Cramps, fasciculations.
- Weakness, nausea, malaise.
- Elevated serum creatinine (rises by 80 mmol/l per day in complete renal failure), urea and potassium; decreased bicarbonate.
- Dipstick test may reveal haematuria or proteinuria.

Treatment

Refer urgently for supportive treatment and treatment of the cause.

Chronic renal failure

There is a progressive decrease in renal function, with an accumulation of waste products. Chronic failure is distinguished from acute renal failure by the duration of the condition.

Presentation

- Pallor, bruising.
- Oedema.
- Hypertension.
- Depression.
- Fatigue, nausea, anorexia, pruritus, insomnia, altered taste.

Aetiology

- Diabetes: 40% of cases.
- Hypertension: 30% of cases.
- Chronic glomerulonephritis: 10% of cases.
- Other: recurrent pyelonephritis, tubular interstitial nephritis (e.g. analgesic nephropathy), vascular disease (e.g. renal arterial disease).

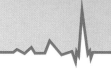

Diagnosis

- Raised urea, potassium, creatinine, uric acid, calcium, phosphate.
- Decreased bicarbonate.
- Raised creatinine clearance.
- Anaemia.
- Midstream urine test: proteinuria, red blood cell casts.
- Renal biopsy (usually avoided if the kidneys are small).
- Renal ultrasound.

Management

Non-drug treatment

- Adequate nutrition and calories, chiefly from carbohydrate.
- Restrict sodium, potassium and phosphate.
- Restrict protein.
- Discontinue nephrotoxic drugs.
- Adjust medication to allow for prolonged half-life.
- Restrict fluid if oedematous.
- Monitor urea and electrolytes, and full blood count.

Drug treatment

- Erythropoeitin 2000–3000 U three times weekly is helpful for anaemia.
- Diuretics (preferably loop diuretics) for fluid overload.
- Correct hypertension with an angiotensin converting enzyme (ACE) inhibitor (but not in hyperkalaemia) or a calcium antagonist.
- Calcium and vitamin D to prevent renal osteodystrophy.

Dialysis or renal transplant

Dialysis or renal transplant is indicated in selected patients. Dialysis is indicated as follows:

- Urgent dialysis: uraemic pericarditis, neuropathy, neuromuscular abnormalities, congestive heart failure, hyperkalaemia, seizure.
- Judgemental dialysis: creatinine clearance 10–15 ml/min, progressive anorexia, weight loss, pruritus, fluid gain with hypertension and congestive heart failure, rising hyperkalaemia.

Renal transplant improves survival: the 2-year kidney graft survival is 70–80% (better for a living donor).

Bladder cancer

- Ranges from low-grade superficial non-life-threatening disease to high-grade invasive disease.
- Field change disease (i.e. the entire urinary endothelium from the renal pelvis to the urethra may be susceptible).
- More common in men over 60 years old.
- Most are transitional cell carcinomas.
- 70% of tumours are localized at presentation.

Presentation

- Gross, painless haematuria.
- Microscopic haematuria.
- Abdominal, flank and groin pain.
- Lymphoedema.
- Renal failure.
- Anorexia.
- Bone pain.

Aetiology

- Cigarette smoking.
- Occupational: azo dyes, textiles, tyres and rubber, petroleum.
- Chemicals: 2-naphthylamine, benzidine, nitrosamines.
- Human papilloma virus type 16.

Squamous cancers are associated with:

- schistosomiasis
- calculi
- indwelling catheters
- bladder diverticulae
- phenacetin
- cyclophosphamide
- radiation
- tuberculosis.

Treatment

- Refer urgently.
- Transurethral resection of tumour.
- Repeat transurethral resection with or without intravesical agents.

- Advanced cases: radical cystectomy or urethrectomy and ileal conduit.

- Occasionally, partial cystectomy if the tumour is in the diverticulum.

- Chemotherapy has palliative and survival benefit.

- Radiotherapy: external beam radiation is sometimes curative (20–30% of cases).

Prognosis

Prognosis depends on the tumour grade, the depth of penetration, multifocality, invasiveness and tumour configuration.

Screening

In the USA it is suggested that people in high-risk professions are screened by means of urine microscopy, dipstick testing or cytology.

DERMATOLOGY

22. Eczema and dermatitis

S Jarvis and WIF Henderson

THIS CHAPTER REVIEWS

- Presentation and differential diagnosis in eczema.
- Complications of eczema.
- Treatment options for the GP.
- When to refer patients.
- Criteria for referral and investigation.
- Follow-up of patients with eczema.
- Prevention of eczema.

Box 22.1 Endogenous eczema

- Atopic
- Seborrhoeic
- Discoid (nummular)
- Pompholyx
- Lichen simplex
- Gravitational (stasis, venous)
- Asteatotic

Eczema is the most common form of inflammatory skin disease encountered in general practice, with approximately 25% of the population developing it at some time in their lives.

The terms 'dermatitis' and 'eczema' tend to be used synonymously, although dermatitis may be used to include all inflammation of the skin – thus all eczema is dermatitis, but not all dermatitis is eczema.[1]

Eczema can be broadly divided into endogenous and exogenous varieties: the former may be inherited and the latter is precipitated by external irritants or allergens (Boxes 22.1 and 22.2).

Diagnosis

People with eczema have a disturbed epidermal barrier function, causing higher transepidermal water loss and lower skin hydration levels.[2] This results in dry skin, which itches, inducing a vicious cycle of itch and scratch; most of the physical changes in the skin are caused by the scratching rather than the eczema.

The clinical appearances of endogenous and exogenous eczema are often similar. Eczema is characterized by:

- itching
- redness
- scaling
- clustered papulovesicles.

Box 22.2 Exogenous eczema

- Irritant
- Allergic
- Photosensitive
- Phytophotosensitive
- Caused by contact with a known irritant or allergen
- Asymmetrical
- Linear
- Clears at weekends or holidays
- Localized to certain parts of the body (e.g. eyelids, hands, feet, perianal area)

Some skin conditions which can mimic eczema are:

- psoriasis
- scabies
- impetigo
- dematophyte infection
- dermatitis herpetiformis
- photosensitivity
- candidiasis
- lichen simplex

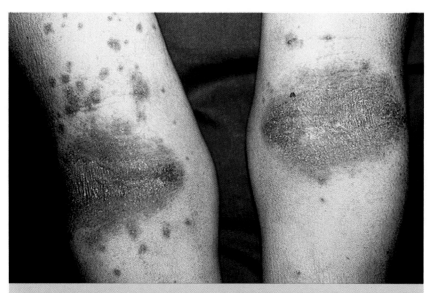

Figure 22.1 Atopic eczema in the flexures of the elbows. Reproduced from Fry, *Update*, 19 August 1999.

- lichen planus
- pityriasis rosea
- Bower's disease
- rosacea.

Types of eczema

Atopic eczema

One of the most common forms of endogenous eczema, especially in children, is atopic eczema. Atopic eczema affects 15–20% of children up to the age of 7 years. A family history of atopy is obtainable in 70% of cases. The aetiology is unknown, although raised levels of immunoglobulin E are common.

The age of onset is 2–12 months in 75% of patients. There tends to be spontaneous improvement throughout childhood, with about half of cases clearing by the age of 13 years. In very few patients lesions fail to resolve by the age of 30 years. There are an estimated 11,000 adults with significant atopic eczema in the UK.[3]

In babies, atopic eczema most often starts on the face, with the extensor aspects of the knees showing signs when the child begins to crawl. From 18 months onwards the areas most commonly affected are the skin flexures of the elbows and knees, and the face and neck (Fig. 22.1). Eczema affecting the ear canal is not uncommon.

The distribution of atopic eczema in an individual tends to be broadly symmetrical. Inflammation and lichenification of affected skin areas are common findings. Scratching may also result in areas of hyper- or hypopigmentation.

GP consultation rates for this condition are high, especially in practices caring for a high proportion of first-generation Asian, Afro-Caribbean and Chinese migrants, in whom the incidence is greatest.

It is worth explaining to parents the likely causes and natural history of their child's eczema. Some may accept that, if their child does not seem upset by the condition, reassurance, simple barrier creams and avoidance of strongly perfumed products is enough.

Seborrhoeic dermatitis

The cause of seborrhoeic dermatitis is unknown. It often presents in the first 3 months of life with cradle cap, an erythematosus scalp eruption which heaps up to form yellowish scales. The scaly rash may spread to involve the neck, the area behind the ears, flexures and the nappy area. Unlike atopic eczema it is not itchy and the child is not disturbed by it.

Mild cases clear with topical emollients, although a mild topical steroid or an emulsifying ointment containing sulphur and salicylic acid may be more helpful for thick cradle cap, as may application of olive oil for a few hours. Mild topical steroids, sometimes combined with an antibacterial or antifungal agent (if secondary infection is present), will usually clear the rash from the trunk.

In adults the forehead, eyebrows and alar folds are commonly affected.

Contact dermatitis

Of the exogenous eczemas, contact dermatitis is probably the most frequently seen in general practice, accounting for 47% of all dermatological consultations.[1] Certain occupational groups are at high risk (Box 22.3).

Contact dermatitis often occurs on the hands, which are most often exposed to irritants. However, irritants which do not cause obvious inflammation on the hands can cause dermatitis when transferred inadvertently to the thinner, more vulnerable skin of the face. Common irritants include detergents and some plants (e.g. hyacinths, giant hogweed and, in the USA, poison ivy and poison oak). Mild exposure may cause dryness, erythema and fissuring, but severe exposure (e.g. poison ivy) may cause blistering, itching, burning and swelling. A history of possible contacts is useful and patch testing may be helpful.

Prevention is difficult. Appropriate gloves, with a cotton layer next to the skin to absorb moisture, may not be feasible for many workers in contact with the public. Barrier creams are of relatively little use.

Treatment of eczema

Loss of the integrity of the lipid barrier is central in the development of eczema. Frequent washing with soap products, many of which contain sodium lauryl sulphate (which has known irritant properties), and conditions of low humidity induce changes in the epidermis, and provide increased opportunity for irritants and allergens to enter the skin. Restoration of barrier function is therefore paramount, together with the elimination of irritants.

The ABC patient leaflet, sponsored by Lever, encourages patients to:

A. avoid soap

B. benefit from emollients

C. control inflammation.

Non-pharmacological treatment

Avoid irritants and trigger factors such as:

- sudden changes in temperature
- irritant substances (e.g. wool, detergents)
- wear pure cotton next to the skin
- trigger foods (unusual for >1 year)
- stress
- allergens and dust
- soap, all together, particularly in children who can wash with emollients (rather as the ancient Greeks washed with olive oil).

In addition:

Box 22.3 Occupations at greater risk of contact dermatitis

Irritant contact dermatitis
- Housewives
- Hairdressers (tints, shampoos)
- Cleaners
- Cooks (citrus peels)
- Bar staff (citrus peels)
- Carpenters
- Rubber industry workers
- Medical personnel (rubber)
- Construction workers (cement)
- Miners

- Farmers (malathion, ragweed)
- Medical personnel (powdered gloves, antiseptics)

Allergic
- Medical personnel (latex)
- Dental technicians
- Jewellery wearers/makers (nickel allergy)
- Photographers
- Electroplating workers
- Chemical workers
- Horticulturists

- A change of job may be helpful if considered early, but patients should be reminded of the need to avoid exchanging one set of allergens for another in a new work environment.
- In allergic dermatitis, avoid allergen. Wash off contacts with plain water and mild soap.

Diet

This can be considered in those who do not respond to topical treatments. The main allergens are cows' milk, egg, soy and wheat, although any food may be implicated. Three to 4 weeks of elimination is usually sufficient to detect a response, but this can be difficult to judge objectively. GPs may find the situation complicated by parents realizing that soya milk is available free on FP10 whereas regular baby milk is not.

Diet is significantly beneficial only in a small proportion of children, usually those under 1 year old.[1] Indeed, excessively restrictive diets devised by mothers keen to avoid potential allergens may pose the risk of dietary deficiency, especially if the intake of calcium and natural fats is limited. In particular, goats' milk can be allergenic. If the diet is restricted, then over the age of 2 years the suspect dietary items should be cautiously reintroduced.

Pharmacological treatment

Emollients

These are the mainstay of treatment. Emollients rehydrate the skin by forming an occlusive barrier, reducing water loss from the stratum corneum. This allows the cells to swell and press against one another, thereby sealing the cracks and fissures. The barrier also reduces the effects of exotoxins produced by *Staphylococcus aureus*.

Emollients are most effective when applied after bathing, when the water content of the skin is higher, and for maximum benefit should be reapplied regularly throughout the day. The key to using emollients successfully is to apply them in sufficient quantity and with sufficient frequency, and to use an emollient non-soap cleanser as an alternative to normal soap. Colloidal oatmeal (Aveeno) in the bath may also be helpful, especially in contact dermatitis.

Hydrating emollients can therefore be used as often as the parent is prepared to apply them. Where skin is very dry, 2-hourly applications are commonly recommended. Frequent application will limit the need for steroids, although emollients are not anti-inflammatory. The British Association of Dermatologists guidelines[3] recommend the application of

Box 22.4 Range of emollients for use in eczema or dermatitis

Lightest

Aqueous cream
Diprobase
E45 (contains lanolin)
Cetamagrogol A
Unguentum Merck
Zinc and castor oil (1 part zinc in 9 parts oily cream)
White soft paraffin 50% and liquid paraffin 50%

Heaviest

250 g/week for a child and 500 g/week for an adult. Regular use of emollients reduces the need for topical steroids; a general rule of thumb is to exceed steroid use by 10:1 in terms of the quantities used.

Since emollients do nothing to reduce inflammation and may make the skin appear temporarily redder, parents often discontinue them at an early stage. An explanation of their barrier role and of the need to apply them regularly will often reassure parents.

In children under about 6 years of age wet-wrapping is an efficient way to 'drive' moisturizer into the skin. If the skin can be rehydrated then the integrity is improved and the sequelae of itching, redness, scratching and skin breakdown and infection can be avoided.

A wide range of preparations, including creams, ointments, soap substitutes and bath oils, is available for use as monotherapy or in combination (Box 22.4). Patient choice is very important. It is therefore useful to let the patient try a variety of emollients and then prescribe the selected one in adequate amounts. Creams with a high water content, such as aqueous cream, are more likely to provide a breeding ground for staphylococci, so if recurrent infection/inflammation is a problem consider switching to a cream with a lower water content.

Topical steroids

Topical steroids should be used where emollients alone fail to control the symptoms (i.e. in the treatment of exacerbations and flare-ups).

It is important to explain the step-up step-down approach to parents and to be familiar with one or two steroid creams and ointments in each class of potency. In general, the least-potent steroid that controls the symptoms effectively should be used. Most dermatologists use the step-down approach (more potent to less potent) for exacerbations in order to get on top of the flare-up quickly.

There are four potency categories in the UK: mild, moderate, potent and very potent. Hydrocortisone is a mild steroid, and is available in concentrations of 0.5–2.5%. Stronger steroids include, in ascending order of potency, Eumovate, Betnovate and Dermovate.

Steroids should be applied twice or once daily (as indicated) to affected areas, and patients and carers should be familiar with the concept of fingertip dosing. A line of cream squeezed from the distal finger crease to the finger tip on the index finger should treat an area the size iof the palmar surface of the hand.

An explanation of the relative strengths and safety of different preparations may greatly improve compliance and cut the risk of inappropriate steroid use. As a rule of thumb, the thinner the skin, the greater the risk of local side-effects such as skin thinning and striation, and the greater the systemic absorption. The thickness of the skin is least on the face and intertriginous areas, and is greatly reduced in younger children and babies. Hydrocortisone 1% cream will not cause significant thinning of the skin on the trunk, not even when used quite regularly.

The British Association of Dermatologists guidelines[3] provide advice to reduce possible side-effects when prescribing topical steroids. As a rough guide, topical steroids should be limited to up to a week for acute eczema and up to 4–6 weeks for chronic eczema. Repeat prescriptions for anything stronger than 1% hydrocortisone (and not even that in children) for eczematous conditions require regular review.

The following considerations will help reduce side-effects when prescribing topical steroids:[3]

- Hydrocortisone 1% cream is sufficient for mild to moderate eczema in most children. Stronger preparations should not be used in the very young. Moderately potent steroids may be given to older children for short periods during flare-ups.
- Hydrocortisone 1% cream should be used on sites with higher absorption rates, such as the flexures and the face.
- Ointments give better skin penetration. Although creams are more cosmetically acceptable, they may contain preservatives, which can cause irritation.
- Most steroids are to be applied no more than twice daily and some of the newer ones are designed for once-daily application.

Oral antihistamines

Oral antihistamines may be of benefit in some cases – they may control pruritis and induce sedation. They are not effective during the day, as the dose required to suppress itch is sedative. Where antihistamines are used at night it is important to use enough. A slightly sedated child is liable to scratch more rather than less. Some paediatricians advise the full daily dose be given at night. Sedative antihistamines can cause other problems – some children will be irritable and overactive the day after taking them.

Topical immunomodulators

Topical immunomodulators are a new addition to the treatment of atopic eczema. These are believed to act selectively on the T-lymphocytes to inhibit the release of inflammatory cytokines, which play a key role in the inflammatory response in eczema. Steroids, however, interfere with Langerhans cells, fibroblasts, blood vessels and T-lymphocytes, potentially causing the side-effects of telangiectasia, skin atrophy and suppression of the hypopituitary–adrenal axis.

Tacrolimus ointment (Protopic) was the first topical immunomodulator to be launched. It is available in two strengths: 0.03% for use in 2–16 year olds and 0.1% for adults with moderate to severe atopic eczema. Application is twice daily, with reduction in strength and/or frequency after 3 weeks until the condition clears.

Pimecrolimus 1% cream (Elidel) is now marketed for primary care use. It is indicated for mild to moderate eczema, although not in children under 2 years old, although studies of both agents are ongoing in children from the age of 3 months. Because of their selectivity and apparent lack of steroid long-term side-effects, these preparations are a useful, although more expensive, addition to the treatment of atopic eczema, especially in sensitive areas such as the face.

It is recommended that prescriptions are made by dermatologists or physicians with extensive experience in the treatment of atopic eczema with immunomodulating therapy', although this covers any GP who prescribes topical steroids.

Antibiotics

Inflamed eczema usually suggests the presence of staphylococci, and nasal carriage in the child is often the source. Treatment with topical antibiotic creams is sufficient for small areas, but oral antibiotics may be necessary where infection is extensive. Oral antibiotics do not reliably eradicate nasal staphylococci, and a course of nasal cream can be extremely helpful in children with recurrently

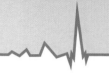

inflamed eczema. Nasal swabs may be taken to confirm the presence of bacteria, but empirical treatment is often a sensible course.

As the most common bacterial infection is *S. aureus*, a 14-day course of flucloxacillin (or, if the patient is penicillin sensitive, a macrolide such as erythromycin) should be given. If this is unsuccessful, a swab should be taken to detect possible resistant strains or an additional streptococcal infection.

Steroid–antibiotic combinations, such as Fucidin H, Fucibet and Betnovate-C, are effective in milder infections.

The use of emollient–antimicrobial preparations to prevent infections is logical, but there are few published data. Oilatum Plus and Dermol 500 have been shown to reduce *S. aureus* colonization.

Complications

The patient with eczema affecting visible skin surfaces may suffer significant distress, and for patients with contact dermatitis or those with eczema affecting the hands who work in the food industry a change of job may be the only solution.

Physical sequelae include vulnerability to secondary infection, particularly by staphylococci, dermatophytes and herpes simplex virus. Herpes simplex virus infection is potentially serious as it can spread rapidly on damaged eczematous skin, causing an extensive vesicular reaction, Kaposi's varicelliform eruption or eczema herpeticum.

Lymphadenopathy is common and usually resolves as the skin improves.

Those with severe eczema may develop severe localized reactions to some immuniations, such as that for tuberculosis, and this was not uncommon with smallpox vaccine in the days when it was widely used.

Where large areas of eczematous skin are exposed to infected bodily fluids there is also a risk of acquisition of blood-borne diseases.

Scarring is not a consequence of eczema, since it involves only the upper layers of skin (spongiform layer) and patients may be relieved to hear this.

Referral and follow-up

Most atopic eczema is managed in general practice. Reasons for referral might include severe disease, apparent failure of treatment and parental request, particularly where

---

Box 22.5 Criteria for referral and investigation

- Refractory eczema despite intensive emollient regimens, topical steroids and antibiotics
- Suspected contact eczema (patch testing indicated)
- Suspected severe infection with herpes simplex virus (eczema herpeticum)
- The eczema leads to severe social or psychological problems (e.g. sleeplessness, absenteeism)
- Diagnostic doubt
- Consideration of second-line therapy (e.g. phototherapy, systemic drugs)

the treatment offered by the GP seems not to have worked. Criteria for referral are given in Box 22.5.

If regular applications of emollient have failed or not been carried out, referral for regular wet wraps may produce dramatic results, breaking the cycle of distress and anxiety for parent and child alike. In many areas specialist dermatology nurses are available to assist parent with wet-wrapping. Severe eczema in a young child can place a heavy burden on families, and involvement of the health visitor is also appropriate.

In any patient whose livelihood depends on use of irritant substances, referral for specialist investigation is appropriate.[1] Even if patients have previously tested negative, a change in symptoms or occupation may warrant re-referral.

The future

Nurses and health visitors could be trained to give advice on appropriate use of emollients and allergen avoidance, as well perhaps as the application of wet wraps. Most models of clinical governance now encompass the practice of the primary care team as well as the GP.[4]

Key points

- **Twenty-five per cent of the population develop eczema at some time in their lives.**
- **The mainstay of treatment is the frequent application of emollients.**
- **A step-up step-down approach to treatment is essential.**
- **There is little evidence for dietary manipulation.**
- **Wet-wrapping is a highly effective way of hydrating the skin in young children.**

- The mildest steroids will not thin the skin.

- Always consider secondary infection and nasal staphylococci when eczema is inflamed.

- Most of the physical changes in the skin are actually due to the scratching.

- Exacerbations should be treated as quickly as possible with the appropriate strength steroids.

- Always prescribe enough topical treatment for the patient.

- Topical immunomodulators are a new addition to the treatment of atopic eczema.

Resources

British Association of Dermatologists, 19 Fitzroy Square, London W1P 5HQ. Tel. 020 7383 0266. Website: http://www.bad.org.uk. The Association provides advice sheets and guidelines on eczema and other dermatological conditions.

British Dermatological Nursing Group (c/o British Association of Dermatologists, see address above). The Group welcomes registered nurses with an interest in skin care and provides education and support.

National Eczema Society, Hill House, Highgate Hill, London N19 5NA. Helpline: 0870 241 3604. Website: http://www.eczema.org. The Society provides a useful support service, information and advice literature for people with eczema and their families.

Primary Care Dermatology Society, Gable House, 40 High Street, Rickmansworth, Hertfordshire WD3 1ER. Tel. 01923 711678. Website: http://www.pcds.org.uk. The Society's aim is to encourage an interest in dermatology in general practice. It also runs regional and national meetings. The Society has developed guidelines for the management of atopic eczema.

Skin Care Campaign, Hill House, Highgate Hill, London N19 5NA. Tel. 020 7281 3553. Website: http://www.skincarecampaign.org. An alliance of skin care groups providing information and advice direct to the public through Skin Information Days.

St. John's Institute of Dermatology, St. Thomas' Hospital, Lambeth Palace Road, London SE1 7EH. Tel. 020 7928 9292. The Institute provides information to GPs on dermatological problems.

References

1. Champion RH, Burton JL, Burns D. Textbook of dermatology, vol. 1. Oxford: Blackwell Science, 1998.

2. Tupker R, Pinnagoda J, Coenraads PJ, et al. Susceptibility to irritants: role of barrier function, skin dryness and history of atopic dermatitis. Br J Dermatol 1990; 123:199–205.

3. National Eczema Society. Management and treatment of eczema. London: National Eczema Society; 1994.

4. Baker R, Lakhani M, Fraser R, et al. A model for clinical governance in primary care groups. BMJ 1999; 318:779–783.

23. Managing acne in practice

M Mead

THIS CHAPTER REVIEWS

- Grading acne in primary care.
- Treatments for acne in primary care.
- Treatment for acne in secondary care.
- When to refer patients.

Acne is a skin disease characterized by comedones (blackheads), papules, pustules, cysts and nodules. It affects about 90% of teenagers and tends to be more severe in boys. Although a disease of teenagers (the peak incidence is at the ages of 14–19 years), it can present for the first time in patients aged 30–40 years. The face is nearly always affected (Fig. 23.1), with lesions also occurring on the back and chest (Fig. 23.2).

The cause is an increase in sebum production and cornification of the sebaceous ducts, with overgrowth of bacteria, such as *Propionibacterium acnes*, and subsequent inflammatory changes.

Severe acne, with pustules and nodules, can cause scarring. It has a considerable psychological impact on the patient. The severity of the psychological effects may determine the aggressiveness of therapy and should be assessed during the consultation.

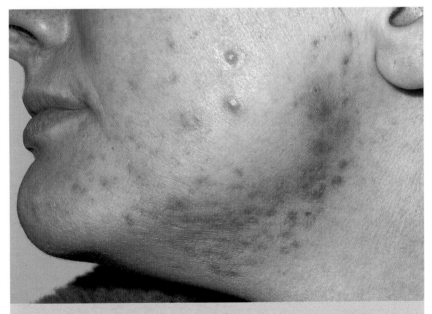

Figure 23.1 Papulopustular acne. Acne lesions usually occur on the face and should be distinguished from rosacea. Reproduced from Avery, *Update*, 14 November 2002, courtesy of Professor W Cunliffe.

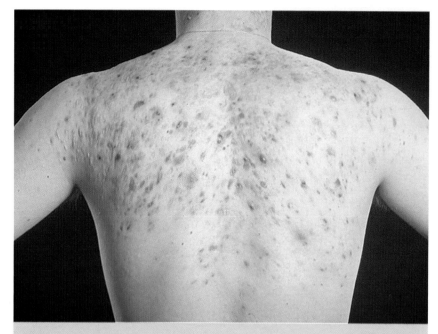

Figure 23.2 The torso may be affected by acne lesions, in particular comedones, papules and pustules. Reproduced from Pywell, *Update*, 24 June 1998.

Differential diagnosis

Acne should be distinguished from rosacea. Rosacea presents only on the face; it consists of erythema, pustules and papules, but no comedones, and usually occurs in women. It tends to affect patients over 30 years old. It is classically made worse by sunlight, topical steroids and drugs or conditions that cause facial flushing.

Diagnosis

The diagnosis is usually obvious clinically, but it is worth assessing the severity of the acne:

- Mild acne: comedones, a small number of papules and only a few pustules.
- Moderate acne: more papules and pustules and a tendency to scar.
- Severe acne: large numbers of papules and pustules, nodular abscesses and scarring.

Management

A simple advice leaflet containing essential points about the management of acne is useful for patients. Include the following advice:

- there is no evidence that changing diet helps
- do not pick or squeeze lesions or spots
- sunlight may ease symptoms (but some acne treatments may photosensitize skin)
- treat dandruff aggressively
- wash twice a day
- use light non-greasy cosmetics
- persist with your treatment, as it can take several weeks before you see any benefit

Treatment

Acne causes significant psychological morbidity. There are effective treatments available and most patients will try drug therapy, often initially using over-the-counter preparations. GPs should enquire about the treatment currently being used before planning a treatment programme. There is no evidence that a change in diet helps. GPs can prescribe a range of topical and oral drug therapies which, over a period of months, may produce excellent cosmetic results.

Guidelines for drug therapy

For mild acne (with comedones, a few papules but little inflammatory material) topical drug therapies may be sufficient, but for moderate acne (with more inflamed papules and pustules) systemic antibiotics (possibly with topical therapy in addition) will be required.

Patients with severe acne (numerous papules, pustules, nodules, cysts and the possibility of scarring) should be referred. The dermatologist may advise oral isotretinoin (Roaccutane) therapy, which can dramatically improve acne and prevent scarring, but is expensive. Remember to make sure of adequate contraception if isotretinoin is prescribed (as it is teratogenic).

Treatment for acne takes about 3 months to begin to have a real effect and more than 6 months (often up to 12 months) to achieve a major improvement. Warn patients of the need to persist with treatment. Patients may need maintenance treatment for 2 or 3 years, or even longer.

The patient should be fully counselled with regard to any anticipated side-effects from the medication and any drug interactions, particularly with the combined oral contraceptive (COC) pill.

Treatment options

There are four main approaches to treatment of acne, including topical and oral drug therapies.

Topical therapy

Topical treatments for acne are summarized in Box 23.1.

For comedones topical retinoids are the first port of call if the patient is not pregnant and is using adequate contraception.

Adapalene (Differin) is a new retinoid-like gel with anti-comedonal and anti-inflammatory actions. An alternative for mild inflammatory acne are benzoyl peroxide preparations, starting at low strength (e.g. initially 2–3 h/day of the 5% strength) and moving upwards to the 10% strength if required. Warn the patient of the possibility of initial skin irritation.

Tretinoin (Retin A), a retinoid, is more effective than benzoyl peroxide in patients where comedones are the main problem, but can also cause similar skin irritation. An effective strategy is to combine the two preparations (benzoyl peroxide and tretinoin) using one in the morning and one at night. A third topical retinoid, isotretinoin (Isotrex), is also available.

Box 23.1 Topical treatments for patients with acne

- Drugs containing benzoyl peroxide:
  - Acnecide
  - Acnidazil
  - Benzamycin
  - Nericur
  - Panoxyl
  - Quinoderm
- Retinoid or retinoid-like drugs:
  - Differin
  - Isotrex
  - Isotrexin
  - Retin-A
- Topical antibiotics containing erythromycin:
  - Benzamycin
  - Stiemycin
  - Zineryt
- Topical antibiotics containing tetracycline:
  - Topicycline
- Clindamycin:
  - Dalacin T
- Azelaic acid:
  - Skinoren

Azelaic acid (Skinoren) is a useful antibacterial topical agent for mild to moderate acne, but treatment is limited to 6 months. Azelaic acid causes less skin irritation than does the benzoyl peroxide and tretinoin combination, but may cause photosensitivity.

Topical antibiotics can be used twice daily for inflammatory acne, but their use is hampered by the development of bacterial antibiotic resistance. This can be partly overcome by alternating topical antibiotics with benzoyl peroxide preparations.

Topical tetracycline fluoresces under disco lights (warn your teenagers!) and there is a rare risk with topical clindamycin of a pseudomembranous colitis. Stop the medication if severe diarrhoea develops.

Oral antibiotics

There are a range of antibiotics to consider (Box 23.2): oxytetracycline 500 mg twice daily, erythromycin 500 mg

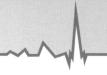

Box 23.2 Oral antibiotics for the treatment of acne

- Tetracyclines:
  - Deteclo
  - Terramycin
  - Tetralysal
- Trimethoprim:
  - Trimopan
  - Ipral
  - Monotrim
- Minocycline:
  - Aknemin
  - Minocin MR
- Erythromycin:
  - Erymax
  - Eryhthrocin
  - Erythroped
  - Isolone
  - Tiloryth
- Doxycycline:
  - Vibramycin

twice daily, trimethoprim 200 mg twice daily, minocycline 100 mg twice daily or doxycycline 50–100 mg once daily. You may need, especially initially, to use doses as high as 2 g/day of erythromycin or oxytetracycline. Tetracyclines must not be given to patients who are pregnant, breast-feeding or under 12 years old in order to avoid interaction with milk and antacids.

Erythromycin generates a high rate of bacterial resistance. Minocycline may cause a greyish black pigmentation as a side-effect and there are other rare side-effects (hepatotoxicity and a systemic lupus erythematosus-like reaction). It can, however, be very effective. Doxycycline can cause photosensitivity. If using a topical antibiotic with a systemic one, ensure both are of the same type (e.g. that both are tetracyclines).

The most likely problem with using systemic antibiotics is candidiasis, although all the usual antibiotic side-effects, including diarrhoea, may occur. Warn patients on the COC pill to take extra contraceptive precautions for the first 4 weeks of antibiotic use. If the patient is taking oral

contraception and the antibiotics are causing diarrhoea, it may be better to use Dianette.

Dianette (ethinyloestradiol and cyproterone)

Dianette is both a contraceptive and an anti-androgen and, as such, is a useful treatment for acne. The GP should remember that contraindications to COCs will apply, as will the need for monitoring along COC lines. Patients can avoid a prescription charge if Dianette is used as a contraceptive.

Isotretinoin (Roaccutane)

The most powerful anti-acne drug is isotretinoin, but it can only be prescribed in secondary care. Apart from being teratogenic (contraception must be 100%) it can cause a rise in liver enzymes and lipid levels, and therefore liver function tests and lipids need to be monitored.

There are a wide range of side-effects, including depression and, in severe cases, even suicidal depression. It is important to remember this significant risk of depression when prescribing isotretinoin.

Monitoring treatment

Acne treatment is slow, and the beneficial effect builds up over months. The patient could be seen after a few weeks of treatment to encourage compliance and gauge side-effects, then at 3 months to check on improvement (if none or minimal, consider changing therapy) and then at 6 months, by which time significant improvement should certainly have occurred.

Referral

The following symptoms indicate that referral to a dermatologist is needed:

- Severe nodulocystic acne; dermatologists may inject individual cysts with triamcinolone.

- Scarring (present or anticipated); dermatologists have a range of new options for the treatment of scarring.

- Moderate acne which is of concern to the patient and is not responding to a drug regimen that has been fully complied with for an adequate length of time.

- Acne in older patients, where treatment is often more difficult.

- Acne causing serious psychological effects.

Key points

- Acne can cause significant psychological morbidity.

- Treatments need to be prolonged and may take up to 6 months to reach their full effect.

- It is important to tailor the treatment choice to the type and grade of acne.

- Some patients with acne should be referred to secondary care (be aware of the criteria for referral).

- A practice formulary for topical and oral acne treatments may be helpful.

- Meetings with local dermatologists to discover who has an interest in acne and what treatments they offer may be helpful.

24. Managing psoriasis in primary care

D Brooks and T Poyner

THIS CHAPTER REVIEWS

- The diagnosis and treatment of psoriasis in general practice.
- Advice on management.
- The importance of discovering how patients feel about their condition and what has prompted them to seek help.
- When to refer those patients who would benefit from secondary care.

Box 24.1 Drugs that can exacerbate psoriasis

- Antimalarials
- Lithium
- Beta blockers
- Quinidine
- Steroids
- Indomethacin
- Tetracyclines
- Captopril
- Chlorthalidone
- Gemfibrozil

Prevalence

Psoriasis is a common inflammatory skin condition affecting approximately 2% of the population. Men and women are equally affected and 30% have a known family history. Psoriasis can develop at any time, although onset is often in early adult life and 75% of cases occur before the age of 40 years.[1]

Most patients have mild disease, but there is evidence of marked variability within individuals over time.[2] There is a 50% chance of a remission, although this is permanent for only 20% of patients.

Diagnosis

Psoriasis is a chronic skin disorder in which excessive proliferation of keratinocytes results in the formation of scaly thickened plaques, itching and inflammatory changes of the epidermis and dermis. The various forms include chronic plaque psoriasis and the guttate, pustular and arthritic variants, and there is strong association with HLA B13, B17 and B27. Men and women are equally affected, and there are peaks of onset in adolescence and around age of 60 years.

The aetiology is unknown, but genetic transmission is dominant, with variable penetrance. Onset and flares may be precipitated by some drugs (Box 24.1) or by streptococcal pharyngitis.

Psoriasis is usually a clinical rather than a histological diagnosis. The well-defined edge of the plaques, their silvery scale and the presence of nail involvement help differentiate psoriasis from the various types of eczema.

Differential diagnosis includes lichen planus, which presents as a very itchy mauve rash, with fine white lace-like scale on its surface (Wickham's striae). Mycosis fungoides presents with plaques, which vary in both colour (red to orange brown) and shape. If mycosis fungoides is suspected the patient should be referred to secondary care, where the diagnosis can be confirmed with biopsies.

Types of psoriasis

Chronic plaque psoriasis

Nail involvement with pitting and onchodystrophy is common, and joint involvement often causes sacroiliitis and spondylitis.

Of the various types of psoriasis the most common is chronic plaque psoriasis (psoriasis vulgaris), representing 85% of cases. The patient presents with a symmetrical rash ▸

on the extensor surfaces of elbows, knees and lower back. The plaques are covered in silvery scale and have a well-defined edge (Fig. 24.1).

Scalp involvement is common and between one-third and one-half of patients have nail involvement. In the scalp there is erythema and scale, but rarely any hair loss (Fig. 24.2). The nail deformity includes pits and separation of the distal nail from its bed (a process known as onycholysis). Psoriasis is also associated with geographical tongue.

Psoriasis can affect the flexures, where the increased hydration predisposes to secondary infection (Fig. 24.3). The friction between the skin surfaces reduces scale, but the well-demarcated edge is preserved. Flexural psoriasis can be mistaken for a fungal infection, and scrapings

should be taken if in doubt. Psoriasis of the nails can be differentiated from chronic fungal infection as psoriasis is usually symmetrical.

Psoriasis can develop on the hands and feet. Some patients (classically middle-aged females) develop palmoplantar pustular psoriasis, with sterile pustules, which are either yellow or brown in appearance.

Psoriasis can also develop at the site of any physical trauma (Koebner's phenomenon).

Guttate psoriasis

Guttate psoriasis usually presents in children and young adults (Fig. 24.4) following a streptococcal throat infection. The rash has a raindrop appearance, with multiple silvery papules developing on the trunk and limbs, and is usually preceded by streptococcal pharyngitis.

Pustular psoriasis

Psoriasis can become unstable; this can be provoked by the sudden cessation of potent topical steroids. The patient develops generalized erythema, which can become

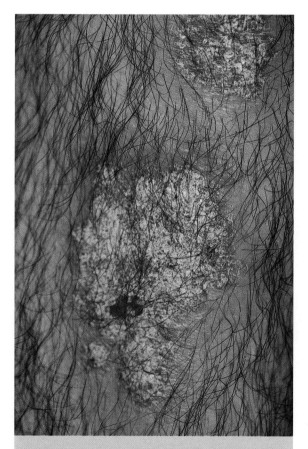

Figure 24.1 Chronic plaque psoriasis accounts for 85% of psoriasis cases in general practice. Reproduced from Poyner, *Update*, 19 December 2002.

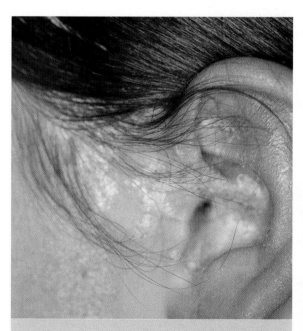

Figure 24.2 Scalp psoriasis. Patients should be reassured that it rarely causes hair loss. Reproduced from Poyner, *Update*, 19 December 2002.

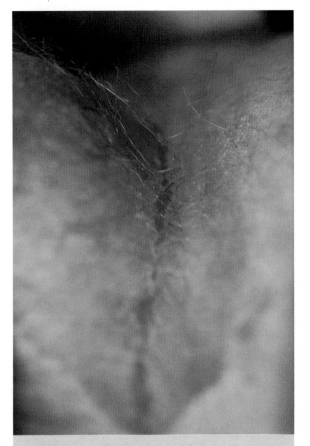

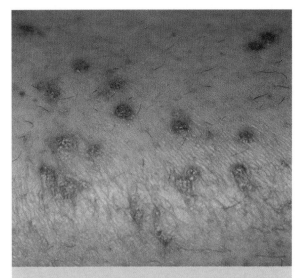

Figure 24.4 Gutatte psoriasis usually presents in children and young adults. Reproduced from Poyner, *Update*, 19 December 2002.

Figure 24.3 Perineal psoriasis. Psoriasis is common in the flexures, where increased hydration can lead to secondary infection. Reproduced from Poyner, *Update*, 19 December 2002.

confluent and is then one of the causes of erythroderma. The rash may be associated with generalized small sterile pustules. The patient with erythroderma or generalized pustular psoriasis is systemically unwell and needs urgent medical attention.

Psoriatic arthritis

Psoriatic arthritis may occur in up to 10% of patients. The pattern is quite variable, although there are a number of classical presentations, which include:

- distal interphalangeal joint involvement and nail dystrophy
- monoarthritis or asymmetrical arthritis
- symmetrical arthritis (similar to rheumatoid arthritis, but the rheumatoid factor is negative)
- spinal arthritis (similar to ankylosing spondylitis)
- arthritis mutilates (a destructive arthritis of the hands).

Patients with psoriatic arthritis are usually managed by a rheumatologist. Non-steroidal anti-inflammatory drugs (NSAIDs) are prescribed, even though they may aggravate the rash. For those with more severe disease, methotrexate (Maxtrex) controls both the rheumatological and the dermatological manifestations.

The consultation

It is important to spend time on the consultation with a patient who has psoriasis. The GP should try to identify why the patient developed psoriasis or presented for treatment when they did. The patient may have taken a drug that could be implicated in an exacerbation. There may be a history of some stressful event or of a recent sore throat.

It is also important to take time to discover how the patient feels about having to contend with psoriasis. Embarrassment, frustration and fear are common. Indeed, most patients will have some psychological disturbance, ▶

which they may or may not handle well, and some patients may have associated depression.

It is helpful to explore the family history and experience of the patient with psoriasis. Such a process helps in identifying not only why a patient has psoriasis at any particular time, but also how it affects their lifestyle, their feelings of self-worth and their expectations of you as a GP and the medical profession as a whole. Only then are we in a position to start managing the patient.

Management

A management plan should be negotiated with the patient and should include:

- perseverance
- reassurance, explanation and advice.

Perseverance is necessary on the part of both the GP and the patient as the right therapy is not usually easy to find, and some treatments are time-consuming.

Empathizing helps build a therapeutic relationship that is more likely to achieve a successful outcome. The GP should explain fully to the patient what psoriasis is, what makes it worse and what can be done about it. Some patients may be concerned that they will infect other people, or that others may believe that they can contract the disease from the patient.

There is no cure for psoriasis and treatment is only suppressive. For the majority of patients psoriasis runs a chronic course. The patient needs to be reassured that the rash is not infectious. About 50% of patients achieve spontaneous remission and 70% are managed entirely in general practice.

It is important to take a positive approach. The patient should be encouraged to tell relatives and friends about the condition and show them lesions in visible areas. The more open the patient is, the less embarrassed he or she will be.

Some patients decide not to treat their rash, while others just want treatment for major flare-ups. The impact of psoriasis on the quality of life of patients is quite variable and is not directly related to the extent of the rash. The patient's age, mobility and social circumstances can affect treatment.

Treatment

The type of treatment chosen is determined by the type of psoriasis, its site, extent and severity, and the patient's medical history, lifestyle, age and sex. In all cases treatment

Box 24.2 Treatment plan for psoriasis

Scalp
- Mild disease: shampoo, such as Capasal
- Moderate disease: add a potent steroid application
- Severe disease: add Cocois ointment for 1 hour

Trunk and limbs
- Mild disease: vitamin D analogue or tar
- Moderate disease: vitamin D analogue in combination with a steroid, or short-contact dithranol

Face and flexures
- Face, mild disease: steroid, tacalcitol or calcitriol
- Flexures, mild disease: steroid cream or mild steroid and antimicrobial (e.g. hydrocortisone and miconazole)

Any site
- Emollients

should start with topical medication, initially moisturizing and descaling preparations, and proceed up the 'ladder' to phototherapy and, finally, systemic medication. A possible treatment plan is given in Box 24.2.

Lifestyle measures

The evidence that diet affects psoriasis is poor, and although the patient may experiment it is probably unwise to encourage this.

Daily baths help to descale the skin and this can be helped by applying moisturizing medication in the direction of the hair growth.

Although sunlight is beneficial in clearing psoriasis, sunburn can be devastating.

GPs should perhaps have a lower threshold for prescribing antibiotics for sore throats in patients with a history or family history of psoriasis in view of the information on the role of the β-haemolytic *Streptococcus*. In this way, it may be possible to prevent, or at least delay, the development of psoriasis in predisposed individuals and exacerbations in individuals with the disorder.

Topical treatments

Patients with limited disease (<20% body area) can be treated with any of the following:

- Soap substitutes, such as aqueous cream, can be useful. For particularly scaly psoriasis, 50% white soft paraffin with 50% liquid paraffin is helpful if used after a bath.

- Topical steroids are one of the most common therapies prescribed for mild or moderate psoriasis. Mild or moderately potent steroid ointments are sufficient for many patients, particularly for sensitive areas. However, potent steroids carry a risk of skin thinning and causing rebound of the disease. They should not be applied to the face.

- Potent steroids can be used on the palms and soles, as the skin is thick and the risk of atrophy is minimal. At other sites one needs to balance the benefits and risks.

- Coal tar is old-fashioned, smelly and certainly messy, but very effective. It can be used overnight or applied in the form of coal tar preparations in the bath water. Coal tar can be made up in various strengths in combination with topical steroids. Tar products are sometimes combined with ultraviolet B (Goeckerman regimen).

Dithranol

This is useful for chronic plaques. It is applied in increasing concentrations in zinc and salicylic acid paste (Lassar's paste), starting with 0.2% applied before bedtime and increasing the strength weekly, depending on sensitivity. The concentration could be increased to 1.0%, but many patients significantly improve long before the maximum concentration is reached.

Initially, the preparation should be left on for 10–60 minutes, but this period can be increased to overnight if the patient does not experience a burning sensation. Patients should be advised to wear old clothes as Dithranol causes purple/brown staining. The hardened paste is wiped off in the morning with arachis oil, followed by a bath. Disadvantages are that the skin is temporarily stained, burning may occur and the tar is smelly. Care should be taken to avoid contact with normal skin, and rubber gloves should be worn when applying it. Success is measured by the absence of scaling and a new smoothness of the skin.

Dithranol is also combined with UVB in some treatment regimens.

Traditionally, dithranol was contained in Lassar's paste, but new formulations of dithranol are more cosmetically acceptable. Dithrocream is available in a number of strengths ranging from 0.1% to 2%. Micanol is a microcrystalline formulation that is available in strengths of

1% and 3%. Micanol needs to be washed off with lukewarm water.

Vitamin D_3 analogues

Vitamin D_3 analogues are used for plaque psoriasis, although not on the face or genitalia. There are no serious side-effects unless they are used in large quantities. Vitamin D_3 analogues can irritate, and alternating them with a topical steroid can reduce this irritation and improve outcomes.

Calcipotriol (Dovonex) is more effective than coal tar and short-contact dithranol.[2] Calcipotriol is available as a cream, an ointment and a scalp formulation. Calcitriol (Silkis) is an endogenous hormonally active form of vitamin D_3 used twice daily on the trunk and limbs. Calcitriol ointment may be used on sensitive areas of the body, such as the face. Tacalcitol (Curatoderm) is another vitamin D_3 analogue; it is used only once daily and can be applied to the face.

A recent development has been the licensing of Dovonex, which combines Betnovate with Dovonex and is more effective than either individually. Separate preparations of Dovonex and Betnovate cannot be mixed as the bases are not compatible, so this represents an advance in treatment for mild to moderate psoriasis.

When using vitamin D_3 analogues one must follow the manufacturer's instructions on how much can be applied without risk of hypercalcaemia (e.g. 100 g Calcipotriol cream or ointment weekly).

Scalp psoriasis responds well to Cocois applied at night and washed off with a tar-based shampoo in the morning. Dovonex and Betnovate scalp solutions are both effective. Dovonex is a little more difficult to use than Betnovate, as the patient needs to try to apply it to the lesions and avoid uninvolved skin

Guttate psoriasis tends to be self-limiting. One can prescribe an emollient or, if the rash is troublesome, refer the patient for a course of phototherapy. One has to rely on intuition and experience, as a systematic review found no firm evidence on how to treat acute guttate psoriasis.[3]

Referral

GPs need to refer patients in whom primary therapies fail, although primary care trusts may in the future need to look at the availability of GP expertise and appropriate therapeutic resources in their own areas so that patients with psoriasis may receive optimum treatment at minimal cost.

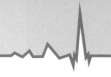

Box 24.3 NICE guidelines for referral

Immediate appointment (within a day):

- if the patient has generalized pustular or erythrodermic psoriasis
- the patient's psoriasis is acutely unstable
- the patient has widespread guttate psoriasis (can benefit from early phototherapy)

Urgent appointment (within 2 weeks):

- the condition is causing severe social or psychological problems
- the rash is sufficiently extensive to make self-management impractical

- the rash is in a sensitive area (e.g. face, hands, feet, genitalia) and the symptoms are particularly troublesome
- the rash is leading to time off work or school, which is interfering with employment or education
- the patient requires assessment for the management of associated arthropathy

Routine appointment:

- The rash fails to respond to management in general practice. 'Failure' is probably best based on the subjective assessment of the patient. Sometimes failure occurs when patients are unable to apply the treatment themselves

---

Failure of therapy, joint involvement or an initially severe form of presentation is an indication for referral. Psoriasis involving more than 20% of the body would normally be considered an indication for referral with view to systemic treatment.

Hospital admission is necessary in severe cases.

Approximately 30% of patients require second-line therapy at some time. Therapies available in secondary care include phototherapy, photochemotherapy and systemic agents. The National Institute for Clinical Excellence (NICE) has produced guidelines for referral to specialist services for psoriasis and on the degree of urgency (Box 24.3).[4] The NICE advice may need modification depending on local circumstances and following input from primary and secondary care.

Follow-up

Follow-up can be either by the GP or a nurse with dermatological expertise.

Prescribing review

Treatment should be reviewed after 1–2 months.[4] The therapies need to be prescribed in specified quantities, as this gives out the message that treatments have to be used very sparingly. At review the patient can bring along unused tubes to check on compliance.

Phototherapy

UVB exposure three times weekly and PUVA (phototherapy with ultraviolet A and psoralens) are both successful

treatments, although they are associated with an increased incidence of skin cancer. In a recent study, the average clearance rate for PUVA was 70%.[5]

Systemic treatments

These include methotrexate (especially for psoriatic arthritis) and cyclosporin, which is very effective (but relapses are common). Synthetic retinoids (etretinate and acitretin) are particularly effective in palmar–plantar pustular psoriasis, but are teratogenic and can cause lipid and liver function abnormalities.

Prevention

Many patients with psoriasis note that stress causes a relapse, and a cognitive–behavioural symptom-management programme is often beneficial.[6] Some patients find it is easier to control their psoriasis if they reduce their alcohol consumption. Smoking is associated with localized pustular psoriasis of the hands and feet; however, cessation of smoking may not affect the natural course of the disease. It is always worth reviewing the patient's other medication, as drugs such as antimalarials, beta blockers, lithium and NSAIDs can aggravate or precipitate psoriasis.

Patients often enquire whether they should embark on home therapy with a sunbed. A controlled study of ultraviolet light and sunbeds found that a short course does improve psoriasis in some patients, but the degree of improvement is small.[7]

It is very difficult to treat nail deformity without resorting to systemic therapies. Keeping the nails short can help prevent onycholysis.

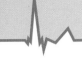

The future

Compliance with therapy is a major problem in psoriasis.[8] Practice nurses may be able to improve compliance. Simple but important issues are: does the patient know how to apply the treatment, and can the patient apply the treatment?

For those patients who come under shared-care arrangements and are on methotrexate, a new blood test, an assay of type III procollagen aminopeptide (PIIINP-0), may go some way to reduce the need for liver biopsies.[9]

Key points

- Topical treatments are indicated in mild to moderate disease.
- Severe disease often requires UV or systemic therapy.
- Psoriasis is a chronic disease and patients may need significant support.
- Psoriasis is common, affecting 2% of the population.
- Psoriasis is chronic, and 80% of patients with psoriasis have a rash at any one time.
- Most cases are mild and the majority can be treated in the community.
- There is no cure, but there are effective treatments.
- Treatment depends on the patients' wishes and the site and severity of the rash.
- Poor compliance is a common problem.

Resources

Fact sheet (No. 26). Royal College of General Practitioners,14 Princes Gate, Hyde Park, London SW7 1PU. Tel. 020 7581 3232.

Health Information Service (Tel. 0800 665544) will supply the latest information and the addresses of self-help groups.

Psoriasis Association, Milton House, 7 Milton Street, Northampton NN2 7JG. Tel. 01604 711129; fax 01604 792894.

References

1. Rees JL, Farr PM. Dermatology. J R Coll Phys London 1997; 31:238–240.

2. Nevitt GJ, Hutchinson PE. Psoriasis in the community: prevalence, severity and patients' beliefs and attitudes towards the disease. Br J Dermatol 1996; 135: 533–537.

3. Chalmers RJ, O'Sullivan T, Owen CM, et al. Interventions for guttate psoriasis (Cochrane Review). In: The Cochrane Library, Issue 4. Oxford: Update Software; 2002.

4. NICE. Referral advice. A guide to appropriate referral from general to specialist services. London: National Institute for Clinical Excellence; 2001, p 20–21.

5. Bandolier, 10 June 1999.

6. Fortune DG, Richards HL, Kirby B, et al. A cognitive–behaviour symptom management programme as an adjunct in psoriasis therapy. Br J Dermatol 2002; 146:458–465.

7. Turner RJ, Walshaw D, Diffey BL, et al. A controlled study of ultraviolet A sunbed treatment for psoriasis. Br J Dermatol 2000; 143:957–963.

8. Richards HI, Fortune DG, O'Sullivan TM, et al. Patients with psoriasis and their compliance with medication. J Am Acad Dermatol 1999; 41:581–583.

9. Bolffa MJ, Smith A, Chalmers RJC, et al. Serum type III procollagen aminopeptide for assessing liver damage in methotrexate treated patients. Br J Dermatol 1996; 135:538–544.

25. Malignant skin conditions

E Warren

THIS CHAPTER REVIEWS

- The importance of early diagnosis and treatment of skin cancer.
- The major features of melanoma.

Prevalence

Skin cancer is not all that common. In 1997, 40,000 new cases were diagnosed in the UK,[1] or just over one case per GP per year. However, the incidence of new cases is doubling every 10 years,[1] an increase attributed to increased sun exposure.[2]

Death from skin cancer is rare. In 1995 there were fewer than 2000 deaths in England and Wales.[3] More than half of theses resulted from malignant melanoma,[3] even though melanoma accounts for only about 1 in 10 of all skin cancers diagnosed.

Most of the lesions that people find on their skin are neither malignant nor premalignant. The publicity about skin cancer has made people more aware of the problem, and they are more likely to consult their GP when they discover a lesion.

Diagnosis

Any skin lesion that occurs in adult life (especially in the elderly) and which grows (however slowly) should be suspected of being malignant until proven otherwise.

A diagnosis may be made from the appearance and history of the lesion. A characteristic case history and/or appearance may help to make the diagnosis, but their absence should not give complete assurance that all is well.

Basal cell carcinomas (BCCs) often ulcerate and show a characteristic raised or rolled pale edge (Fig. 25.1). They may begin as a persistent pearly nodule and are typically on the face. They can occasionally be pigmented.

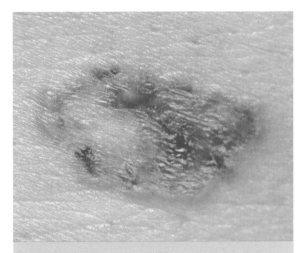

Figure 25.1 Basal cell carcinoma, showing a raised rolled edge with a pearly appearance and ulceration and bleeding from the central area. Reproduced from Price, *Update*, 22 April 1999.

Squamous cell carcinomas (SCCs) commonly form on areas of sun-damaged skin, commonly on the pinna, scalp, back of the hands or lip. The lesion often has a scaly erythematosus surface macule or plaque, and central ulceration may also occur (Fig. 25.2).

As far as malignant melanoma is concerned, the average GP has about a 50% chance of making the diagnosis just on the appearance of the lesion (Fig. 25.3), compared with the 90% accuracy which a dermatologist ought to be able to achieve.[4] It is not practicable to refer, excise or biopsy every skin lesion, so a fail-safe method of detection is needed. A lot of work has been done on the diagnosis of malignant melanoma (Boxes 25.1 and 25.2). A GP will want a diagnostic test with high sensitivity; a test with low specificity is more of a problem for the dermatologist.

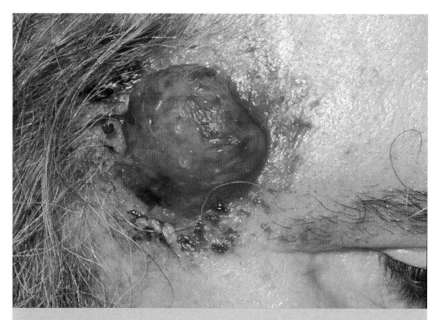

Figure 25.2 Squamous cell carcinoma. This tumour has the appearance of a 'wet strawberry'. Reproduced from Price, *Update*, 22 April 1999.

A few other rare skin cancers such as T-cell lymphomas and Kaposi sarcomas will present very rarely to the GP, but remind us that lesions we do not recognize which do not resolve should be referred.

Prevention

Exposure to sunlight is the only known alterable risk factor for skin cancer. A number of public health campaigns around the world have attempted to point out the dangers of too much sun, while at the same time trying to alter the notion that a suntan is healthy. Even so, in 1995, 40% of people aged 16–24 years in England reported an episode of sunburn in the previous 12 months, and 40% regarded having a suntan as being important to them.[3] This is of particular concern, as episodes of sunburn predispose to melanoma[4] and BCC,[1] while cumulative exposure to the sun is a stronger predictor of SCC.[1] Reasonable recommendations on sun exposure are given in Box 25.3. A recent Australian campaign called for patients to slop on the sun cream, slip on a shirt and slap on a hat.

In fact, it is not proven that sun creams protect against skin cancer, but it is plausible that they should.[1] More and more retired people are wintering abroad, and many of the men

have little scalp protection if they do not wear a hat (Fig. 25.4). A further increase in solar keratoses, and hence SCC, can be expected.

In addition to encouraging prevention, primary care workers are involved in the early detection and treatment of skin cancers when they have arisen. All GPs should be prepared to check skin lesions if their patients request it. The clinical appearance and history will be reassuring in most cases. Seborrhoeic warts are very common in the elderly, and often look as though they ought to be malignant (Fig. 25.5). The 'stuck-on' appearance and greasy texture confirm the diagnosis.

Ordinary skin moles usually appear in the second and third decades of life, a time when skin cancer is virtually unknown. The adolescent concerned about the emergence of a few moles can be similarly reassured.

Management of suspected skin cancers

If the GP thinks that a lesion might be cancerous, urgent referral is mandatory. Sometimes, early BCC is difficult to distinguish from other things that cause little lumps in the skin; watching for a few weeks will clarify the situation

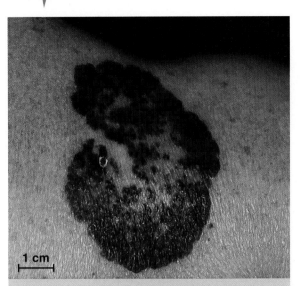

1 cm

Figure 25.3 Malignant melanoma. This rapidly growing lesion had bled on several occasions. Other signs suggestive of melanoma in this case are the irregular coloration and outline, and a diameter greater than 7 mm. Reproduced from Price, *Update*, 22 April 1999.

Box 25.1 Major features of malignant melanoma[5]

- A pigmented lesion that changes in size
- A pigmented lesion that changes in shape
- A pigmented lesion that changes in colour

One feature present: sensitivity 100%, specificity 37%
Two features present: sensitivity 65%, specificity 96%

Box 25.2 Key questions for the GP

- How long has the lesion been present?
- Has the lesion altered in size, shape or colour?
- Does the lesion look malignant or premalignant; is it of a recognizable form?
- Is the patient at risk, either through age, skin type, past history or sun exposure?
- Are there facilities for managing this condition in the practice?
- What does the patient want?
- Will a period of watchful waiting clarify the diagnosis or could it worsen the prognosis?
- Can the lesion be safely excised in general practice?
- How worried is the patient?
- How worried is the doctor?

Box 25.3 Recommendations for avoiding overexposure to the sun[2]

- Avoid the sun between 11 a.m. and 2 p.m. Observe the shadow rule: do not go out in the sun when your shadow is smaller than you are
- Wear a hat and long-sleeved clothing
- Use a high-factor sun cream, and re-apply after swimming, even if the cream is claimed to be waterproof

without worsening the prognosis. Similarly, solar keratosis has such a small chance of progressing to SCC that emollients and sun protection, together with regular review, may be appropriate. However, if there is any doubt, involve a specialist.

Secondary care treatments for BCC and SCC are well established. BCC should be treated early because it may become locally invasive (but rarely metastatic), while SCC may metastasize if neglected.

Melanoma is an altogether more aggressive cancer (Fig. 25.6). The chance of being alive 5 years after diagnosis is 75% for women and 52% for men.[6] Once a melanoma has spread, the 5-year mortality is 95% and the median survival time is only 6 months.[4]

Sometimes, delays in securing treatment occur because the patient does not present early enough; indeed, patients who fear cancer the most are more likely to present later.[7] Other delays have resulted from the poor quality of some GP referral letters: in one series of suspected melanoma, 22% of the letters did not use the word 'pigmented' and 56% did not request an urgent appointment.[8]

A GP who undertakes to remove skin lesions in the surgery must be sure that he or she has suitable experience. A survey of melanomas operated on by GPs showed that a quarter had been incompletely excised, compared with only 7% operated on by specialists. Only 40% had been correctly diagnosed beforehand.[9] In the same study, less than a third of GPs routinely sent all excised skin specimens for histology.

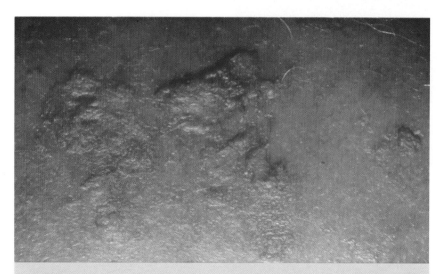

Figure 25.4 Multiple solar keratoses on the forehead, the most common site in men. Reproduced from Price, *Update*, 22 April 1999.

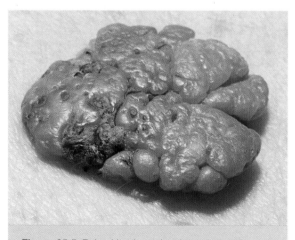

Figure 25.5 Raised benign seborrhoeic keratosis (seborrhoeic wart). These are often covered by a thick layer of warty, grey keratin. Reproduced with permission from Stevens & Lowe, *Pathology*, Mosby, 2000.

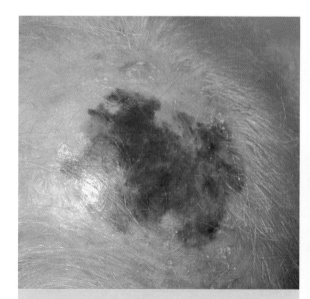

Figure 25.6 Lentigo maligna: a large patch of irregular pigmented skin with surface change into melanoma in situ. Reproduced from Price, *Update*, 22 April 1999.

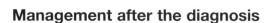

Management after the diagnosis

Solar keratosis

Solar keratoses can be treated by cautery, cryotherapy or a cream containing a chemotherapeutic drug. The physical treatments may leave a scar and the cream irritates. The vulnerable skin should be checked periodically even though the chance of progression to cancer is small. The same treatments also work for Bowen's disease, but excision may also be necessary. Regular checks for recurrence are also needed.

Basal cell carcinoma

BCC can also be excised, curetted or treated with cryotherapy. In addition, radiotherapy may be offered, and this carries the extra side-effects of erythema, crusting and systemic disturbance (e.g. nausea). However, the prognosis, except for neglected lesions, is good.

Squamous cell carcinoma

SCC should always be excised because the chance of metastasis is greater. A good prognosis is less certain for SCC than for BCC.

Malignant melanoma

A diagnosis of malignant melanoma is a distressing one. It is inappropriate to be too optimistic about the prognosis, and this issue will require sensitive handling by the GP, who may have to manage the manifestations of the patient's grief at the prospect of death (denial, anger and depression).

The melanoma will need to be surgically excised, and a skin graft may be needed. Other treatment will depend on the thickness of the melanoma and whether or not it has spread. Any recurrence is usually within the 5 years after diagnosis,[10] but late recurrence is not uncommon. Further excisions are sometimes needed. Metastatic disease may require chemotherapy or radiotherapy.

Training and organizational implications

All the clinical members of the primary care team need to be aware of the basic features of skin cancer and the seriousness of the condition. Skin cancers occur very rarely, and a periodic review in the practice of the clinical features of skin cancer will help. It is an area that lends itself well to the use of photographs. Dermatology textbooks are invariably written by consultants working in hospital clinics, and the photographs they contain may bear no relation to the odd little lesions that GPs are asked to diagnose.

A system should be in place to ensure urgent referral to a dermatologist when skin cancer is suspected. Most hospitals now have 'pigmented lesion' or 'suspected melanoma' clinics to deal rapidly with such cases.

Although the urgency of referral for BCC and SCC may not be quite as great as for melanoma, they are all cancers. being diagnosed with any sort of cancer is distressing for the patient, and cancers that occur in exposed areas are also potentially disfiguring. Patients expect that their GP will be able to provide prompt diagnosis and treatment.

Government guidelines suggest that all patients with suspected cancer should be seen within 2 weeks – in the case of melanoma this is too long to wait, in the case of BCC a longer wait is not inappropriate, but in the eyes of the patient any wait at all is fraught with anxiety.

It is tempting for the primary care trust to improve access by negotiating walk-in dermatology clinics for suspicious lesions, but experience from overseas is not encouraging. While around 5% of suspicious lesions referred by British GPs turn out to be malignant, in the USA and The Netherlands, 0.4% and 0.2%, respectively, of people who self-refer to open-access skin clinics have cancer.[11]

Key points

- All suspected skin cancer should be referred.
- Skin cancer is still rare in UK general practice.
- All members of the primary care team need to be aware of suspicious signs in skin lesions.
- A very short spell of waiting and reviewing can be sensible management in SCC and BCC, but is not appropriate where melanoma is suspected.

References

1. Do sunscreens prevent skin cancer? Drug Therapeut Bull 1998: 36:49–50.

2. Price CJ. Skin cancer: the GP's role. Update 1999; 58:777–782.

3. Ness AR, Frankel SJ, Gunnell DJ, et al. Are we really dying for a tan? BMJ 1999; 319:114–116.

4. Taylor A, Gore M. Melanoma: detection and management. Update 1994; 48:209–219.

5. Healsmith MF, Bourke JF, Osborne JF, et al. An evaluation of the revised seven-point checklist for the early detection of cutaneous malignant melanoma. Br J Dermatol 1994; 130:48–50.

6. Austoker J. Melanoma: prevention and early diagnosis. BMJ 1994; 308:1682–1686.

7. Helman CG. Culture, health and illness, 3rd edn. Oxford: Butterworth Heinemann; 1994.

8. Dunkley MP, Morris AM. Cutaneous malignant melanoma: an audit of the diagnostic process. Ann R Coll Surg Engl 1991; 73:248–252.

9. Khorshid SM, Pinney E, Newton Bishop JA. Melanoma excision by general practitioners in North East Thames region. Br J Dermatol 1998; 138:412–417.

10. Malignant melanoma of the skin. Drug Therapeut Bull 1988; 26:73–75.

11. Mackie RM. Clinical recognition of early invasive malignant melanoma. BMJ 1990; 301:1005–1006.

26. The herpes viruses and morbidity in primary care: chickenpox, shingles and herpes

N Higson

THIS CHAPTER REVIEWS

- The range of herpes virus infections.
- The long-lasting latency and ability of the viruses to cause disease after primary infection.
- The need for early and appropriate treatment.
- Screening of pregnant women for varicella to prevent neonatal infection.
- Which antiviral to prescribe.
- The need for polypharmacy in preventing postherpetic neuralgia.

Box 26.1 The seven herpes viruses known to infect humans

- Herpes simplex type 1 (sensory nerve ganglia): cold sores, conjunctivitis, corneal ulcers, herpetic whitlow, genital herpes, encephalitis
- Herpes simplex type 2 (sensory nerve ganglia): genital herpes, encephalitis, congenital or neonatal herpes
- Varicella zoster virus (sensory nerve ganglia): chickenpox, shingles
- Cytomegalovirus (leucocytes, epithelial cells): congenital infection, mononucleosis, pneumonia, choroidoretinitis
- Epstein-Barr virus (B lymphocytes): infectious mononucleosis (glandular fever), lymphoma and nasopharyngeal carcinoma
- Human herpes virus 6 (T lymphocytes): erythema subitum
- Human herpes virus 7 (T lymphocytes): morbidity not known

The herpes viruses are an intriguing family that comprises more than 100 members, seven of which infect man (Box 26.1). They have an encapsulated DNA structure and after a primary infection they persist in a non-pathological state

---

Box 26.2 Complications of varicella

Common

- skin and soft tissue infections
- pneumonia
- hepatitis (common in immunosuppressed individuals; many normal children develop reversible changes to their liver enzymes during an attack)

Rare

- acute cerebellar ataxia
- encephalitis
- acute transverse myelitis
- hemiparesis
- foetal varicella syndrome following maternal infection in the first 20 weeks of gestation (hypoplasia of the skin; cicatricial lesions of the skin; mental retardation; abnormalities of the CNS, urological and gastroenterological systems)
- death (routine vaccination in the USA has reduced the death rate from 40 per annum in the early 1990s to 3 per annum in 1997)
- severe congenital neonatal infection can arise from maternal chickenpox around the time of delivery

---

until reactivated, a trait known as 'latency'. The three most common herpes infections seen in general practice are herpes simplex 1 and 2 and varicella zoster.

Varicella zoster

Although varicella zoster (chickenpox) can strike at any age, in the past few years there has been a worrying shift towards more adults experiencing primary zoster infections. This may be a result of increased isolation of primary chickenpox in children, preventing it spreading in schools and to other groups. Varicella is usually a mild disease in children and adolescents. However, adults and those with a deficient immune systems may experience severe pneumonitis or secondary skin infections (Box 26.2).

Chickenpox is endemic throughout the West and the highest incidence is in winter and spring in the UK. Family members of a primary case are highly susceptible and mortality increases from 2 per 100,000 in children to 25 per 100,000 in adults. There is a risk of foetal damage throughout pregnancy (overall risk 0.7%) and a 2–5% risk of foetal damage if the infection is contracted between the 13th and 20th weeks of pregnancy.

Varicella is highly infectious, with an infectivity rate of 96% in non-immune family members within 1 month of exposure. It is infectious for 2 days before the typical vesicular rash (Fig. 26.1) appears and for a further 3 days afterwards. Symptoms can last between 10 and 14 days, and the skin may be permanently scarred.

In adults the illness tends to last longer than in children and irritation can be severe. Males show a tendency to more severe chickenpox than females, and asthma is a risk factor for children but not for adults. The virus does not infect other species.

After a primary zoster infection such as chickenpox, the virions remain dormant until the individual's natural immunity wanes or is put under stress, at which point the virions replicate again to initiate an attack of 'shingles' (herpes zoster). An individual with no previous chickenpox history can become infected after significant contact with a patient with zoster. Shingles itself cannot be caught, it is a secondary manifestation of zoster.

Treatment

The virus is rapidly killed by soap and water: a soapy bath is a good means of decreasing morbidity and infectivity.

Adults and older teenagers should routinely be considered for treatment.

Oral aciclovir is effective if started within 24 hours of the rash appearing. For treatment of acute varicella zoster (chickenpox), the *British National Formulary* recommends that adults should take aciclovir 800 mg five times daily for 5 days, while children should take aciclovir at 20 mg/kg (maximum 800 mg) four times daily for 5 days.

A seriously ill child or adult will require hospital admission. Aciclovir in high doses intravenously is indicated for severe infection in the immunocompromised, in neonates and in those with varicella pneumonitis. Immunosuppressed children, neonates or those with significant respiratory disease should be considered for admission to hospital.

Prophylactic administration of varicella zoster immunoglobulin (VZIg) early in the incubation process can

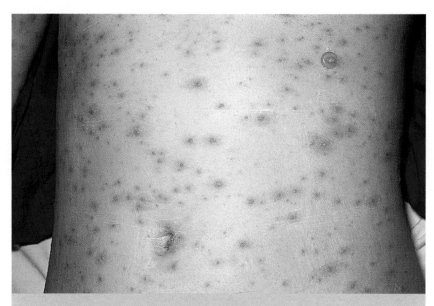

Figure 26.1 Chickenpox. Reproduced with permission from Haslett et al, *Davidson's Principles and Practice of Medicine*, 18th edn, Churchill Livingstone, 1999.

prevent or alter the disease process in those at risk of severe illness with zoster. Local guidelines will determine the use of VZIg.

Pregnant women should have a risk analysis in consultation with the obstetrician because treatment is outside the licence for aciclovir in the UK

Pregnancy and chickenpox

Pregnant women who have no history of chickenpox or who have no immunity to varicella zoster virus (immunoglobulin G negative) should seek medical advice if significantly exposed to chickenpox.

The local pathology laboratory, on advance telephoning by the GP, can usually offer same- or next-day immunoglobulin results, indicating whether the woman is in fact immune. If she is not, and contact seems likely, they will then instruct on local protocol, which is dependent on the stage of pregnancy.

Women at high risk of varicella pneumonitis should be referred to a consultant unit for management. Risk factors for pneumonitis in pregnancy include smoking, pre-existing lung disease, immunocompromise and an extensive or haemorrhagic rash.

Women who develop chickenpox in pregnancy and who present within 24 hours of the rash appearing should be considered for aciclovir therapy (800 mg five times daily for 5 days). If the patient has had appropriate counselling and has given her consent, she may be prescribed aciclovir. Although outside its approved use, aciclovir is thought to be safe and effective in limiting the chance of pneumonitis in pregnant women.

It is particularly important to reduce the chance of neonatal varicella. Maternal varicella during the week before delivery or within the first 2 days after delivery is likely to lead to severe neonatal varicella infection. Maternal varicella occurring between 4 days before and 2 days after delivery carries a 5% infant mortality rate. The infant may be well at birth, but close supervision is advisable for up to the first 16 days of life. There is a case for screening all pregnant women for varicella zoster immunity at the antenatal booking appointment.

Shingles

Shingles is associated with high morbidity, the most problematic symptom being post-herpetic neuralgia.

After a primary chickenpox infection, latent varicella zoster virions may be reactivated within the posterior root (sensory

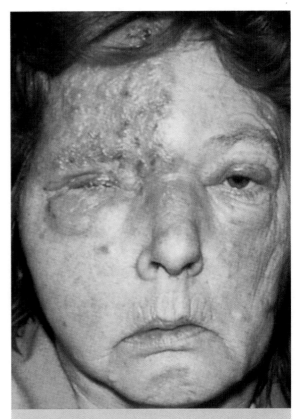

Figure 26.2 Herpes zoster ophthalmicus (shingles). Reproduced with permission from Maclean, *The Eye in Primary Care*, Butterwort-Heinemann, 2002.

nerve) ganglia and cranial nerve ganglia. The virus is reactivated within the ganglia and migrates along the length of the sensory nerve to cause the shingles rash. Some spread may also occur to adjacent ganglia, affecting more than one dermatome.

Changes within the sensory nerve cause pain, burning or paraesthesia before the rash. Unexplained pain or sensory change should raise the suspicion of shingles even before the pathognomic rash is identifiable (Fig. 26.2). This is the prodromal phase, which may cause the patient to feel 'fluey' or below par.

Stress and exposure to the sun have been linked to the onset of shingles. However, most attacks seem to be triggered by increasing age and decline of immune defences to the varicella virus.

Repeat attacks are possible in patients with impaired immunity. A viraemia can also result in widespread vesicles ▷

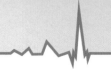

that mimic chickenpox. Recurrent attacks of shingles should prompt investigation for an underlying immune disorder.

Treatment

Management of shingles is not just a matter of treating the cause, but also of managing the complications (Box 26.3). Many patients suffer long-term pain in the affected dermatome, caused by permanent damage to the sensory nerve. Early identification of the condition is paramount for effective treatment. In particular, patients who have ophthalmic shingles should be referred to a specialist for an assessment of corneal damage. Protective measures for the cornea should be considered, such as a combination of topical and parenteral antiviral drugs.

Oral aciclovir, famciclovir or valaciclovir should be started as early as possible, preferably within 48 hours of the appearance of the rash. A prescribing policy for shingles is outlined in Box 26.4. This is effective in decreasing the replication rate of the virus and also limits further damage to the efferent nerve. Intravenous aciclovir may be appropriate for immunosuppressed patients or for those seriously compromised by the extent of the herpetic

---

Box 26.3 Complications of shingles

Common
- Pain
- Postherpetic neuralgia (particularly in the elderly)
- Secondary infection
- Scarring
- Persistent visceral dysfunction (particularly in the absence of a rash)
- Loss of sight with corneal scarring (particularly secondary to ophthalmic herpes)

Rare
- Ramsay–Hunt syndrome
- Transverse myelitis
- Meningoencephalitis
- Motor nerve damage including:
  - ocular nerve dysfunction
  - urinary retention
  - erectile dysfunction
  - paralysis of limbs, diaphragm and trunk muscles (less common)

Box 26.4 A prescribing policy for shingles

- Aciclovir 800 mg at 2-hour intervals five times daily; or famciclovir 250 mg three times daily for 1 week

Plus
- Co-dydramol two tablets four times daily

Plus
- Benzydamine cream applied up to six times daily

Plus
- Amitriptyline 10–25 mg at bedtime for 1 week, increasing by 10–25 mg/week to a maximum dose of 75 mg for a minimum of 6 weeks

---

damage. Topical ocular therapy may be combined with oral therapy for ophthalmic shingles to prevent damage to the cornea.

Amitriptyline can decrease the damage to the sensory nerve. This must be started early and maintained for a minimum of 6 weeks. Amitriptyline should be started at a low dose (10–25 mg/day at bedtime) and increased to a maximum of 75 mg/day over the first 4 weeks.

Gabapentin is a suitable alternative, where the treatment is not tolerated.

Analgesia should be offered to the patient to be taken regularly. Topical analgesics may also be effective. Persistent pain associated with zoster may require referral to a pain management unit for specialist advice. Possible treatments include:

- capsaicin cream
- transcutaneous electrical nerve stimulation
- acupuncture and hypnotherapy.

Educating patients

Shingles can be managed effectively if it is accurately diagnosed and effective therapies are prescribed in adequate dosages. Postherpetic neuralgia is less likely if shingles is diagnosed early.

The practice team has a role in educating all patients, particularly the elderly, about the importance of presenting early. Early initiation of antivirals means less cellular damage and better preservation of organ function.

The practice team must encourage patients to recognize the shingles rash and to report unexplained pain or sensory changes that may pre-date its onset. If a patient telephones the practice, saying that he or she believes that shingles has started, the receptionist should offer an emergency appointment.

Careful explanation of the need to take appropriate antiviral medication will result in better compliance and fewer complications. Patients should be aware of why amitriptyline is being used and that it is being used as a nerve protector rather than an antidepressant.

Genital herpes

Genital herpes is caused by an infection with herpes simplex virus type 1 (HSV-1) or type 2 (HSV-2). HSV-2 is the main cause of genital herpes, while HSV-1 is the main cause of cold sores although it is implicated in at least 10% of genital herpes.

The incidence of genital HSV ranges from 1% to 80% in adult populations.[1,2] Recurrent genital HSV infections can be devastating psychologically for the normal adult; it can be a progressive antiviral-resistant complication for an immunocompromised patient. From 1983 to 1993 the frequency of diagnosis in genitourinary medicine clinics rose in real terms by 28%.[3] An average GP list will have five new cases of genital herpes every 2 years.

The virus infects cells through mucous membranes and the virions are transported to nerve cell bodies where they lie dormant. Reactivation occurs from time to time, often in relation to a specific stressor, such as hormonal changes, emotional stress or even trauma (including sexual intercourse). Once activated, the virions migrate to the skin, initiating a secondary attack of active virus replication. Despite having had a primary attack of herpes, some individuals are asymptomatic and others may have attacks which vary in intensity.

The first episode of genital herpes is usually severe, with a duration of some weeks (as with other herpetic diseases). There is a prodromal phase of up to a week before vesicular lesions appear. The vesicles last up to 8 days (Fig. 26.3), during which time the mucous membrane can break down to form a superficial ulcer which is active for 14 days, healing and forming a crust over a further 7 days. The initial vesicular stage is characterized by severe pain and may be complicated by:

• herpes pharyngitis

• meningitis

• dysuria

• urinary retention.

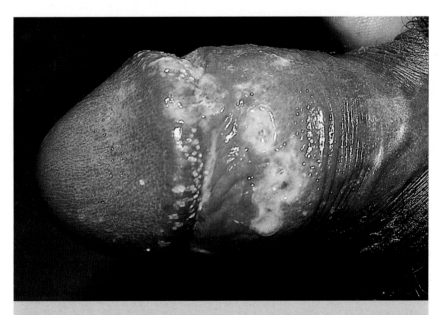

Figure 26.3 Acute ulcers of primary genital herpes. Both herpes simplex virus types 1 and 2 can cause genital herpes. Reproduced with permission from Swash, *Hutchison's Clinical Methods*, 21st edn, Saunders, 2001.

Some 60% of patients will experience at least one further attack of herpetic pain or lesions following the primary episode. If herpes simplex is passed from mother to neonate during natural childbirth it may result in a widely disseminated infection with serious complications and even neonatal death.

Genital herpes should be suspected in any patient with true dysuria or with any form of genital ulcer. Herpes is more likely when there are multiple painful ulcers. Diagnosis is further strengthened by a prodromal illness of discomfort and sensory changes in sacral nerve dermatomes. Swabs of the vesicles will confirm the disease, but treatment should not be delayed.

Treatment

Genital herpes requires oral therapy, as topical antivirals do not provide an adequate tissue concentration of antiviral drugs. Aciclovir and famciclovir are both effective in the treatment of acute genital herpes. Prophylactic treatment or suppression is also possible.

Famciclovir 250 mg three times daily for 5 days is given for the first attack of genital herpes; subsequent attacks are treated with 125 mg three times daily for 5 days. When used for suppression, famciclovir is given for up to 6 months at a dose of 250 mg twice daily. Aciclovir is given in a dose of 200 mg five times daily for 5 days for treatment, or 400 mg twice daily for long-term suppression (for up to 6 months).[4]

Patients must be fully informed about the diagnosis and management of genital herpes. Not only will they be extremely distressed to learn that they have a lifetime propensity to further attacks, but they will also feel anger towards the person from whom they contracted the virus. It is usually appropriate to refer patients for specialist care at the local genitourinary medicine clinic.

Herpes simplex

Herpes simplex (cold sore) is a recurrent infection with HSV-1. Initial infection is usually by oral contact with a relative or partner who has active infection.

The initial infection does not cause the typical cold sore lesion on the buccal or nasal mucosa, but creates an ulcerative disease, often within the buccal cavity (herpetic gingivostomatitis). This is painful but self-limiting and is often not recognized for what it is. Nevertheless it can occasionally necessitate hospital admission due to an inability to eat or drink, particularly in children. Some time

thereafter the secondary outbreaks result in the typical cold sores, which start with a prodromal phase of slight discomfort and become tingly in sensation before erupting as a blister. The blister lasts for up to 10 days, going through the typical herpetic process of blistering and scabbing before resolution.

Cold sores can be treated with topical aciclovir (five times daily for 5 days) or penciclovir (2-hourly for 4 days). Severe or recurrent cold sores are better treated with oral aciclovir 200 mg every 2 hours for 5 days.

Key points

- Shingles is commonly treated inadequately in primary care.
- Early treatment with viral inhibitors is essential to prevent secondary morbidity.
- Screening for varicella can prevent foetal damage.
- Chickenpox can cause considerable morbidity to foreign students coming from the Far East to study in the UK.
- Genital herpes is increasing in incidence.
- Topical treatment of herpetic infections is unlikely to affect the disease process. Oral antiviral drugs affect replication and tissue damage.
- Aciclovir, famciclovir and valaciclovir are effective provided that treatment is appropriate, early and adequate.

Resources

A printable patient information leaflet on chickenpox can be downloaded from the toolkit on the DoctorUpdate.net website: http:// www.doctorupdate.net/du_toolkit/leaflets/l10.pdf

Collier L, Oxford J. Human virology, 2nd edn. Oxford: Oxford University Press; 2000.

Timbury M. Notes on medical virology. Oxford: Churchill Livingstone; 1997.

American official website offering chickenpox advice: http:// www.cdc.gov/ncidod/srp/varicella.htm

American official website on shingles: http://www.nlm.nih.gov/ medlineplus/shinglesshe

References

1. Johnson RE, Nahmias AJ, Madger LS, et al. A seroepidemiologic survey of the prevalence of herpes

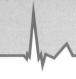
simplex virus type 2 infection in the US. N Engl J Med 1989; 321:7–12.

2. Corey L, Adams HG, Brown ZA, et al. Genital herpes virus infections: clinical manifestations, course and complications. Ann Int Med 1983; 98:958–972.

3. Department of Health Statistics Division. London: HMSO; 1994.

4. British Medical Association, Royal Pharmaceutical Society of Great Britain. British national formulary. London: BMJ Press; 2000.

27. Acute fever in childhood

M Coren

THIS CHAPTER REVIEWS

- The physiology of fever.
- How to assess when fever in childhood is dangerous, and when can it be managed in primary care.
- The measurement of temperature in children.
- The differential diagnosis of childhood fever.
- Convulsions associated with fever.
- Fever with no apparent source.
- Prolonged pyrexia of unknown origin/fever in returning travellers.

Those who care for young children tend to consider fever to be a bad thing in itself, as well as a sign of illness. In reality, the fever response is almost certainly a beneficial part of the host response to infection.

Physiology of fever

Fever is an elevation of the temperature set point. This is why there may be shivering when temperature is rising and sweating as the fever breaks.

There is no single endogenous cause of fever; rather it results from the production of a number of cytokines in response to infection.[1,2] Animal studies have shown an increase in mortality when the fever response is blocked.[2]

Children tend to have higher fevers than adults because of their relative immune immaturity, leading to a larger load of infecting organisms. However, very young infants, especially premature babies, may have a minimal or absent fever response to infection and the reason for this is unclear. In fact, in the youngest babies hypothermia may be a sign of sepsis as normal temperature regulation fails with the stress of infection.

Measurement of temperature

Normal body temperature is 36.4–36.9°C. There is a variation of about 0.3°C during the day, with the highest temperature being in the evening. Body temperature has traditionally been measured orally or rectally, but in recent years alternative methods have become popular. Unfortunately, while these are easy to perform, they lack accuracy. These include axillary temperature measurement by means of small chemical thermometers with dots that change colour (e.g. Tempa-DOT), liquid crystal forehead thermometers (e.g. FeverScan) and electronic thermometers for measuring the temperature at the tympanic membrane. FeverScan tends to read high, but Tempa-DOT performs better.[3] Tympanic membrane devices perform adequately if properly used;[4] they have a slightly lower normal range than conventional mercury thermometers.

Differential diagnosis of acute fever in a child

The spectrum of disease associated with fever in childhood is very wide. The most important thing to assess at the outset is whether the child is reasonably well or ill, and what associated symptoms are present.

Common causes

The most common causes of acute fever are upper respiratory tract infections, including pharyngitis/tonsillitis and otitis. Urinary tract infection (UTI), pneumonia and meningitis all may lack overt physical signs, especially in very young patients.

The common viral causes must be considered and the diagnosis is often apparent from a skin eruption. Roseola infantum, in which the fever precedes the rash, may present with fever without apparent source. The skin, lymph nodes, bones and joints must be carefully examined if the focus of infection is still not apparent.

▸

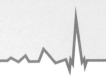

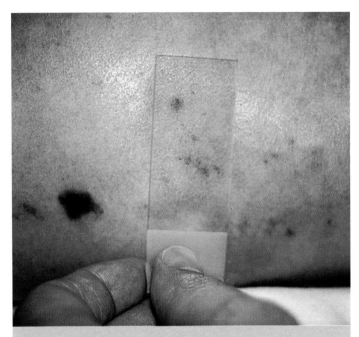

Figure 27.1 The glass test for meningococcal purpura. Parents are advised to suspect meningococcal disease if their child is febrile and has a rash that does not blanche when pressed under a glass. Reproduced with permission from Lissauer & Clayton, *Illustrated Textbook of Paediatrics*, 2nd edn, Mosby, 2001, courtesy of Dr Parviz Habibi.

Meningococcal disease is at the forefront of every GP's mind. The rash is not invariably present and not invariably purpuric, but a non blanching rash (Fig. 27.1) in an unwell and pyrexial child should be considered reason for urgent admission and intravenous or intramuscular penicillin given.

Some key areas in the history will help in rapid assessment (Box 27.1).

Fever without apparent source

In 20% of children with fever there is no apparent source, despite a full history and examination.[5] Most of these patients are under 3 years old and they create anxiety both in primary care and in accident and emergency departments.

Whether a child requires invasive investigation with, or without, empirical antibiotics pending culture results, depends on the balance between risk factors (Box 27.2).[6]

Box 27.1 Rapid history taking: key discriminatory questions

- Duration of fever and associated symptoms
- Previous health, growth and development
- Health of the rest of the family
- Immunization and any travel history
- Contact with other infected individuals

Occult bacteraemia

About 3% of these children have occult bacteraemia. Patients appear non-toxic and have no clinical evidence of sepsis.[7]

The major concern is with fever in infants <3 months old, in whom the incidence of bacteraemia has been found to be up to 10%.[8] In most paediatric units in the UK, infants

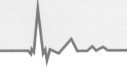

Box 27.2 Investigations in febrile infants

Factors favouring investigation and empirical treatment

- Age <2 months
- High fever
- Known predisposition to infection (e.g. immunodeficiency)

Factors reducing the need for investigation and empirical treatment

- Older child (especially if >2 years)
- Looks well
- Low-grade fever
- Localized minor illness (e.g. upper respiratory tract infection)

<3 months of age with confirmed fever are fully investigated for bacterial sepsis (blood, urine, and cerebrospinal fluid culture; chest x-ray), and are given empirical intravenous antibiotics for 48 hours while awaiting culture results.

A fever of >39°C is another concern; with less severe fevers there is a much lower risk of a serious occult bacterial infection.[5]

Since the widespread uptake of Hib immunisation, *Streptococcus pneumoniae* causes the majority of cases of occult bacteraemia in febrile children. Most occult bacteraemias clear spontaneously, but the adverse consequences of missed occult bacteraemia can be severe. Some 3–6% of cases of *S. pneumoniae* bacteraemia result in meningitis, with approximately 10% mortality and adverse neurological sequelae in 30% of those affected.[7]

Neisseria meningitidis is a rare cause of fever in apparently well children; however, some 25% or more of children who subsequently develop overt meningococcal disease are initially discharged home after evaluation. Once again children <2 years old form much the largest group of those affected.

It is now routine practice in the USA to vaccinate babies with a conjugate vaccine protecting against seven common *S. pneumoniae* serotypes. This significantly reduces the likelihood that a child with acute fever without focus has an occult bacteraemia. This vaccine (Prevenar) now has a European licence and is to be launched in the UK. It remains to be seen whether it will become part of the routine UK schedule of vaccination.

Box 27.3 Kawasaki disease: key facts

- The cause is still unknown, although an infectious process seems overwhelmingly likely
- It is rising in incidence in the UK (partly due to increased awareness and diagnosis)
- Serious complications include coronary artery aneurysms and sudden death
- Prognosis is greatly improved by the use, as early in the disease process as possible, of high-dose intravenous immunoglobulin and high-dose aspirin

Clinical features:

- fever for >5 days

plus 4 out of 5 of

- conjunctival infection
- inflamed lips and tongue
- cervical lymphadenopathy
- polymorphous rash (often vivid)
- oedema of the hands and feet, with later peeling of the skin

---

Box 27.4 Causes of prolonged fever in childhood

Bacterial infection

- Occult infection (abscess, osteomyelitis)
- Enteric fevers (typhoid and paratyphoid)
- Tuberculosis
- Brucellosis
- Leptospirosis

Viral infection

- Epstein–Barr virus
- HIV
- Hepatitis viruses

Parasitic diseases

- Malaria
- Leishmaniasis
- Schistosomiasis
- Toxoplasmosis

Other important possibilities

- Kawasaki disease (see Box 27.4)
- Juvenile idiopathic arthritis (systemic onset type)
- Malignancy, especially lymphoma

Urinary tract infections

Young infants with a UTI usually have no specific symptoms and the diagnosis must be considered in the evaluation of a febrile young child. A UTI is present in 6–8% of febrile girls and in 2–3% of boys <12 months old (although it is rarer in circumcized boys). A very high fever increases the chance of a UTI being present.[5]

The younger the baby the more the possibility of occult UTI must be considered and excluded. Taking a urine sample is difficult but, due to skin contamination, bag urine can only ever exclude a UTI, it cannot be used to make a confident positive diagnosis.

Febrile convulsions

Up to 5% of children experience at least one febrile seizure during childhood. Fever can be a cause of convulsions rather than simply a precipitant in children between the ages of 6 months and 5 years.

Certain infections, classically human herpes virus (HHV6) and *Shigella* spp., are strongly associated with febrile seizures,[9] whereas seizures are extremely uncommon in association with enteric fevers despite the very high temperatures. However, despite these differences, it is the fever itself which is the major triggering factor in most cases.[10]

Prolonged fever

Significant fever in a child, with or without other signs, that persists for more than a week almost always warrants further investigation. Kawasaki disease (see Box 27.3) is rising in incidence in the UK and should not be overlooked as a possible cause of fever. Possible causes of prolonged pyrexia are listed in Box 27.4.

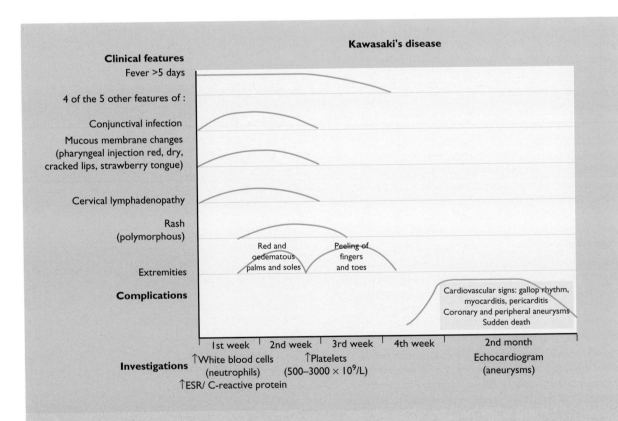

Figure 27.2 Clinical features and investigations in Kawasaki disease. Reproduced with permission from Lissauer & Clayden, *Illustrated Textbook of Paediatrics*, 2nd edn, Mosby, 2001.

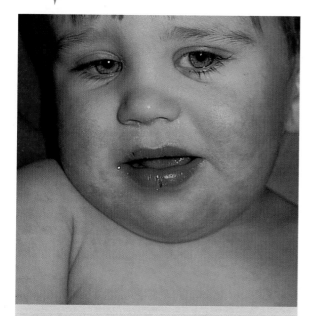

Figure 27.3 Kawasaki disease. Red and cracked lips and conjunctival inflammation. Reproduced with permission from Lissauer & Clayden, *Illustrated Textbook of Paediatrics*, 2nd edn, Mosby, 2001.

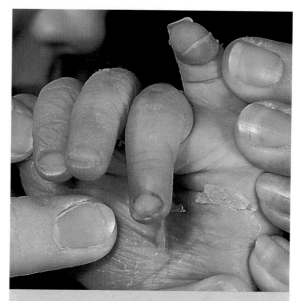

Figure 27.4 Kawasaki disease: Peeling of the fingers, which developed on the 15th day of the illness. Reproduced with permission from Lissauer & Clayden, *Illustrated Textbook of Paediatrics*, 2nd edn, Mosby, 2001.

The history, especially of any travel and any associated symptoms, must be taken very carefully. Examination must be thorough and it is likely that this will need to be repeated. Investigations will be guided by the history and examination and the likely diagnoses. A period of admission to hospital is usually required.

Kawasaki disease

The pathophysiology of this disease, first described in Japan in 1969, represents a major activation of the immune system such as occurs in toxic shock syndrome, although the activating antigen in Kawasaki disease has not been identified.

Early diagnosis and admission is imperative (Box 27.4 and Figs 27.2 to 27.4). Potentially fatal coronary artery aneurysms are a late complication (10 days or more) and may be avoidable if treatment is started in time.

Conclusion

Most children with fever have a benign, self-limiting illness, but some have more sinister pathology, such as occult bacteraemia or UTI. It is important to identify and treat the cause of fever in children, and to be alert to the possibility of convulsions associated with fever in susceptible patients.

Key points

- Fever is part of the adaptive response to infection but is associated with convulsions in susceptible children.
- Most fevers are caused by mild upper respiratory infections.
- In children with fever with no apparent source, there is a 3% incidence of occult bacteraemia.
- The threshold for investigation of children with fever is lowest in the youngest patients.
- UTI is an important cause of fever.
- Prolonged fever always requires investigation and Kawasaki disease should be considered.

References

1. Kluger MJ. Fever revisited. Pediatrics 1992; 90:846–850.

2. Kluger MJ, Kozal W, Conn C, et al. The adaptive value of fever. Infect Dis Clin North Am 1996; 10:1–21.

3. Morley C, Murray M, Whybrew K. The relative accuracy of mercury, Tempa-DOT and FeverScan thermometers. Early Hum Dev 1998; 53:171–178.

4. Childs C, Harrison R, Hodkinson C. Tympanic membrane temperature as a measure of core temperature. Arch Dis Child 1999; 80:262–266.

5. Baraff LJ. Management of fever without source in infants and children. Ann Emerg Med 2000; 36:602–614.

6. Kupperman N. Occult bacteraemia in young febrile children. Pediatr Clin North Am 1999; 46:1073–1079.

7. Baker MD. Evaluation and management of infants with fever. Pediatr Clin North Am 1999; 46:1061–1072.

8. Lissauer T, Clayden G. Illustrated textbook of paediatrics. London: Mosby; 1997, p 36–37.

9. Rantala R, Uhari M, Hietala J. Factors triggering the first febrile seizure. Acta Paediatr 1995; 84:407–410.

10. Suga S, Suzuki K, Ihira M, et al. Clinical characteristics of febrile convulsions during primary HHV-6 infection. Arch Dis Child 2000; 82:62–66.

28. Childhood respiratory and ENT infection

JE Thistlethwaite and M Tarlow

THIS CHAPTER REVIEWS

- Diagnosing common respiratory infections in children.
- Why parents seek medical advice.
- The presentation and management of croup and bronchiolitis.
- When to admit patients with croup and bronchiolitis.
- Prescribing in otitis media.
- Tonsillitis and gingivostomatitis.
- The differential diagnoses of persistent problems, including inhaled foreign bodies, tuberculosis, asthma and cystic fibrosis.

Box 28.1 Why parents seek advice about children's respiratory infections

- Not sure about the diagnosis
- Concern about serious illness, such as meningitis
- Child or other children previously ill and needing antibiotics
- Previous prescription issued for self-limiting illness
- Unusual or prolonged symptoms
- Disabled child or child with chronic illness
- Going on holiday soon
- Advised to see a doctor by a family member, friend or teacher
- Child causing disruption to family routine (e.g. nocturnal cough)
- Child refusing to eat

Prevalence

Respiratory infections are common in childhood, and range from the simple 'common cold' to the more serious bronchiolitis or pneumonia. A normal child can expect to have about eight colds a year. Although 90% of childhood respiratory infections are caused by viruses, many parents seek medical help for various reasons (Box 28.1).[1]

About one-third of consultations in childhood are related to symptoms caused by respiratory infections, and parents living in areas with more economic deprivation seek medical help for children with colds more often than parents from more affluent backgrounds.[2]

Diagnosis

Diagnosis becomes easier the older the child.

Colds make children miserable, but not acutely ill. The main sign is nasal discharge, which may be clear or purulent, but is bilateral (a unilateral discharge is highly suggestive of a foreign body). The child may complain of a stuffy nose and aching limbs. There may be a cough, although the chest will usually be clear on auscultation. A sore throat may be the result of pharyngitis or tonsillitis.

It is difficult to distinguish between viral and bacterial infections of the throat on examination. Young children may have enlarged tonsils anyway, and exudates are found in both types of infection.

Earache is a common symptom and may be caused by referred pain from the throat. It is prudent to examine the ears of every child who presents with signs of an upper respiratory infection or unexplained fever. A bright red, bulging eardrum is diagnostic of otitis media. If the drum has burst, the canal may be full of an offensive discharge.

Croup

Croup is a frightening viral laryngotracheobronchitis, diagnosed on finding inspiratory stridor in children with an upper respiratory tract infection. The onset is often marked by a barking cough and then inspiratory stridor begins. In ▸

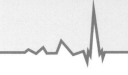

mild croup the stridor is apparent only when the child is upset or hyperventilates. Airway obstruction at rest, accompanied by subcostal and intercostal recession, is a more serious sign, especially when there is also tachycardia and lethargy.

Croup typically presents in the winter and affects children aged 1–2 years. There is often a barking cough. Symptoms are worse at night. Foreign bodies inhaled into the upper airway will also produce stridor, and this should be considered when making the diagnosis.

Any children with more than mild airway obstruction (Box 28.2) should be observed in hospital.

Although most cases of croup settle without any major problems, one or two children each year will be admitted to the intensive care unit. The differential diagnosis is based on the elimination of acute epiglottitis, which is a severe systemic illness associated in almost all cases with septicaemia.

Management at home

Reassurance and support of the patient are all that are necessary. Traditional humidification treatment with steam kettles is of little value, and may lead to accidents. There is no role for antibiotics in croup, which is a viral infection.

Oral and inhaled steroids improve croup and, although their use is generally reserved for the more severe cases, some GPs now give oral prednisolone or dexamethasone.

Box 28.2 Symptoms of airway obstruction in croup

Mild airway obstruction
- Happy child behaving normally
- Not using accessory muscles of respiration

Moderate airway obstruction
- Child becoming tired at times
- Using accessory muscles of respiration
- Child worried by breathing difficulty

Severe airway obstruction
- Child exhausted
- Restless or decreased level of consciousness
- Pallor
- Tachycardia
- Cyanosis

Bronchiolitis

Bronchiolitis is a clinical illness characterized by cough, crepitations and hyperinflation (usually with a wheeze), occurring in infants usually <6 months old. Most cases are caused by the respiratory syncytial virus (RSV), but any of a number of other viruses may also be responsible.

Bronchiolitis occurs in epidemics in the winter. The illness characteristically starts with a cold, followed within 1 or 2 days by wet coughing and wheezing. The chest is hyperinflated and there are widespread crepitations throughout both lung fields. The respiratory rate rises, causing difficulty in feeding. A pyrexia >38°C in bronchiolitis is a predictor for secondary infection and for needing support.

Management at home

Management in the home is essentially expectant. Recovery can be expected over a period of 5–7 days. More prolonged illness should raise the possibility of secondary infection, pneumonia or lobar collapse, and should be an indication for hospital review.

It is felt, on balance, that steroids and beta agonists do not have a role in simple bronchiolitis. Antibiotics do not have a part to play in uncomplicated bronchiolitis.

Babies <6 months old who were premature and were ventilated are particularly likely to need hospital admission.

The indications for hospital admission for bronchiolitis are given in Box 28.3. Most hospital management is supportive. Children with feeding difficulties are generally tube fed for a few days, and occasionally patients may need to be ventilated if the illness is particularly bad.

The antiviral agent ribavirin has a limited but definite effect in bronchiolitis caused by RSV. It is, however, extremely

---

Box 28.3 Indications for hospital admission for bronchiolitis

- Difficulty in feeding
- Apnoeic spells
- Tachypnoea
- Age <3 months
- Co-existing problems:
    - congenital heart disease
    - prematurity
    - chronic lung disease (e.g. cystic fibrosis)
    - Down's syndrome

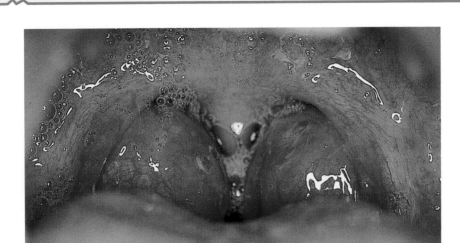

Figure 28. 1 Acute tonsillitis. The tonsils are swollen and acutely inflamed, almost meeting in the midline. Reproduced with permission from Stevens & Lowe, *Pathology*, Mosby, 2000.

expensive, and its use is generally restricted to children with a severe underlying illness such as cyanotic congenital heart disease or cystic fibrosis.

Pneumonia may cause a similar picture to bronchiolitis, although sometimes older children may appear only mildly unwell with a persistent cough. Abdominal pain is occasionally a feature of pneumococcal pneumonia, although pleuritic pain is more common.

Epiglottitis

Children with epiglottitis are very ill, often pale, and may drool because they have difficulty in swallowing. Direct examination of the throat in epiglottitis can precipitate total respiratory obstruction. If there is any possibility of epiglottitis, the child should be referred immediately to hospital where systemic antibiotics can be started, prophylactic intubation or tracheostomy performed, and the throat examined under controlled conditions. Most cases of acute epiglottitis are caused by *Haemophilus influenzae* B. However, since the introduction of the Hib vaccine this is fortunately now very rare.

Otitis media

Almost every child has at least one episode of otitis media before the age of 5 years. Those who have their first attack before 6 months of age constitute a high-risk group, who tend to get recurrent episodes of otitis. The peak incidence is in the toddler age group.

Optimum treatment of acute otitis media is still debated. Some studies have shown that antibiotics provide short-term relief,[3] reducing the pain and fever caused by the infection,[4] but have no long-term benefits. In other studies, no benefits have been shown,[5] although this may partly reflect doctors' diagnostic uncertainty when treating infants.[6] Many of these conflicting reports are from The Netherlands, some from the same workers. Doctors in The Netherlands adopt a 'wait and see' policy for children with otitis media, prescribing antibiotics if symptoms and signs do not resolve within a few days. The incidence of acute mastoiditis is reported to be no higher in The Netherlands than in the UK. Most cases of otitis media cure themselves spontaneously.

Acute tonsillitis/pharyngitis

About one-third of cases of acute tonsillitis are caused by group A haemolytic streptococci and one-third are caused by viruses. In the final third, no aetiological agent can be identified. The appearance of the throat (Fig. 28.1) does not provide any clue as to the aetiology, and exudates on the tonsils can be found in viral as well as bacterial tonsillitis. Enlarged tender cervical nodes are, however, more common in streptococcal infections, and cough or coryzal symptoms favour a viral aetiology. Children <3 years old seldom get streptococcal tonsillitis. In these children an adenoviral aetiology is most likely.

Penicillin V has long been considered the drug of choice in bacterial pharyngitis or tonsillitis, but there is increasing evidence that cephalosporins or the newer macrolides are even more effective.

Hospital referral is only indicated for complications. Acute rheumatic fever is now rare in the UK, but this or acute glomerulonephritis may occasionally follow bacterial pharyngitis with group A streptococci.

Acute gingivostomatitis

Herpes simplex virus causes the common acute gingivostomatitis seen in children (Fig. 28.2). It typically occurs in children between 1 and 3 years of age. There may be a 24–48 hour prodromal illness, with fever, and the total length of the illness before healing begins is usually about 1 week. Ulcers appear on the lips, tongue, gums and hard palate, usually sparing the back of the mouth. Lymphadenopathy is common, and this, together with absence of a vesicular rash on the hands and feet, differentiates herpetic stomatitis from hand, foot and mouth disease.

Aciclovir is not usually necessary, except in patients with eczema (in whom the virus can spread, leading to Kaposi's varicelliform eruption) or with very severe disease or immune defects. To be effective, aciclovir needs to be started very early in the clinical course of the disease. A few children need to be hospitalized, largely because of refusal to feed or drink during the acute phase.

Inhaled foreign body

Consider this in any child with a possible history. Often the history is only of a sudden episode of coughing, which has ceased by the time the child sees the GP. There may be no chest signs initially, and initial x-rays may be negative if the item does not show up. Have a high index of suspicion and refer to accident and emergency for assessment.

If symptoms do not resolve and the child re-presents, reconsider the possibility of an inhaled foreign body. Subsequent x-ray will sometimes show the classical hyperinflation beyond the obstruction.

Examining the child

Some children are difficult to examine and the skilful doctor will have ways to put them at ease. The parent needs to be shown the correct way to hold the child when the ears are

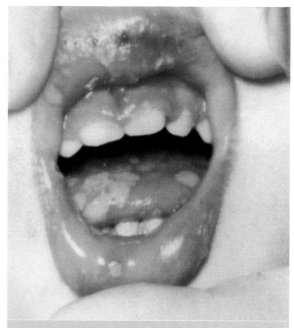

Figure 28.2 Primary herpes simplex type 1 (gingivostomatitis). Reproduced with permission from Kumar & Clark, *Clinical Medicine*, Saunders, 2002.

to be examined. If epiglottitis is suspected the throat should not be examined because of the risk of precipitating complete respiratory obstruction.

When examining the chest, remove enough of the child's clothes to allow a good view of the rib cage; it is then possible to assess the degree of respiratory effort, which is often a more reliable indicator of the child's condition than the sounds heard on auscultation. Wheezing is common in bronchitis and bronchiolitis; there may be no added sounds when the child has pneumonia.

Investigation of respiratory problems

In most cases the diagnosis will be made after taking the history and examining the child. Only when the diagnosis is in doubt, because of unusual features in the history or examination, or when a child suffers from recurrent infections, will investigations be necessary.

If an infection is slow to resolve with standard treatment, take swabs from the appropriate sites (e.g. a sore throat, a discharging ear). If glandular fever is suspected, consider a monospot test. A persistent cough in a child may be caused by catarrh following on from a cold, but a cough that remains productive may indicate lung disease. In such cases a chest radiograph is indicated.

Is there anything in the history that suggests an inhaled foreign body? A wheezy or nocturnal cough suggests asthma, particularly in a child from an atopic family. The cough may be precipitated by exercise. A teenager may have started smoking.

Has the child been immunized against whooping cough? Healthy children cough, on average having 11 bouts/day, but these bouts are neither nocturnal nor prolonged.[7]

Tuberculosis is increasing in incidence. Cystic fibrosis also needs to be excluded in a child with recurrent chest infections associated with poor growth.

Management of viral respiratory infections

Upper respiratory infections are usually self-limiting and, as the causative agent is almost certainly a virus, antibiotics are not required. However, the decision to prescribe antibiotics is not always made on clinical grounds alone, although they are necessary if the clinical picture suggests chest infection.

GPs often face tremendous pressure to prescribe from parents, particularly if the child's nasal discharge is green, thick or has been present for more than a few days. A child who coughs all night disrupts the normal sleeping patterns of the whole household, and there is then the argument that 'a cold always goes on his chest' unless antibiotics are dispensed. There is no evidence that treating an upper respiratory tract infection prevents pneumonia or shortens the infection.[8]

Parents' inappropriate health beliefs are fostered by irrational prescribing. Deciding not to treat means that the GP will need to spend time explaining this decision, and warning parents what signs in the child require a further consultation. These include apathy, persistent poor appetite and a raised respiratory rate at rest.

Advice should also be given about simple remedies, which include making sure the child is well hydrated and comfortable. Infants with nasal obstruction who have difficulty sucking and taking fluids may be helped by cleaning the nostrils gently with a moistened cotton bud before feeds. Parents are often more worried about a child with a raised temperature than one with a raised breathing rate.[9] Paracetamol is advisable, particularly if a child is

prone to febrile convulsions. It is more effective than sponging alone and more acceptable to parents.[10]

Role of the practice team

Parents should be encouraged to give up smoking, or at least not to smoke in the same environment as their children.[11] Practice nurses and health visitors can give advice about smoking at well-baby clinics and on home visits. They should also emphasize the benefits of breast-feeding, as this reduces the frequency and duration of respiratory infections in the first 6 months of life.[11]

Some practices have nurse-run clinics where children can be seen and parents advised about self-limiting infections.

Key points

- Croup typically presents in the winter and affects children in the toddler age group.
- Epiglottitis is rare in the UK due to HiB immunization, but should not be forgotten.
- Bronchiolitis is characterized by cough, crepitations and hyperinflation. Infants <6 months of age are most commonly affected.
- Use of antibiotics in childhood respiratory infection usually produces no benefit, but reinforces parental beliefs about the need for future prescriptions.
- Pus on the tonsils does not prove that tonsillitis needs antibiotics, but enlarged cervical lymph nodes may suggest streptococcal infection.
- The use of antibiotics in acute otitis media is controversial.
- Acute gingivostomatitis is caused by herpes simplex virus and is usually self-limiting.

References

1. Chan CSY. What do patients expect from consultations for upper respiratory tract infections? Fam Pract 1996; 13:229–235.
2. Edwards A, Pill R. Patterns of help seeking behaviour for toddlers from two contrasting socio-economic groups: new evidence on a neglected topic. Fam Pract 1996; 13:377–381.
3. Van Balen FA, De Melker RA, Touw-Otten FW. Double-blinded randomized trial of co-amoxiclav versus placebo for persistent otitis media with effusion. Lancet 1996; 348:713–716.

4. Burke P, Bain J, Robinson D, et al. Acute red ear in children: controlled trial of non-antibiotic treatment in general practice. BMJ 1991; 303:558–562.

5. Appleman CLM, Claessen JQPJ, Touw-Otten FW, et al. Co-amoxiclav in recurrent otitis media: placebo-controlled study. BMJ 1991; 301: 1450–1452.

6. Froom J, Culpepper L, Grob P, et al. Diagnosis and antibiotic treatment of acute otitis media: report from the International Primary Care Network. BMJ 1990; 300:582–586.

7. Munyard P, Bush A. How much coughing is normal? Arch Dis Child 1996; 74:531–534.

8. Gadomski AM. Potential interventions for preventing pneumonia among young children: lack of effect of antibiotic treatment for upper respiratory infections. Pediatr Infect Dis J 1993; 12:115–120.

9. De Melker RA, Van der Velden J, Kuvenhoven MM. House calls for respiratory tract infections: family medicine pure and simple? Fam Pract 1995; 12:284–298.

10. Kinmouth A-L, Fulton Y, Campbell MJ. Management of feverish children at home. BMJ 1992; 305:1134–1136.

11. Colley JRT, Holland WW, Corkhill RT. Influence of passive smoking and parental phlegm on pneumonia and bronchitis in early childhood. Lancet 1974; ii: 1031–1034.

29. Common infectious diseases of childhood

M Tarlow

THIS CHAPTER REVIEWS

- The symptoms and treatment of various childhood infectious diseases.
- Erythema infectiosum.
- Roseola infantum.
- Chickenpox.
- Infant gastroenteritis.

Erythema infectiosum (fifth disease or slapped cheek disease)

Although erythema infectiosum has been known to doctors for generations, its cause (parvovirus B19) has only recently been discovered. It affects older children of school age and occurs in highly infectious outbreaks.

The illness is characterized by a bright red erythema of the cheeks (Fig. 29.1), which later spreads to the limbs and then the trunk as a fine maculopapular rash, which resolves over a few days. The illness lasts about 1 week. Some older patients may develop arthritis.

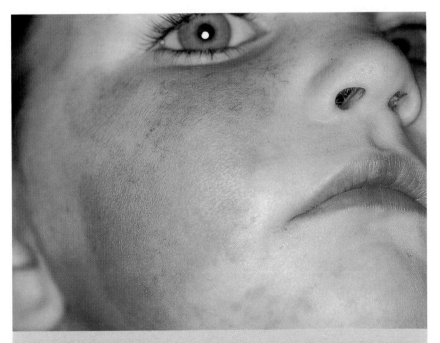

Figure 29.1 Erythema infectiosum is characterized by a bright red erythema of the cheeks. Reproduced with permission from Burkitt & Quick, *Essential Surgery*, 3rd edn, Churchill Livingstone, 2001.

PAEDIATRICS

The virus damages red cell precursors in the bone marrow. This does not matter in normal children, who may have only a mild anaemia, but in patients with shortened red-cell survival (e.g. those with sickle cell anaemia or hereditary spherocytosis) it can cause serious bone marrow infection. Infection in pregnancy can damage the developing foetus.

Roseola infantum

Roseola infantum affects up to 30% of infants or toddlers. Until recently, the aetiology was unknown. Research over the past few years has shown that it is caused by the previously unrecognized human herpes virus 6 (HHV-6).

The illness is characterized by a high fever (often up to 40°C) lasting about 4 days and with no obvious focal infection. The fever resolves and, as it does so, a widespread maculopapular rash appears, which is more marked on the body than on the extremities (Fig. 29.2). The rash is not itchy and usually lasts 2–3 days. The illness is sporadic and does not need specific treatment.

Chickenpox

Chickenpox affects almost everyone during infancy and childhood, but those who escape early infection are likely to be more severely affected when they are

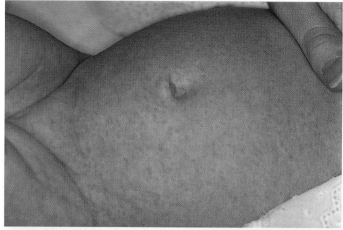

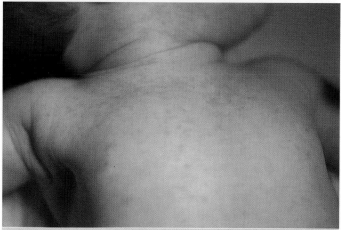

Figure 29.2 Roseola infantum. As the temperature falls, a transient pink eruption, similar to the measles rash, appears, and disappears within 24 hours. Reproduced from Bailie, *Update*, 3 February 2000.

infected by the virus for the first time in adolescence or adult life.

By the time the rash appears (Fig. 29.3), the child's most infectious period has passed, and infection has already spread rapidly by respiratory droplets. Most cases are caught from other children with chickenpox, but contact with shingles can occasionally lead to chickenpox in susceptible children. Immunity is usually lifelong, but second attacks have been reported on very rare occasions.

Children should be isolated for a minimum of 5 days after the onset of the rash, when no further vesicles should be developing and all existing vesicles should be dry and crusted over. It is no longer considered necessary to isolate patients until the dry crusts have fallen off.

Management

Symptomatic treatment alone is sufficient in most cases. The itching can be treated with calamine lotion; crotamiton (Eurax) is also widely used and safe.

Daily baths, using soap and water, are recommended. The virus has a lipid envelope, which is rapidly destroyed by soap and other detergents.

Diphenhydramine (Caladryl lotion) can be absorbed through the skin in chickenpox, leading to toxicity. Other topical preparations containing antihistamines should similarly not be used in chickenpox.

Aciclovir

Aciclovir (Zovirax) has a small but definite effect in shortening the illness and alleviating the symptoms in normal children with chickenpox.[1] There is an argument for treating secondary cases of chickenpox within a family when the disease occurs in an adolescent, as both these factors are associated with more severe disease.

Indications for hospital referral

Indications for referral of a child with chickenpox are listed in Box 29.1.

Between 1% and 4% of cases of chickenpox are complicated by secondary bacterial infection. This is almost always with *Staphylococcus aureus* or group A β-haemolytic streptococci. Cellulitis is frequent, and overwhelming shock can occur associated with specific toxic-shock toxins, which are produced by both organisms.

Bullous varicella is seen when the vesicles of chickenpox progress into large bullae. It is caused by secondary infection with staphylococci, which produce a specific toxin

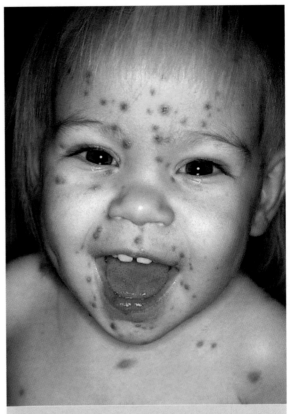

Figure 29.3 Chickenpox rash. Reproduced with permission from the Mike Wyndham Picture Collection.

Box 29.1 Indications for referral to hospital of a child with chickenpox

- Secondary skin or soft tissue infections (if systemic symptoms are present)
- Bullous varicella
- Chickenpox pneumonia
- Acute cerebellar ataxia

and should be treated promptly with antibiotics. It may heal with scarring.

Chickenpox pneumonia accounts for about one in eight hospital admissions with chickenpox and is usually caused by secondary bacterial infection as a result of the initial viral illness.

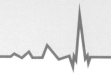

Acute cerebellar ataxia is the most common neurological complication of chickenpox. It occurs about 1 week after the onset of the disease, lasts about 7–10 days, and the prognosis is very good. Some evidence suggests that it may be caused by direct viral invasion of the central nervous system.

Immunosuppressed or immunodeficient patients

Chickenpox can be fatal in immunosuppressed or immunodeficient patients. Extreme care should be taken to prevent contact with known or potential cases. If contact does occur, immediate treatment with γ-globulin is necessary to attempt to abort or ameliorate the infection. If any rash appears, however atypical, the patient should have immediate hospital treatment and high-dose aciclovir.

Infant gastroenteritis

Gastroenteritis is one of the most common infectious illnesses in childhood. It accounts for 10% of all paediatric admissions to hospital. Every GP sees about 18 cases a year, and many others are managed at home without medical consultation.

Most cases in Britain are viral. In infants and pre-school children, rotavirus is far more common than all other viruses put together. Gastroenteritis occurs in epidemics in the winter months, when as many as 70% of all infant admissions to some hospitals may be caused by rotavirus.

In most cases the systemic illness caused by the infection is minimal. The clinical problems, however, result from fluid losses and consequent dehydration, to which the infant is susceptible. A 10% fluid loss in an infant will result in severe dehydration with clinical shock (10% of a 4-kg baby is

400 ml – only two cupfuls of fluid). A baby with severe and frequent diarrhoea and vomiting can lose this amount of fluid very rapidly, and be transformed within hours from a healthy child to one at death's door.

Viral diarrhoea is always watery. Bacterial enteritis in infants is much less common. *Campylobacter* spp. is one of the most frequent organisms, followed by *Salmonella* spp. and *Shigella* spp. Bacteria invading the large gut produce a dysenteric illness, with blood and mucus in the stool. *Campylobacter* spp. and some strains of *Escherichia coli* may produce dysentery, but do not necessarily do so.

Indications for admitting an infant with gastroenteritis to hospital are given in Box 29.2.

Management of uncomplicated gastroenteritis

The cornerstone of management is oral fluid and electrolyte therapy during the acute stage, followed by reintroduction of milk feeding. Most vomiting can be overcome by frequent small feeds.

The fluids used should be either proprietary glucose–electrolyte mixtures (such as Dioralyte or Rehidrat) or sodium chloride and glucose compound mixture, BP. In most situations the diarrhoea will settle in less than a week. Continuing illness, particularly if accompanied by systemic symptoms, or failure to gain weight, should be an indication for hospital referral.

In many infants, some looseness of stools persists for a week or two after an episode of acute gastroenteritis. This is caused by damage to the gut mucosa, which leads to transient lactose intolerance and, consequently, to osmotic diarrhoea on milk challenge. Management is by reassurance alone if the child is otherwise well and gaining weight. If there is marked parental anxiety, a low-lactose diet can be used for up to a week. Continuing diarrhoea should lead to a hospital consultation.

Box 29.2 Indications for hospital admission of an infant with gastroenteritis

- Any degree of dehydration
- Inability to take sufficient oral fluids
- Persistent vomiting
- Parental anxiety
- Doubt about the diagnosis, especially if a surgical emergency such as intussusception is a possibility
- Any neurological disturbance or disturbance of consciousness
- Blood and mucus in the stools

Key points

- **Erythema infectiosum is characterized by a bright red erythema of the cheeks, which later spreads to the limbs and then the trunk; it resolves over a few days.**

- **Roseola infantum is characterized by a high fever lasting about 4 days. As fever resolves, a widespread maculopapular rash appears, usually lasting 2–3 days.**

- **By the time the rash of chickenpox appears, the child's most infectious period has passed.**

- Indications for hospital referral of children with chickenpox include: secondary infection if systemic symptoms are present, bullous varicella, chickenpox pneumonia and acute cerebellar ataxia.

- If an immunodeficient patient is in contact with chickenpox, immediate treatment with γ-globulin is necessary.

- Rotavirus is the most common cause of infant gastroenteritis.

- Indications for hospital admission in infant gastroenteritis are: any degree of dehydration, inability to take sufficient oral fluids, diagnostic doubt, neurological disturbance or disturbance of consciousness, and blood and mucus in the stool.

- In many infants some looseness of stool persists for a week or two after acute gastroenteritis; this is caused by a transient lactose intolerance.

Reference

1. Dunkle LM, Arvin AM, Whitley RJ, et al. A controlled trial of aciclovir for chickenpox in normal children. N Engl J Med 1991; 325:1539–1544.

30. Meningococcal disease

M Selby

THIS CHAPTER REVIEWS

- The pathophysiology of meningococcal disease.
- Who is at risk of meningococcal disease.
- The presentation and treatment of meningococcal disease.
- The rationale behind prophylaxis during an apparent outbreak.

Prevalence

Neisseria meningitidis can affect any age group, but is the leading infectious cause of death in childhood in the UK.[1]

Highest attack rates are in infancy and in children <5 years old, with another peak at 15–19 years of age, where group C mortality is highest. Early recognition and treatment can significantly reduce mortality, and missing meningococcal disease is every GP's dread.

The incidence of meningococcal disease has increased over the last 5 years, with winter peaks. The three common presentations are meningitis alone (50%), septicaemia alone (10%) and combination of the two (40%). Septicaemia alone has the highest fatality rate (20%).

The meningococcus

There are at least 13 meningococcus subgroups. Subgroups B and C are commonest in the UK. Group B accounts for around 60% of cases of invasive disease and group C for almost 40%. Group A is rare in the UK, but is the epidemic strain elsewhere in the world.

There is no reservoir other than humans, and the organism dies quickly outside the host. Transmission is by droplet spread, or by direct contact with carriers or those in the early stages of the infection.

Nasopharyngeal carriage is widespread. About 10% of us carry one of a number of strains, many of which are not virulent. Carriage rates are lowest in young children (2%) and highest in teenagers and military recruits (around 25%). The rate of carriage is increased in smokers. Carriage of *Neisseria lactamica*, which is believed to confer protection, is highest in young children.[2]

The process of infection

Acquisition of the meningococcus is followed by either a variable period of carriage (mean 9 months) or by invasive disease, which usually develops within a week. It is rare for identified carriers to develop invasive disease.

Recognition

GPs will see meningococcal disease rarely, but must retain a high index of suspicion.

The classical presentation is of an unwell patient with a non-blanching rash (Fig. 30.1) and signs of septicaemic shock and/or meningitis (Box 30.1). The characteristic purpuric lesions are irregular in size and outline, have a necrotic centre and may be extensive (purpura fulminans), making the diagnosis obvious. However, isolated petechiae may appear, and it is important to search the whole body in good light for further marks.

A petechial or purpuric rash in a febrile patient is a medical emergency, as there is a significant chance of invasive meningococcal disease. All such patients should be given penicillin and sent urgently to hospital.

However, the rash is not invariably present (Fig. 30.2). While 80% of bacteriologically confirmed cases will develop purpura or petechiae, the rest have either a maculopapular rash (13%) or no rash (7%), and these patients may also develop severe disease.[3]

Uncertainty

The real problem for GPs is that early disease may present when the patient is still relatively well. Early signs may be non-specific. Onset can be mild or sudden; at first the rash ▶

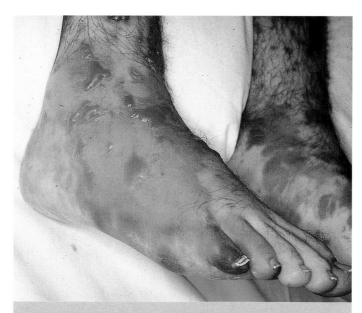

Figure 30.1 Large areas of haemorrhage and skin infarction. Reproduced from Welsby, *Update*, 29 November 2001.

may be maculopapular and blanching, or there may be no rash. As so often in general practice, a degree of uncertainty is therefore unavoidable in the large number of febrile children without purpura that are seen. GPs have to use their clinical judgement to assess their degree of suspicion (Box 30.2), and then choose between referring to hospital, with or without penicillin, arranging later review or offering later review at the parents' instigation.

It is always important to empower parents to seek immediate help should the clinical situation worsen, by giving them information on symptoms and signs to watch for, including the tumbler test (Box 30.3), and promising immediate review if there is further concern.

Box 30.1 Signs of meningococcal disease

- 80% develop purpura or petechiae
- 13% have only blanching maculopapular rash
- 7% have no rash

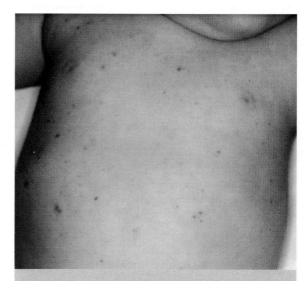

Figure 30.2 This baby was febrile when admitted, and had no signs of meningeal irritation or rash. The rash developed 1 hour later. Reproduced from Welsby, *Update*, 29 November 2001.

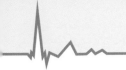

Box 30.2 Clinical features of meningitis and/or septicaemia

Septicaemia

- Pyrexia, rigors
- Vomiting/abdominal pain/diarrhoea
- Difficulty walking/standing
- Myalgia/arthralgia
- Drowsiness/impaired consciousness
- Petechial or purpuric rash or blood blisters
- Tachypnoea/tachycardia
- Cold peripheries and increased capillary refill time (>4 seconds)
- Hypotension (late sign)

Meningitis

- Vomiting
- Headache, photophobia, neck stiffness
- Pyrexia
- Drowsiness/impaired consciousness
- Signs of raised intracranial pressure:
  - hypertension with bradycardia

  - unequal, dilated or poorly responsive pupils
  - papilloedema
  - focal neurological signs, seizures
  - abnormal posturing
  - Brudzinski's sign (neck flexion when supine causes flexion of the knees and hips)
  - Kernig's sign (pain on knee extension when supine with the hips and knees flexed)

Suspicious clinical features in babies

- Mottled skin (poor perfusion)
- Staring
- Poorly responsive or lethargic
- Irritable or floppy when handled
- High-pitched cry
- Poor feeding
- Increased or decreased tone
- Abnormal posturing
- Tense or bulging fontanelle
- Neck stiffness and back arching (late signs)

Box 30.3 The tumbler test for parents

If a tumbler is pressed firmly against a petechial rash it remains visible through the glass and does not fade

Box 30.4 Immediate dose of benzylpenicillin

- Adults and children ≥ 10 years: 1200 mg (2 vials crystapen)
- Children aged 1–9 years: 600 mg (1 vial crystapen)
- Children <1 year: 300 mg (0.5 vial Crystapen)

Give intravenously if possible (the intramuscular route is less effective in shocked patients)

Where there is a history of penicillin anaphylaxis:

- Adults: chloramphenicol 1.2 g
- Children <12 years (avoid in newborns and the premature): 25 mg/kg

Acute anaphylaxis following penicillin injection is rare (0.002% of exposed patients)

Initial treatment

Mortality is significantly reduced by early antibiotic therapy (Box 30.4). Give an immediate intravenous (if possible) or intramuscular penicillin bolus and arrange transfer to hospital by the quickest available means. Penicillin-resistant *N. meningitidis* is rare in the UK, but an alternative is cefotaxime 80 mg/kg intravenously or intramuscularly, which covers other bacterial diagnoses.

In known penicillin anaphylaxis use chloramphenicol. Consider accompanying a very sick patient to hospital.[4]

Accompanying children to hospital

Occasionally, the GP might opt to accompany an extremely sick child to hospital. On the way you should give oxygen (particularly if there are signs of shock) and be prepared to administer cardiopulmonary resuscitation, remembering that in very young children it is important not to hyperextend the neck, which can occlude the airway. If you feel able to obtain intravenous access, and this does not delay transfer, then intravenous fluids may help prevent circulatory collapse (in children give a 20 ml/kg bolus).

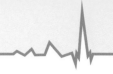

Pathophysiology

Threat to life in invasive meningococcal disease is either from shock or raised intracranial pressure.

Shock results from loss of circulating blood volume due to increased vascular permeability, and impaired myocardial function caused by acidosis, inflammatory mediators and hypoxia.

Hypoperfusion of the CNS causes decreased consciousness.

There may be pronounced peripheral oedema due to capillary leak, and the characteristic purpura result from disseminated intravascular coagulation (DIC).

Hypotension is a late stage in children, who compensate well at first.

Hyperventilation may be due to hypoxia, or be a late stage due to pulmonary hypoperfusion or oedema.

Public health implications

Confirmation and notification

Confirmation of disease usually takes place in hospital, so the hospital will notify the Consultant in Communicable Disease Control (CCDC) who will advise on contact treatment and monitor case clustering.

If parenteral penicillin has been given then blood culture is rarely positive, but throat swabs give a positive yield of 50%. Rash aspirates, antigen detection, paired serology and polymerase chain reaction tests on blood and CSF may also confirm diagnosis, but many cases are unconfirmed.

Positive throat swabs of household contacts are likely to show the same strain as the index case, especially if it is a child, so you may find that the CDC department has swabbed family members to help identify it. It is important, to forestall feelings of guilt, to explain to the family that this is to try to prevent them catching the disease.

Chemoprophylaxis and prevention of spread

Chemoprophylaxis and immunization are offered to all appropriate contacts, and while the CDC department will advise on who to treat, it is helpful for GPs to know how decisions are taken, as surgeries are frequently inundated with calls from anxious parents wanting antibiotics after a case.

There is evidence of increased risk (around 1% chance of invasive disease) for those in the same household. This is

---

Box 30.5 Recommended chemoprophylaxis for meningococcal disease

Rifampicin

- Adults and children >12 years: 600 mg twice daily for 2 days
- Children – approx doses of rifampicin 100 mg/5 ml:
  - 0–2 months, 20 mg (= 1 ml twice daily for 2 days)
  - 3–11 months, 40 mg (= 2 ml twice daily for 2 days)
  - 1–5 years, 1150 mg (= 7.5 ml twice daily for 2 days)
  - 6–12 years, 300 mg capsule twice daily for 2 days

Contraindications: jaundice, hypersensitivity to rifampicin

Interactions: anticoagulants, oral contraceptive (reduced efficacy), staining of contact lenses

Alternatives

- Ciprofloxacin 500 mg orally, single dose (not licensed)
- Intramuscular ceftriaxone 250 mg (adult), 125 mg (children)

Pregnancy options

1. No prophylaxis
2. Rifampicin or ceftriaxone (rifampicin is used in pregnancy in the USA)
3. Throat swab and treat only if positive for the same strain

Contacts should be vaccinated if appropriate when the strain is known

---

highest for the first 7 days, and is probably a combination of increased rate of exposure and genetic susceptibility.

The risk of linked cases outside the household is low.

Chemoprophylaxis (Box 30.5) aims to eliminate carriage from the network of close prolonged contacts and is given to those who have been in the same household for 1 week prior to the illness.

Childminders may be part of the extended household, but nurseries and playgroups are not (Box 30.6). There is no evidence that chemoprophylaxis prevents further cases in nurseries. Children in this age group are also more likely to be carrying the protective N. lactamica, so treatment could be counterproductive. Healthcare workers need prophylaxis if they have given mouth-to-mouth resuscitation.

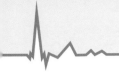

Box 30.6 Information for schools and nurseries

- A case has occurred
- The chance of another is very small
- Antibiotics are not given after one case, as there is no evidence that further cases are prevented and it may do harm by eradicating protective bacteria
- Signs and symptoms of meningococcal disease and the tumbler test
- Information leaflets are available from
  - National Meningitis Trust, Tel. 01453 751738
  - Meningitis Research Foundation, Tel. 01454 281811
  - Department of Health, Tel. 0800 555777

Prophylaxis should ideally be given within 24 hours of the index case presentation. Supplies should be available at the admitting hospital out of hours. Rifampicin is the drug of choice. Penicillin does not consistently eradicate nasal carriage, and the index case should receive eradication treatment when they are able to take oral medication.

Conjunctivitis

Eye swabs may occasionally grow virulent strains of meningococcus. This is potentially invasive and should be notified and contacts treated in the same way as above.

Clustered cases

The CCDC will advise. Who to treat depends on many factors (e.g. whether the strain is the same, whether it is vaccine preventable, what links are established between cases, feasibility, level of public concern).[3]

Vaccination

The meningococcal conjugate group C vaccine gives long-term immunity and is now in widespread use. In 1998–1999 there were 1530 group C cases, with a mortality of 10%.

Meningococcal plain polysaccharide A&C vaccine is still available and has a 90% response, but there is little response to group C under the age of 18 months or to group A under 3 months. Immunity lasts only a few years, and less in young children. It is still the most appropriate vaccine for travellers, where the danger is mainly from group A.[5]

Key points

- *Neisseria meningitidis* is the leading infectious cause of death in childhood in the UK.
- Nasopharyngeal carriage is widespread.
- Carriage of *Neisseria lactamica*, which is believed to confer protection, is highest in young children.
- Acquisition of the meningococcus is followed by either a variable period of carriage (mean 9 months) or by invasive disease, which usually develops within a week.
- In invasive disease 80% develop purpura or petechiae, but 13% have only a blanching maculopapular rash and 7% have no rash.
- The disease is easily missed in the early stages and yet can progress rapidly.
- Educating parents on the tumbler test and other worrying signs will help cover uncertainty in the febrile child.
- Febrile children with purpuric rashes should be admitted, even if well.
- Chemoprophylaxis aims to eradicate carriage.
- Mortality is significantly reduced by early antibiotic therapy.
- Meningitis C immunization has had an impact on the incidence of the disease, but meningitis B remains a threat.

Resources

Meningitis Research Foundation. Website: http://www.meningitis.org/gpsympt.html.

References

1. Platt M. Child health statistical review. Arch Dis Child 1997; 77:542–548.
2. Gold R, Goldschneider I, Lepow ML, et al. Carriage of *N. meningitidis* and *N. lactamica* in infants and children J Infect Dis 1978; 137:112–121.
3. PHLS Meningococcal Working Group and Public Health Medicine Environmental Group. PHLS communicable diseases report, vol 5, No 13, Dec 1995. Available at: http://www.phls.org.uk/publications/cdr/CDRreview/1995/cdrr1395.pdf
4. Meningitis Research Foundation Guidelines. Guidelines 2000; 11: 178–180.
5. Salisbury DM, Begg NT (eds). 1996 i mmunisation against infectious disease. London: HMSO; 1996.

31. Childhood urinary tract infections

JE Thistlethwaite

THIS CHAPTER REVIEWS

- The signs that should make you suspect a UTI in a baby.
- The best method of obtaining a urine specimen from a baby or child.
- The significance of pyuria and bacteriuria.
- The first-line treatment of UTI in children.
- The importance of detecting UTIs.
- Which children to refer.
- The management of children with renal scarring following a UTI.

Box 31.1 Factors predisposing to UTI

- Urethral valves
- Vesicoureteric reflux
- Renal calculi
- Bladder dysfunction
- Incomplete voiding during micturition
- Constipation

Urinary tract infections (UTIs) in early childhood can result in renal scarring and lead to serious illness in later life. It has been estimated that at least 8% of girls and 2% of boys will develop a UTI during childhood.[1] As untreated infections may result in damage to the undeveloped kidneys and subsequent reduced renal function or hypertension, it is important that the condition is recognized and treated as soon as possible.

The diagnosis of a UTI in older children is usually straightforward. They have similar symptoms to those of adults (i.e. pain on passing urine and increased frequency), with possibly incontinence or enuresis returning in a previously dry child. Diagnosing a UTI in a baby is more difficult, and the condition should be suspected in any sick baby with an unexplained fever.

Urinary tract infections in infants

UTIs in children most commonly occur before the age of 1 year. They occur more frequently in boys before 3 months of age and after that the incidence is almost twice as high in girls.[2] The rate in circumcized boys is very low.

Young children are at particular risk of renal damage compared with older children. Such renal damage increases with recurrent infections.

Factors predisposing to UTIs are listed in Box 31.1. Infections are likely to be caused by urinary stasis due to obstruction of the urinary tract, and thus UTIs are often a marker of obstructive anomalies or vesicoureteric reflux (VUR). Urinary tract abnormalities occur most frequently in children under the age of 2 years.

Accurate diagnosis is important in infants and young children, both to permit identification, treatment and evaluation of children who are at risk of kidney damage, and to avoid unnecessary treatment and investigation of children who are not at risk.

Diagnosis

A UTI should be suspected if the child cries while passing urine, if there has been a change in the pattern of urination or if the urine is foul smelling. Vomiting is common in UTI. However, symptoms in infants can be non-specific (e.g. failure to thrive or irritability).

A UTI should be considered in all young children with unexplained fever, although it is important to bear in mind that there is often no fever. A UTI can be a cause of prolonged jaundice in newborn infants.

Box 31.2 Methods of obtaining a urine sample

- Clean-catch urine specimens
- Adhesive bags
- Absorbent pads in nappies
- Tapping over the bladder (infant)
- Container attached to front of potty
- Dip slides (urine voided onto slide)
- Urethral catheters
- Direct aspiration from bladder

Collecting urine samples

Ideally, all children with suspected UTI should provide a urine sample for testing. Older children, with the help of parents, should be able to follow instructions on how to collect an uncontaminated midstream urine (MSU) specimen. Obtaining a sample from babies and younger children is, however, a difficult task.

Before collecting urine the perineal area should be washed with soap and water, then rinsed with clear water and dried. Urine can then be obtained by one of the methods described in Box 31.2; however, all have their drawbacks.

Clean catch specimens take time but this method is preferable to get an uncontaminated sample.

Urine collected in an *adhesive bag* is easily contaminated and, when urine has been passed into one, it should be decanted into a sterile container as soon as possible. Using a syringe to aspirate urine from *absorbent pads in nappies* is relatively simple but, again, the sample is often contaminated, although less frequently than with adhesive bags.[3]

In hospital, more invasive methods are used, such as *suprapubic aspiration*.

When a clean specimen has been obtained, it should be tested at the microbiology laboratory, within a few hours if possible and certainly the same day. Dipstick testing may help in the diagnosis, particularly when looking for nitrites, but microscopy and culture are mandatory for an accurate diagnosis.

If the sample shows no significant growth of bacteria, the child does not have a UTI.

Interpreting the MSU results

Bacteriuria combined with white cells (pyuria) in the urine specimen is highly indicative of a UTI.[4] White cells alone are not diagnostic and may be caused by systemic viral infections, foreign bodies, threadworms or non-infective renal disease.

An infection may be present without any white cells being found in the urine at all, particularly in the early stages. The local laboratory should comment on the significance of the growth of bacteria and give some indication as to whether this growth is considered significant or is likely to be the result of contamination. Commonly, a pure growth of more than 10^5 organisms/ml is taken as proof of a UTI, although lower counts of bacteria may be clinically important, especially in boys.[5]

Management

If the GP is highly suspicious that a child's symptoms are caused by a UTI, treatment should be started as soon as possible. Evidence suggests that delaying treatment may be associated with increased rates of renal scarring.[4] Treatment can be modified as necessary when the result of the urine test is known.

The doctor must also decide if the child is well enough to be managed at home. Very sick children should be admitted to hospital for intravenous treatment. Admission is also necessary if the diagnosis is in doubt. Infants are particularly at risk of toxicity and dehydration, and thus hospital admission is usually recommended.

As the most likely organism precipitating the UTI is *Escherichia coli*,[6] the first-line drug of choice is trimethoprim, which is given twice daily. It is rare for this antibiotic to cause any side-effects, and it can be given to children of all ages. *Proteus* sp. is also common in boys, accounting for about 30% of cases.

Antibiotics should be given for 7–10 days, as this is more effective than short courses.[7] With such a lengthy treatment, there may be problems with compliance, particularly when the child is well.

Referral

It is important to diagnose, treat and investigate UTIs in children because they lead to renal scarring in 5–15% of children infected.[8] It is impossible to predict which children will develop complications later in life.[9] Renal scarring can lead to poor renal growth, recurrent pyelonephritis as an adult, impaired kidney function, early hypertension and renal failure.[10] Children with established renal scarring require prophylactic antibiotics to prevent further infections, as damage increases with each infection.

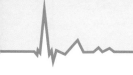

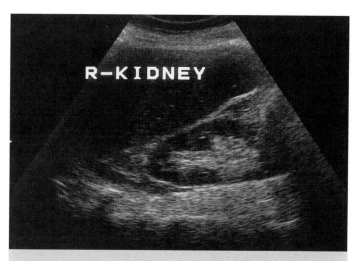

Figure 31.1 Renal ultrasound. Reproduced with permission from Jacob, *Atlas of Human Anatomy*, Churchill Livingstone, 2001.

As children at increased risk of morbidity cannot be identified, it is common practice to investigate all children who have had a proven UTI. However, the evidence that such routine diagnostic imaging improves overall outcome is poor.[4] The highest rates of renal scarring after an episode of pyelonephritis occur in children between the ages of 1 and 5 years,[11] so children in this age group probably do need investigation. After the age of 4 years the risk of developing scarring is very low.[12]

Who should be scanned?

The ultrasound examination is used to pick up structural abnormalities that predispose to infections, and the DMSA is used to look for renal damage. DMSA scans look at renal parenchymal function and are carried out 3–6 months after the last known infection

Ultrasound is non-invasive and picks up some structural lesions, such as hydronephrosis, dilatation of the distal ureters and hypertrophy of the bladder wall (Fig. 31.1), although it does not detect all abnormalities, such as VUR or renal scarring. Isotope scans (DMSA) do detect renal scarring and demonstrate functioning renal tissue (Fig. 31.2).

GPs should check their local guidelines, but the following are typical.

Children <2 years old

Infants under 2 years old with a proven UTI should have an ultrasound and a DMSA scan. Indeed, as UTI in young

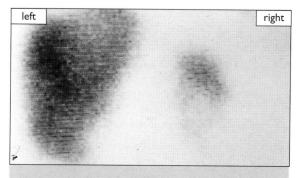

Figure 31.2 DMSA scan showing a small scarred right kidney and scars at the upper and lower poles of the left kidney. Reproduced with permission from Lissauer & Clayden, *Illustrated Textbook of Paediatrics*, 2nd edn, Mosby, 2001.

children serves as a marker for abnormalities of the urinary tract, imaging of the tract has been recommended in every infant with an unexplained fever.[13]

In addition, since ultrasound does not pick up all cases of VUR, boys <1 year of age should have a micturating cystourethrogram (Fig. 31.3) and girls under 1 year of age should have an isotope cystogram.[14] Children between 1 and 2 years of age do not need cystograms unless the scans are not normal.

Infants with a UTI are best referred for further management to a paediatrician, if they have not already been admitted to hospital. If there is open access to scans, an older child only needs to be referred if abnormalities are found. A summary of the commonly recommended investigations is given in Table 31.1.

Children >2 years old

Some authorities suggest that all children aged between 2 and 7 years who have had one proven UTI should be investigated by both ultrasound and DMSA scan,[15] whereas older children have a low risk of new scar formation and so only need ultrasound after recurrent UTIs.[16] However, other research has led to recommendations that DMSA scans are needed if children >2 years of age present with a fever or have had a previous UTI.[13] Guidelines in some areas also suggest that the GP orders an ultrasound scan and an abdominal plain x-ray (to look at the renal outline) in children >3 years but <10 years old.

Prophylaxis

Prophylactic antibiotics are prescribed to minimize the risk of further UTI and renal damage in children with urinary tract abnormalities such as VUR. Antibiotics are prescribed for children whose kidneys are already damaged by scarring. The evidence suggests that this helps to prevent recurrent UTIs during treatment, although the long-term benefits are unclear.[17] The optimum duration of treatment is undefined.[4]

Prophylaxis should be started as soon as acute treatment is finished. The antibiotic can be stopped if the subsequent investigations are normal. If symptoms of a UTI recur while a child is taking antibiotics, the urine should be cultured

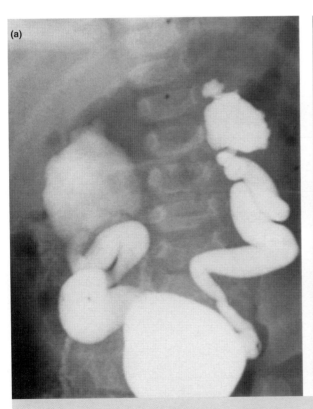
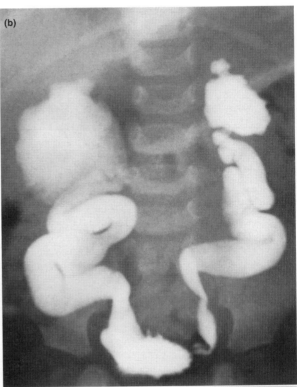

Figure 31.3 Micturating cystograms. (a) The bladder has been filled by contrast medium through a urinary catheter. Even before micturition there was gross vesicoureteric reflux into widely distended ureters and pelvicalyceal systems. (b) The bladder is now empty except for a small residual pool, but contrast medium is retained in both collecting systems. Reproduced with permission from Haslett, *Davidson's Principles and Practice of Medicine*, 18th edn, Churchill Livingstone, 1999.

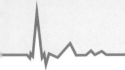

Table 31.1 Recommended investigations for children with UTI

Age of child (years)	Investigation	Rationale
<1	US, DMSA, MCUG	Check for structural scarring, VCR
1–2	US, DMSA	MCUG usually only if abnormality on US or DMSA
2–7	US, DMSA	As above
7	US	Only if infection is recurrent

DMSA, DMSA isotope scan; MCUG, micturating cystourethrogram; US, ultrasound

Table 31.2 Antibiotics used in the treatment and prophylaxis of UTI

Drug	Acute dosage	Prophylaxis dosage	Notes
Trimethoprim	8 mg/kg/day twice daily	1–2 mg/kg at night	Maximum 400 mg, 200 mg single dose
Nitrofurantoin (only for children >3 months old)	3 mg/kg/day four times daily	1 mg/kg at night	Maximum 200 mg, 50–100 mg single dose
Amoxycillin	25 mg/kg/day three times daily	–	Maximum 750 mg, 1.5 g/day
Cephalexin	25 mg/kg/day four times daily	–	Maximum 1.5 g
Nalidixic acid	50 mg/kg/day four times daily	12.5 mg/kg at night	Maximum 2–4 g, 500 mg single dose

and the child treated appropriately. Commonly used antibiotics are listed in Table 31.2.

Other treatments

Surgical treatment of urinary tract abnormalities is considered for children with severe VUR whose condition is unlikely to resolve spontaneously.[18] Bilateral moderate to severe VUR and unilateral severe or non-resolving VUR are common indications. Less severe VUR resolves in the first few years of life.

Follow-up

Children with known renal scarring should have their blood pressure measured every 6–12 months and their urine tested for proteinuria. If complications arise and they are not already being followed up in outpatients, children should be referred to a specialist paediatrician.

Key points

- A UTI should be suspected in any sick baby with an unexplained fever.
- Urine samples are difficult to obtain, but should be collected before treatment starts.
- Laboratory testing is the surest method of diagnosis. Usually a pure growth of >100,000 organisms/ml is proof of a UTI, but lower bacteria counts may be clinically important, especially in boys.
- Trimethoprim should be the first-line treatment.

- UTIs may be a result of urological abnormalities and can lead to renal scarring in children.

- Investigations are carried out to look for abnormalities and to detect renal damage.

- Children with renal damage are predisposed to renal disease and hypertension in later life.

- Children with urological abnormalities and/or renal scarring should receive prophylactic antibiotic treatment.

- Children with renal scarring should be followed up because of the risk of developing renal disease and hypertension. If complications arise they should be referred to a specialist paediatrician.

Resources

American Academy of Pediatrics. The diagnosis, treatment and evaluation of the initial UTI in febrile infants and young children. Pediatrics 1999; 103:843–852.

Larcombe J. Urinary tract infection in children. BMJ 1999; 319:1173–1175.

Useful websites with good patient information leaflets:
US National Institutes of Health: http://www.niddk.nih.gov/health/urology
American Academy of Family Physicians: http://www.familydoctor.org/handouts/272.html

References

1. Stark H. Urinary tract infections in girls: the cost-effectiveness of currently recommended investigative routines. Pediatr Nephrol 1997; 11:174–177.

2. Ginsberg CM, McCracken GH Jr. Urinary tract infections in young infants. Pediatrics 1982; 69:409–412.

3. Feasey S. Are Newcastle urine collection pads suitable as a means of collecting specimens from infants? Paediatr Nursing1999; 11:17–21.

4. Hoberman A, Wald ER. Urinary tract infections in young febrile children. Pediatr Infect Dis J 1997; 16:16–17.

5. Larcombe J. Urinary tract infection in children. BMJ 1999; 319:1173–1175.

6. Honkinen O, Lehtonen O-P, Ruuskanen O, et al. Cohort study of bacterial species causing urinary tract infection and urinary tract abnormalities in children. BMJ 1999; 318:770–771.

7. Moffatt M, Embree J, Grimm P, et al. Short-course antibiotic therapy for urinary tract infections in children: a methodological review of the literature. Am J Dis Child 1988; 142:57–61.

8. Dick PT, Feldman W. Routine diagnostic imaging for childhood urinary tract infections: a systematic overview. J Pediatr 1996; 128:15–22.

9. Greenfield SP, Ng M, Gran J. Experience with vesicoureteric reflux in children: clinical characteristics. J Urol 1997; 158:574–577.

10. Berg UB. Long-term follow-up of renal morphology and function in children with recurrent pyelonephritis. J Urol 1992; 148:1715–1720.

11. Benador D, Benador N, Slozman D, et al. Are younger patients at risk of renal sequelae after pyelonephritis? Lancet 1997; 349:17–19.

12. Vernon SJ, Coulthard MG, Lambert HJ, et al. New renal scarring in children who at age 3 and 4 years had had normal scans with dimercaptosuccinic acid: follow-up study. BMJ 1997; 315:905–908.

13. Rickwood AMK, Carty HM, McKendrick T, et al. Current imaging of childhood urinary tract infections: prospective survey. BMJ 1992; 304:663–665.

14. American Academy of Pediatrics. The diagnosis, treatment and evaluation of the initial urinary tract infection in febrile infants and young children. Pediatrics 1999; 103:843–852.

15. Royal College of Physicians Research Unit Working Group. Guidelines for the management of acute urinary tract infection in childhood. J R Coll Phys London 1991; 25:36–42.

16. Coulthard MG, Lambert HJ, Keir MJ, et al. Occurrence of renal scars in children after their first referral for urinary tract infection. BMJ 1997; 315:918–919.

17. Garin EH, Campos A, Homsy Y. Primary vesico-urethral reflux: a review of current concepts. Pediatr Nephrol 1998; 21:249–256.

18. Smellie JM. Commentary: management of children with severe vesicoureteric reflux. J Urol 1992; 148:1676–1678.

32. Managing the child with enuresis

M Selby

THIS CHAPTER REVIEWS

- The causes of enuresis.
- The treatment of enuresis.

Definition and prevalence

Nocturnal enuresis is usually defined as failure to achieve night-time bladder control, wetting at least 50% of nights, by the age of 5 years. It affects about 15% of 5 year olds, and there is a spontaneous cure rate of around 15% each year among all age groups. Ten per cent of bed-wetters also wet during the day. At age 10 years, about 1 in 15 children wets the bed, as do about 1% of 30 year olds.[1] Enuresis is more common in boys, where there is a family history, and in children with other behavioural problems.[2]

Bed-wetting can cause considerable distress, with feelings of shame, poor self-esteem and a sense of social isolation. Children with the problem tend to avoid staying with friends or going away on school trips. Parents bear the burden of changing sheets several times a night, the cost of washing them, ruined mattresses and smelly bedrooms, although parents who have a history of enuresis themselves are usually sympathetic and tolerant.

Achieving bladder control is a development–maturation linked process. A three-systems model for enuresis has been described, involving:[3]

- bladder instability or small capacity (normal bladder capacity = 30 ml + (age × 30 ml))
- deficient nocturnal release of antidiuretic hormone (ADH)
- inability to wake on full-bladder sensation.

Although one of these problems may predominate, more than one may be involved.

Managing the consultation

There are three important elements in the consultation: the history, the examination and providing reassurance.

History

- Determine whether this is primary or secondary enuresis (in secondary enuresis, exclude urinary tract infection).
- A family history of enuresis is significant, as are recent stresses and family conflict.
- Ask what parents have done so far. Parents who lift their child to the toilet at night but allow them to void when half awake may be reinforcing voiding when asleep.
- Questions about fluid intake may reveal a high level in the evening. In many cases this is because the child's school allows little access to drinks during the day.
- Exclude constipation (which may affect bladder capacity and cause unstable bladder contractions).
- Does the child ever wake to urinate?
- Does the child have several episode of bed-wetting per night?
- Does the child soak the bed or just void small amounts?

Examination

If the history suggests it will be useful, examine:

- the urethra, for inflammation or infection
- the anus, for poor tone
- the abdomen, for constipation and renal abnormalities
- the spine, for spina bifida occulta.

Reassurance and explanation

Reassure the child that he or she is not alone with the problem. Explain that in an average class of thirty 10 year olds there will be two who wet the bed.

Discuss with the parents and/or child any secondary gain (e.g. being taken into the parents' bed) and why this needs to stop.

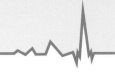

It may be helpful to offer a description of the bladder as a muscular balloon. The three-systems model can be used to explain the problem to the child and the parents. It illustrates how the problem is assessed and treated, helps compliance and, most importantly, takes the blame away from the child.

About a third of children achieve dryness after one consultation, with an explanation of bladder function and enuresis coupled with reassurance, and there is a low relapse rate in this group.[4]

Bladder instability

About a third of children with nocturnal enuresis have uninhibited bladder contractions.[5] This is suggested by:

- frequent daytime voids (more than seven)
- urgency
- low or variable bladder capacity
- multiple wetting at night.

Treatments to consider

A simple explanation that the bladder is like a balloon which needs to be stretched may help the child to understand and tackle the problem.

Twice-daily bladder training can be helpful. This involves the child drinking, hanging on 'to bursting' and then a few minutes more.

Anticholinergics such as oxybutynin are not first-choice treatment, but can be useful in some cases.

Consider referral for daytime wetters, those with poor stream or those with evidence of urinary tract infection.

ADH deficiency

ADH is released throughout sleep in a pulsatile fashion.[6] It reduces nocturnal urine production, so that most non-enuretic children sleep all night but do not have to void until morning. Some children with enuresis lack this circadian rhythm, and have high nocturnal urine production that exceeds bladder capacity.[7]

ADH deficiency is suggested by:

- wetting soon after going to sleep
- large wet patches
- some dry nights because the child wakes and voids
- family history.

Treatment to consider

Desmopressin is a synthetic ADH analogue which decreases urine production. It results in immediate cessation of wetting in 65–75% of patients, and can be useful for school trips and stopovers (Box 32.1).[8] The response is related to the child's ADH level. Both normal and very low ADH levels are associated with a poor response.

Desmopressin is given as 0.2 mg tablets or a nasal spray. Children using the tablets should be given 0.1–0.4 mg at bedtime, or 1 hour beforehand for early wetters. The spray must be kept in the fridge, and the dose is 10–40 µg at night. Fluid intake needs to be restricted after administration.

Treatment usually has to be maintained for several months, and there is a high relapse rate if it is discontinued abruptly.

Not waking to void

Children need to wake to void only if they have bladder instability or ADH deficiency. Most children with nocturnal enuresis are unable to rouse from sleep when their bladder reaches maximum capacity. The problem is not heavy or deep sleep, more a difficulty with waking, and this is something that children can learn to control. It is important to establish with the child that they can easily wake themselves up when it is important, such as early on Christmas morning. Sometimes this is sufficient.

Treatment to consider

Enuresis alarms (see Box 32.1) are usually not suitable for children aged <7 years. When used in older children they are 70% effective.[9] The alarm alerts and sensitizes the child to respond quickly to a full bladder, converting the signal to wake from urination to the inhibition of urination. Enuresis alarms may be loaned by specialist enuresis clinics, usually provided by the community paediatrics service.

An alarm will work only if the child wants to be dry. When it sounds, the child must wake, get out of bed, finish voiding in the toilet, assist in changing the sheets then reset the alarm. This needs the child's cooperation and the support of the family.

Combination approach

Most children with nocturnal enuresis have low ADH secretion and low arousability. Although it is best to start with one treatment, two may be useful, particularly in the

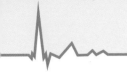

Box 32.1 Treatment options

Desmopressin

Better for:

- older children
- those with fewer wet nights
- those with a family history of bed-wetting

Treatment of choice when:

- there is family stress or intolerance
- the child has low self-esteem
- the child is too young or immature for an alarm
- behavioural problems may sabotage an alarm
- the family needs help for nights away
- there is more than one bed-wetter in the family
- the child has a learning disability

Alarms

Better where:

- there are no perceived behavioural problems
- there is no daytime wetting
- there are no family difficulties or disharmony
- the child does not share a bed

Tricyclic antidepressants

- Success rate of about 50% reported for imipramine and amitriptyline
- Worries about the effect on learning skills, risks of overdose and cardiac arrhythmia
- Not recommended

older child. Behavioural methods such as star charts can be helpful for children >10 years old, but they can be confusing.

Relapse

About 30% of bed-wetting children relapse after using the alarm, and 50% or more relapse as soon as medication is abruptly withdrawn. Part of the problem is that the child attributes success to the treatment method, and therefore expects to relapse when it is withdrawn.

Overlearning, in which the child tries to learn bladder control even after a large evening drink, may help older individuals, although it can lead to despondency if it causes an increase in wetting.

One approach is to try to make the child assume responsibility for the success, supported by gradual withdrawal of medication. For example, the dose of desmopressin spray can be reduced by 10 µg every 4 weeks, unless wetting occurs, in which case the child should go back to the previous successful dose.[10] This approach reduces the relapse rate to about 25%.[3]

Children <5 years old

Nocturnal enuresis is usually considered normal among children <5 years old, but it can be a sign of distress or infection. Neither medication nor training is usually appropriate, but the parent can be offered a contact number for the Enuresis Resource and Information Centre and advice on waterproof sheets, lifting the child, scheduled lifting and social services support.

Child abuse

Some persistent bed-wetters will be victims of child sexual abuse.[11] Abused children may become dry only when they feel safe and protected.

Key points

- A good history and a logical approach often point to the best treatment.
- Some children respond to the first consultation alone. With persistent follow-up, dryness can be achieved and maintained in most children.
- The main treatment options are explanation and reassurance, desmopressin and enuresis alarms.
- About a third of children achieve dryness after one consultation, with an explanation of bladder function and enuresis coupled with reassurance, and there is a low relapse rate in this group.

Resources

Enuresis Resource and Information Centre, Old School House, Britannia Road, Kingswood, Bristol BS15 2DB. Tel. 0117 960 3060 (10 a.m. to 4 p.m.). Website: http://www.eric.org.uk

References

1. Blomfield JM, Douglas JWB. Bedwetting: prevalence among children aged 4–7 years. Lancet 1956: i:850–852. ▸

2. Hobbs CJ, Hanks HGI, Wynne JM. Child abuse and neglect. Edinburgh: Churchill Livingstone; 1999.

3. Butler RJ. Night wetting in children: psychological aspects. J Child Psychol Psychiatry 1998; 39:4453–4463.

4. Dische S. Management of enuresis. BMJ 1971; 2:33–36.

5. Watanabe H, Kawauchi A. Nocturnal enuresis: social aspects and treatment perspectives in Japan. Scand J Urol Nephrol 1994; 163:29–38.

6. Wood CM, Butler RJ, Penney MD, et al. Pulsatile release of AVP and its effect on response to desmopressin in enuresis. Scand J Urol Nephrol 1994; 31:7–10.

7. Norgaard JP, Pedersen EB, Djurhuus JC. Diurnal ADH levels in enuretics. J Urol 1985; 134:1029–1031.

8. Rittig S, Knudsen UB, Norgaard JP, et al. Abnormal diurnal plasma vasopressin and urinary output in patients with enuresis. Am J Physiol 1989; 256: 664–667.

9. Houts AC, Berman JS, Abramson H. Effectiveness of psychological and pharmacological treatments for nocturnal enuresis. J Consult Clin Psych 1994; 62:737–745.

10. Ribaconna M, Oswald J, Glauninger P. Long term vs a tapered dose reduction of intranasal desmopressin in the treatment of enuretic children. Br J Urol 1981; 53(suppl):317–323.

11. Bentovim A, Boston P. In: Child sexual abuse within the family. London: Wright; 1988, ch 2.

33. Developmental disorders in children

M Selby

Child development is the result of the interaction of genetic potential and the environment. The normal range is very wide, both in timing of achievement of milestones and in patterns of development, making early identification of the abnormal difficult. Nevertheless, early detection of problems gives the best chance of management to correct or modify the course of any underlying condition.

The challenge for the GP is to identify those children who require referral for further assessment, and to reassure (but also arrange an appropriately timed review) for those who still fall within the normal range.

Diagnosis

Diagnosis is usually by a specialist, often after multidisciplinary assessment. There are a huge range of conditions, many having no clear diagnostic definition, and no GP could be aware of all of them, nor assess them in a 10-minute appointment.

Children with an uncomplicated neonatal history (i.e. not already under specialist services) with developmental problems often present to their GP or health visitor. GPs therefore need a working grasp of normal development, a feel for abnormal development patterns, an awareness of indications for urgent assessment and a reassuring manner when they are sure that referral is unnecessary.

The wide range of normal

Development can be divided into hearing, vision, language comprehension, language expression, fine motor skills, gross motor skills, social skills and behavioural development. Clearly, problems with some of these may impact on others.

The normal range for each is a widely distributed curve, but children more than two standard deviations from the mean for a particular milestone fall in the bottom 2% and are more likely to include many children with underlying problems. For example, at 12 months of age 50% of children will be walking, with under 1% emulating Peter the Great, Tsar of all the Russias, by walking before 8 months of age, and 90% walking by 15 months. However, some of those who have not walked by 18 months may have an underlying problem, such as muscular dystrophy, and referral is recommended.

Assessment

Antenatal and birth history

When assessing a child with a query over development, antenatal and birth history are essential. A history of problems, or being one of a multiple birth, should lower referral thresholds. Premature birth affects development. Children develop according to their developmental age not their chronological age, although this becomes less significant by the age of 2 years.

Social history

Parental occupation may give a clue to genetic potential, and any concerns about parenting skills and environment also form part of the assessment. Child abuse may cause episodes of regression and recovery resulting in overall delay, together with behavioural and social problems at a very early age. Children who are overprotected may also show delays; for example, children who are never allowed to tumble because they are constantly in baby walkers or strapped in chairs may walk late.

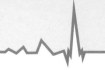

Previous milestones

Parents will remember any previous concerns about their baby's development, even if they are not able to give accurate milestone dates.

Significant medical history

Chronic disease or prolonged or repeated spells in hospital are likely to affect specific or global development.

Familial delay and family history

When assessing a child whose parents are concerned, it is important to ask about other siblings and more distant family members such as cousins. Delayed speech development, clumsiness and delay in walking are often familial, but so are muscular dystrophy, tuberous sclerosis and, occasionally, autism.

Pattern recognition by the GP

The pattern of development is not fixed. Not all children crawl before they walk and patterns of social development vary widely. However, some patterns are clearly abnormal. The child whose social skills have ceased to progress, avoids eye contact and does not attempt verbal or non-verbal communication is clearly not in a normal phase of development; the GP might suspect autism or a neurological disorder.

Regression

Regression of developmental skills is always important and requires urgent referral for investigation. Problems that might cause global regression include abuse of any kind, space-occupying lesions, autism and neurodegenerative conditions. Duchenne's muscular dystrophy may cause regression of motor skills and usually presents at the age of 3–6 years. Regression of motor milestones is also seen in various neuromuscular and muscular disorders, including spinal muscular atrophy and the myopathies.

Speech delay may be caused by chronic glue ear. However, most conditions causing neurological deafness in children are not present at birth, but appear and are progressive in the first 5 years of life. Language regression may be caused by neurological or hearing disorders. Regression of skills is always of concern.

Other abnormal signs: gait disturbance and posturing

Abnormal tone and posturing in early infancy is suggestive of cerebral palsy, although this can present late with motor delay. Asymmetric tone or reflexes or hand preference in children <12 months old may signify hemiparesis. An affected arm often pronates and flexes, and scissoring of the legs may be seen. Infants with gait or posturing abnormality should be referred urgently. Strange posturing is sometimes seen in older children with autistic spectrum disorder, particularly tiptoe walking and hand-flapping.

Box 33.1 Health surveillance checklist for the supine infant

- Social/behavioural skills: responsive smiling (50% achieve this by 6 weeks, refer by 8 weeks as absence may signify a neurological or visual problem)
- Fine motor skills/vision: eyes show conjugate movement when following an object with no squint or nystagmus
- Gross motor skills: normal muscle tone, not floppy, able to raise head to 45° when prone; all four limbs move symmetrically; asymmetry or abnormal posturing needs urgent referral
- Language and hearing: normal crying; response to sounds

Box 33.2 Health surveillance checklist for the sitting child

- Social/behavioural skills: puts solid food in mouth by 6 months; holds and chews a biscuit by 9 months; can tell strangers from familiar people by 9 months
- Gross motor skills: sits unsupported by 6 months; pulls to standing at around 9 months (but the opportunity is necessary)
- Fine motor skills: reaches for small objects and passes them between hands
- Vision: should not squint; fixes immediately on interesting small objects within 15–30 cm by 6 months; reaches for them with one hand by 9 months
- Hearing: turns to a voice by 7 months; the 8–10 months distraction test has a high false-positive rate
- Language: vocal babbling by 10 months; shouts for attention by 9 months

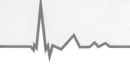

Examination

The examination is general, including inspection for suspicious skin lesions, which may point to conditions such as tuberous sclerosis and neurofibromatosis. Look for dysmorphism. The younger the child the greater the possibility that a syndrome such as trisomy 21 (Down's) has been missed. Examination of gait, reflexes and tone may suggest cerebral palsy or neurological problems.

Child surveillance

Child surveillance examines children at five stages: the newborn, the supine infant (6–8 weeks), the sitting infant (6–9 months), the mobile toddler (18–24 months) and the communicating child (3–4 years). Boxes 33.1 to 33.4 give checklists for the last four stages. About 98% of children should have achieved the milestones by these ages.

Box 33.3 Health surveillance checklist for the mobile toddler

- Social skills: symbolic play is appearing (e.g. with miniature toys); lack of symbolic play is one of the characteristics of autism
- Behavioural: feeds him- or herself with a spoon (if has been allowed to try); asserts his or her wishes; points to named body parts
- Gross motor skills: walks with normal gait by 18 months; if not, refer. Duchenne's muscular dystrophy often presents with delayed walking and there is eventually regression of motor skills. The most common cause of non-regressive motor impairment in children is cerebral palsy, which usually presents before the age of 12 months and is often associated with learning impairment, squint and global developmental delay
- Fine motor skills: scribbles with a pencil by 14 months; builds a tower of three cubes by 18 months and of six cubes by 24 months. Delay in acquiring fine motor skills can be familial, but refer the child to exclude global problems and neurological deficit
- Language/hearing: uses two-word combinations by 20 months; pivotal grammar (one main word, e.g. 'give', with others attached) by 24 months; no parental concern about hearing. Speech delay may be familial or associated with hearing problems. Autistic spectrum children often show normal speech development until 9 months, with little progression after this and often no words at all by 2 years of age
- Vision: manipulates small objects; no parental concerns about vision; no squint

---

Box 33.4 Health surveillance checklist for the communicating child

- Social/behavioural skills: sophisticated skills (can name a friend, wash hands, brush teeth, eat with cutlery); vivid pretend play; likes stories; shows sympathy
- Gross motor skills: hops on one foot and walks on tiptoe; manages stairs (two feet at a time by 3 years, one foot at a time by 4 years); stands on one foot (momentarily at 3 years, for 3 seconds at 4 years); normal gait. If gait or ability is abnormal, consider late-presenting mild cerebral palsy or muscular dystrophy. The latter usually presents at 3–6 years of age; look for Gower's sign and pseudohypertrophy of the calves, and regression of motor skills
- Fine motor skills: can copy a circle by 3 years, a square by 4 years
- Vision: no squint; parents happy
- Language/hearing: gives first and last name; asks 'Why?', 'Where?', 'What?' questions; large intelligible vocabulary; listens to, and likes, long stories

---

The neonate

In developmental terms, look mainly at tone and head control, at symmetry of primitive reflexes and antigravity movement of all four limbs. Also look for response to sound (the infant becomes still to hearing a voice, startles at loud noises) and if the infant is looking at the mother's face.

Significant concerns at this stage should be referred back to the hospital. In particular, if parents feel their child is dysmorphic, urgent assessment is required as bonding can be seriously affected and a syndrome may have been missed.

If you suspect dysmorphism, but the parents have raised no concerns, refer the patient, but be careful how you explain this as the suggestion will be very distressing and you may be wrong.

When to reassure

No GP can remember a mass of milestones, and a full developmental assessment takes far longer than 10 minutes. The Sheridan tables listing developmental milestones for children aged from 1 month to 5 years can be used as a checklist to define the child's developmental age in each area.[1] Obviously, however, this is not an exact science.

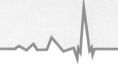

Referral

Indications for referral are:

- serious concerns on the part of the health visitor or parents
- dysmorphism with delay
- severe delay in one developmental area
- milder but global delay
- regression in any area
- abnormal patterns (e.g. motor asymmetry or gait disturbance)
- abnormal behaviour patterns (e.g. posturing or social withdrawal)
- your gut reaction is to refer.

The referral threshold may be lowered by:

- a history of perinatal problems
- being one of a multiple birth
- a positive family history
- social services concerns.

Where adverse circumstances are having a significant impact on development, referral for a full assessment is essential for child protection, both to define baselines and to examine how to change things.

Late-presenting conditions

Some conditions may not present until the child is of school age. Examples of such conditions are dyslexia, dyspraxia, attention deficit and hyperactivity disorder and Asperger's syndrome. Dyslexia is assessed by the local authority educational psychologist. Other conditions need specialist assessment, usually by a consultant in child development.

The future for GPs

Some conditions, particularly attention deficit and hyperactivity disorder and autism, are causing increasing referrals. Improved survival of very premature babies and of children with disorders such as Duchenne's muscular dystrophy, who often now survive to young adulthood, also have funding implications, and the costs of the service can only increase.

After the child has reached school age most costs are borne by the education system, but there are grey areas over who should fund equipment and care. There is surprisingly little support for families of severely disabled children who are not in residential care. Equipment grants are small, and specialized wheelchairs cost thousands of pounds.

Community paediatrics has traditionally been managed by community trusts, but with the advent of primary care trusts some community paediatrics will come under the umbrella of these, and GPs may have be involved in making funding decisions.

Key points

- **Children develop at different rates – there is a wide range of normal.**
- **Mild delays in one area are less likely to be significant than is global delay.**
- **Global delay or severe delay in one area merits referral.**
- **Suspicion of dysmorphia merits referral, usually urgently.**
- **Around half of children with severe problems will never have a specific diagnosis.**
- **The aim of treatment is usually management and modification.**
- **Many rare conditions present in early childhood.**

Resources

Harvey D, Kovar I. Child health – a textbook for the DCH. London: Churchill Livingstone; 1991.

Lissauer Y, Clayden G. Illustrated textbook of paediatrics. London: Mosby; 1997.

References

1. Sheridan M. Charts illustrating the developmental progress of infants and young children. Report on public health and medical subjects, No. 102. London: HMSO; 1960, revised 1975.

34. Child abuse: non-accidental injury

M Selby

THIS CHAPTER REVIEWS

- The need to be alert for signs of child abuse.
- The prevalence and seriousness of abuse.
- When and how the GP should raise suspicions of non-accidental injury.
- The importance of documentation.

Child abuse has existed for as long as there are records of human societies, yet its prevalence is hard to estimate. Perception of what constitutes physical abuse may be subjective – community studies have shown that 9 out of 10 children are physically hit by their parents.[1] Ninety percent of abusers are parents or carers.

Most professionals agree that a child may be at risk if visible physical injury is caused. The risk is not only to the health and happiness of the child. Without intervention, the abused may one day become the abuser, and so the pattern is perpetuated in the next generation.

Presentation

Presentation may be by the child, a parent or by an interested third party such as a schoolteacher. The case may be brought to the GP as a cry for help by the abusing or the non-abusing parent.

Handicapped children are more likely to be abused, and nearly half of all abused children are firstborn. However, the risk is greater in large families and those with adverse social circumstances.

The GP should be on the lookout for worrying signs (Fig. 34.1 and Box 34.1), and be ready to seek further information (Box 34.2).

Examination and documentation

If you are concerned for the child or unhappy about what the parent says, refer the case to a paediatrician specializing in child abuse.

Keep full contemporaneous notes and be ready to describe to the paediatrician what you have seen. If the child is subsequently concealed you may be the only person who has seen the injuries.

Dealing with parental denial

Parents often deny abuse. They may deny there was an injury or conceal the child until injuries heal. They often say: ▸

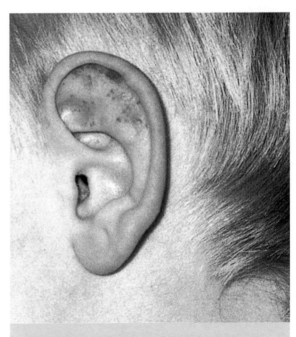

Figure 34.1 Pinching to ear. There are paired marks on the back of the pinna. The child had similar injuries to the other ear and bruising elsewhere on his body.

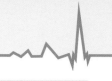

Box 34.1 Possible signs of non-accidental injury

- Repetitive pattern:
  - recurrent visits
  - repeated injuries
- Injuries that are not consistent with the story:
  - too many
  - too severe
  - wrong place or pattern
  - child too young for the activity described
- Any bruising to a young baby
- Multiple injuries

- Fractures in children under 3 years old
- Head injury
- Fractured ribs
- Concurrent failure to thrive
- Suggestion of sexual abuse
- Factors in parental behaviour:
  - delay in seeking advice
  - minimization or denial of symptoms
  - refusal to allow admission or proper treatment
  - aggression

'If I had done that, would I have brought the child to you?'. Denial is a coping mechanism for reducing the distress of the diagnosis. If the presenting parent is not the perpetrator there may be a terrible conflict of loyalty. Admitting that abuse is a possibility means implicating another loved one. Denial is dangerous because it prevents intervention and change.

Explain your concerns to the parent. Be honest. I say: 'I have heard what you have told me about these marks, but to me they look as if they were caused by ...'. I generally explain that I am not making any suggestion about who might have done it, but that I feel we both need further advice from the child protection team as to whether someone might have caused harm, whether intentionally or otherwise. Indeed it is my duty to ask the team's opinion if I'm worried. I say that I know I am sometimes wrong. Attempting to proceed without this degree of openness will lead to a breakdown of trust.

Most parents are cooperative with child protection procedures. Abusers may be relieved – they may love their children and be desperate for help. However, there are exceptions, and some parents will continue to deny abuse passionately even in the face of very damning evidence. If they are not cooperative you should be very concerned.

Involving the child protection team

Any child in immediate danger should be admitted to hospital at once for assessment and observation. No one gets it right all the time. At some point in your career you will either fail to pick up on abuse or refer a child who has not been abused. The latter error is the safe one. By alerting the appropriate agencies you may upset the family,

---

Box 34.2 Questions to ask

- Clarify the story. What are the details of time, place, persons, actions?
- Is the story the same from everyone?
- Are there any trigger factors – difficult child, crying, bed-wetting, behavioural problems, handicap, recent family crisis?
- Were the parents abused themselves, or in care?
- Who can the parents turn to for help?
- Do the parents have unrealistic expectations of the child?
- What is the child's history? Have there been previous concerns about accidents, growth or development?

---

but you are not harming them. You are arranging assessment of a possible need for help.

Remember that an injury seen by the GP may be the only visible crisis in a long history of violence against the child. If no one intervenes it will go on. In most of the headline cases in recent years there has been professional involvement, but the interventions have not been adequate enough to protect the child, usually because only the tip of the iceberg was seen and the degree of risk was underestimated.

Patterns of injury

Bruises

Bruises are present in 90% of physically abused children, but they are also common in non-abused children.[2] As a rule of thumb, up to 12 bruises may be considered to be casually acquired.

In a study of 400 non-abused children, most of those aged >1 year had at least one bruise, mostly on distal limbs, buttocks and bony prominences.[1] Only 0.5% of non-abused children had genital bruises and there was a clear explicable history in every case (Fig. 34.2).

In cases of non-accidental injury, 60% have facial bruising, and the chest and back are common sites for fingertip injuries. Bruises to the pinna also suggest non-accidental injury, as the outer ear is protected during accidental falls by the protective triangle of the shoulder, the base of the neck and the skull.

Bruises are uncommon in children <9 months old and should raise extreme concerns in babies <3 months old.[2]

Unusual bruises

In children with non-accidental injury there may be:

- implement marks
- signs of impact on a hard object
- bite marks, which can be forensically matched to the perpetrator

- signs of kicking
- bizarre marks
- hand marks (fingertip bruises, slap marks with a stripe effect, marks from jewellery)
- pinch marks (paired crescents), poking marks and fist marks (diffuse and severe)
- petechiae on the face, which may be due to strangulation
- scalp haematoma due to severe traction on the hair.

Consider the differential diagnoses – idiopathic thrombocytopenic purpura, clotting disorder, leukaemia and meningococcus – but remember that such conditions do not necessarily exclude non-accidental injury. They may co-exist.

Fracture and bony injury

Bony injuries are simpler for the GP to deal with as they are referred to accident and emergency. Injuries of this sort in normal bones suggest considerable force. Absence of associated bruising does not exclude non-accidental injury.[2,3]

Fractures are often found in cases of fatal abuse. They are sudden and painful, and no child ever continues to play normally afterwards. Parents who say the child did not

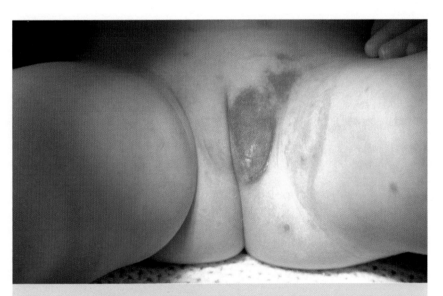

Figure 34.2 Accidental bruising to the labia in a 7-year-old girl with chickenpox. She woke in the night to go to the bathroom and slipped on her bed guard. Her mother found the injuries next morning and presented her at once. The social worker recognized the significance of the bed guard when she went to inspect the child's bedroom after the interview. Reproduced from Selby, Update, 11 October 2001.

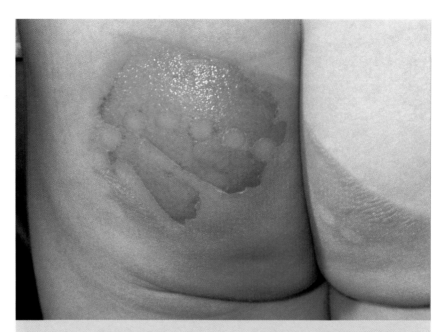

Figure 34.3 Contact burn in a toddler due to a domestic iron. The boy's mother initially said he brushed past the edge of the iron, but clearly this injury is from the flat of the iron and not the edge. Reproduced from Selby, Update, 11 October 2001.

seem distressed are either lying or were not there when the injury occurred. Pain is worst immediately. If presentation is late, loss of function may be the only symptom. In one study, 95% of abusive fractures were in children <3 years and 85% of non-abusive fractures were in children >5 years.[4]

Skin injuries

Most burns and scalds occur in pre-school children. They may be due to brief lapses in protection or neglect, or they may be deliberate (Fig. 34.3). Burns and scalds are always extremely painful and there is an association with sexual abuse.[2]

Children with burns should be referred to accident and emergency unless there is a clear history and the burn is superficial and smaller then a 5 pence piece.

Cigarette burns

Cigarette burns may be found anywhere, but particularly on the hands (Fig. 34.4), forehead and upper trunk. Such a burn needs 1–2 seconds of contact; in an accident with a cigarette a child would pull away in 1–2 ms. Cigarette burns are circular, 5 mm across with a flat base. There may be a 'tail' burn made as the child pulls away or escapes. If

neglected burns may become infected. The burns may then be difficult to distinguish from primary impetigo. Look for other healed lesions.

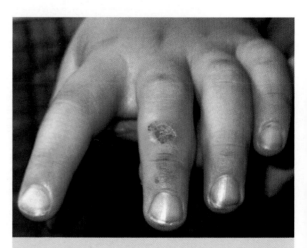

Figure 34.4 Cigarette burns in a toddler. Note the punched appearance and circular shape. Reproduced from Selby, Update, 11 October 2001.

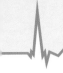

Worrying features again include delay in presentation and denial of the child's pain. Differential diagnoses include bullous skin disorders, insect bites, drug reactions, chicken pox, impetigo and other infection.

Cot death

The reduction in cot death since the campaign on infant sleeping positions has controversially highlighted the fact that there is a link with abuse in a subgroup of these fatalities.[5] A previous cot death in the family of a child with a suspicious injury should therefore lower the GP's threshold for concern.

The GP's options

The main difficulty comes from uncertainty, and uncertainty is unavoidable when a child has a suspicious injury. If uncertain, then you must seek advice. Confidentiality cannot override the welfare of the child in suspected child abuse. If you have concerns they must be raised with the appropriate agencies, whatever the wishes of the parents, and even though you know that you may be wrong. Whatever course of action the GP takes, it is essential to be straight with the parents.

In cases of suspected physical abuse the GP has three choices:

- Admit the child to hospital. This ensures immediate safety, may avoid direct confrontation with the parents and allows investigation of any other injuries and the differential diagnosis.

- Ask the duty social worker to see the child. This professional will interview the family and may ask for a paediatric opinion. Again, the investigation will be largely out of the GP's hands.

- Contact the local paediatrician who specializes in child abuse. These specialists usually advise referral to social services, but may offer to see the child without this if the GP's index of suspicion is very low.

A wait and see approach is not an option. In most cases of fatal child abuse in the UK, a professional has at some point decided to wait or trust the carer.

Each week, one or two children are killed by their carers in the UK, and this may be an underestimate.[6] Many will have come to the attention of child protection services in the past. The risk of death is greatest for babies and declines with increasing age.

What happens next?

Referral to social services is usually followed by an investigation and case conference. The key people are police, social workers and the examining paediatrician, who decide what action best serves the interests of the child. The most common outcome involves agencies working with the child and the family. The GP has a role in supporting the family and maintaining a relationship through this process.

Key points

- **Make sure you are alert to the signs of possible non-accidental injury.**

- **Confidentiality does not override your duty to the child if you suspect child abuse.**

- **In cases of suspected physical abuse the options are to admit to hospital, to ask the duty social worker to see the child or to discuss the case with your local paediatrician.**

- **Referral to social services is usually followed by an investigation and case conference.**

- **Never decide to adopt a wait and see approach to non-accidental injury.**

References

1. Smith SM. A community study of physical violence to children in the home. Presented as a poster at the ISPCAN 5th conference on child abuse and neglect, Norway. 1995.

3. Taitz LS. Child abuse – some myths and shibboleths. Hospital Update 1991; 5:400–405.

4. Worlock P, Stower M, Barber P. Patterns of fracture in accidental and non-accidental injury in children. BMJ 1986; 293:100–102.

2. Hobbs CJ, Hanks GI, Wynne JM. Child abuse and neglect: a clinician's handbook. London: Churchill Livingstone; 1999, chs 1–6, 15, 17, 18.

5. Green MA. Time to put cot death to bed? BMJ 1999; 319:697–700.

6. Home Office. Criminal statistics for England and Wales, 1993. London: TSO; 1994.

35. Sexual and emotional abuse in children

M Selby

THIS CHAPTER REVIEWS

- The estimated prevalence of child sexual abuse.
- The consequences of child sexual abuse.
- Presentation as the tip of the iceberg.
- The role of the GP when faced with a suspicion.
- The role of the GP when faced with a disclosure.
- Emotional abuse and failure to protect.

Children usually survive sexual abuse, emotional abuse, neglect or failure to protect, but they suffer irretrievable harm. Sexual and emotional abuse frequently co-exist, and are often chronic. Moreover, children who are abused may go on to become abusers themselves in later life.

Failure to protect is present in most cases of abuse, as another carer with responsibility may stay silent and fail to take steps to prevent harm.

Child sexual abuse

Child sexual abuse (CSA) is difficult to detect because it is often clinically silent. Even when a child does disclose sexual abuse, the truth may seem too unpleasant to contemplate.

Acknowledging sexual abuse within the family causes terrible disruption and trauma. It may involve implicating a loved one or accepting the unacceptable. Denial is usually much easier, but it is dangerous as it impedes change. In a sense we all fail to protect if we do not keep the possibility of abuse somewhere among our alternative diagnoses in every paediatric consultation.

CSA can be described as the involvement of children and adolescents in the sexual gratification of adults. Informed consent is not involved and the social taboos of families are often violated.

It is a major cause of morbidity and is certainly substantially under-reported.

Patterns of CSA

Sexual abuse ranges from showing pornographic material, inappropriate touching of and by the child, to actual oral, vaginal, anal or urethral penetration. Progression is often stepwise, with penetration achieved very carefully and over a prolonged period to avoid acute signs and acute distress, thereby avoiding detection. There is no act that is never perpetrated on a child, and nothing that children have reported is too bizarre or awful to have happened. The GP must always keep a very open mind.

Effects on the child

CSA is most damaging when it is repeated, when there is actual physical contact and when it involves a family member. It is unpleasant, harmful, frightening and painful. Children, even those old enough to experience sexual pleasure, generally do not like it and wish it to stop.

Emotional trauma increases in proportion to the invasiveness of the act. There are short-term and long-term consequences that do not simply reverse when the abuse stops (Box 35.1). Abused children should always receive long-term specialist counselling.

Who abuses?

CSA most often takes place within the family or household, although organized sex rings and paedophiles are sometimes involved. There have been many cases of families giving birth to children purely to supply victims for abuse and of families selling children for abuse. Police have found websites devoted to the abuse of babies.

The perpetrator is most commonly the father or father figure, but mothers, siblings and babysitters also abuse. The abuser may be another child, usually older, and probably themselves a victim of abuse. Recruitment into sex rings may be via adults or other abused children.

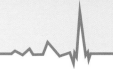

Box 35.1 Consequences of child sexual abuse

Immediate effects
- Pain
- Local trauma, bleeding, scarring
- Fear (of punishment, further abuse, rejection)
- Guilt (reduced self-worth, feelings of dirtiness)
- Pregnancy
- Sexually transmitted infection

Short-term effects
- Behavioural disturbance (soiling, wetting, self-harm)
- Abnormal emotional states (withdrawal, anxiety, depression)
- Educational disturbance
- Distorted social relationships (the child may relate only to adults of one sex and be unable to form bonds with peers)
- Alienation from other children because of sexual behaviour

Long-term effects
- Mental health problems
- Sexual problems and marital difficulties
- Parenting difficulties
- Social dysfunction

Prevalence

In 1995 there were 35,000 children on the UK at-risk register, and 24% of these for CSA. This gives a prevalence of 0.75 per 1000, but is an index of level of suspicion rather than incidence.

A MORI poll of a representative sample of 2019 men and women showed that 10% had been abused before the age of 16 years. Of these, 23% said they had been repeatedly abused, some by multiple perpetrators. Half of cases involved physical contact; 5% involved penetration.

Children of both sexes and any age, including babies, are sexually abused. About two-thirds on the register for CSA were girls.

Covering up and adjustment

Abusers always deny. At first they deny the act itself. After admitting it, they deny the harm and the consequences.

To prevent disclosure, children are threatened with withdrawal of love, loss of family or with being 'taken away'. This is often very successful. If children cannot trust their own guardians, how can they trust anyone else with the truth? In any case, young children may not even be able to understand what the truth is.

Children can appear to be happy, developing an adjustment pattern to cope with and rationalize the abuse. This produces a pattern of secrecy, helplessness, delayed disclosure, non-disclosure or disclosure followed by retraction. Victims may also accommodate abuse by holding themselves responsible for the acts.

Detection

CSA is a silent and, for the most part, carefully hidden practice. What is certain is that many cases of abuse are undetected, and most unrecognized victims see a member of the primary care team at some point, often for an unrelated problem. It is essential to be alert to possible signs, and never to dismiss disclosure.

Warning signs and disclosures do sometimes present in primary care. However, the GP has no chance of picking them up without an awareness of patterns of CSA and an acceptance that abuse is not ruled out simply because the family is 'nice', the child seems happy and healthy or the story is just too grotesque.

Presentation and disclosure

CSA can present with disclosure by the child, suspicion by an adult such as a teacher or social worker, or with symptoms and signs that may or may not relate directly to the abuse (Boxes 35.2 and 35.3). Consider whether there are any risk factors in or around the family (Box 35.4).

Disclosure is more likely in some circumstances:
- an overwhelmingly impossible situation at home
- presence of a sensitive friend or teacher
- loss of contact with the abuser
- exposure to education strategies
- accessible telephone helplines.

A repeatedly abused child may offer disclosure only once. If the story is rejected the child may give up.

What the GP should do

Investigation of possible CSA needs a team approach, involving social services, police and specialist paediatricians. It cannot be attempted by a lone GP.

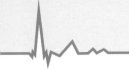

Box 35.2 Suspicious symptoms

Physical symptoms
- Discharge, itch or soreness: external inspection is warranted; bear in mind other common causes of vulvovaginitis
- Constipation or soiling: perform an external anal inspection only for fissures and soreness
- Recurrent dysuria
- Recurrent genitourinary infections
- Rectal or vaginal bleeding: indicates a high probability of CSA; defer genital inspection to a paediatrician
- Foreign object in vagina: indicates a high probability of CSA; young children rarely insert objects unless taught

Psychosomatic symptoms
- Recurrent abdominal pain
- Recurrent headache
- Eating disorders
- Enuresis, encopresis

Behavioural symptoms
- Sexual play or precocity (reflected in drawings, language)
- Substance abuse, truancy, depression, running away, self-harm, suicide (teenagers)
- Children with learning difficulty may show sexualized behaviour or disturbed behaviour, and attempts at disclosure may not be understood

Box 35.3 Possible suspicious signs

- Fingertip bruising on inner thighs or inner knees
- Grip marks on hips or upper arms
- Any injury in the genital area
- Discharge: sexually transmitted diseases are diagnostic of CSA; *Streptococcus* and *Candida* infection are common in non-abused children
- Indications of partial suffocation: petechiae around the orbit, linear marks around the neck
- Anal fissures (may be due to constipation); multiple fissures are worrying
- Warts: before 2 years of age they are probably perinatally acquired, after 3 years of age they can indicate CSA; certain types of wart are more likely to be associated with CSA
- Physical abuse, neglect
- Non-accidental burns
- Bites, especially on the neck and breasts
- Pregnancy

Box 35.4 Risk factors for CSA

- A parent who was abused
- Previous incestuous abuse within the family
- Other forms of abuse (physical, emotional)
- Presence in the home of a male with a record of sexual offences
- High alcohol use
- Loss of maternal libido
- Paedophilic orientation of adult family member (may be evident from use of pornography)

Do not question very young children yourself. You might jeopardize the chance of discovering the truth by putting words into the child's mind or going over things too often. Write down what is said verbatim, including anything the child tells you spontaneously. Other facts and observations to record in suspected cases of CSA are listed in Box 35.5.

Because physical signs are commonly inconclusive, the history from the child, taken by an expert, is extremely important. Do not dismiss anything as impossible. The child's interpretation of events may be confused and inaccurate, but that does not mean that nothing happened. Descriptions of pain or semen are very worrying.

Avoid genital or hymenal examination if you already suspect abuse. Full genital examination will be performed by the specialist paediatrician and it is unfair to do this more often than necessary.

Who to involve

If you are concerned, if the child makes a disclosure or if someone else alleges abuse, you should always involve social services, who will in turn involve police family units. They are the experts at interviewing children without leading them. Confidentiality does not apply. Referral is urgent if the child is still at risk, and if there is a suggestion of abuse within the previous 7 days (because there may be forensic evidence).

If there has been no allegation or disclosure and your suspicion is low, for example if the child has recurrent

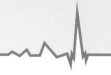

Box 35.5 What to record in notes

- Full history of incidents or explanation of injuries
- Who is present at any examination
- Who gives consent for the child to be examined
- Details of growth and development
- Behaviour
- School history and truancy
- Previous illnesses or accidents
- Previous attendance pattern
- Genitourinary and bowel symptoms
- Previous problems within the family
- If the child is on the at-risk register
- Any risk factors
- Whether a registered sex offender lives in or is closely involved with the household (social services have a statutory obligation to make carers aware)

Box 35.6 Effects of emotional abuse and neglect

Physical effects

- Failure to thrive, short stature
- Recurrent, persistent minor infections
- Frequent attendance at accident and emergency
- Severe nappy rash
- Microcephaly
- Unkempt, dirty appearance

Psychological effects

- Attachment disorders
- Anxiety
- Emotional problems
- Behavioural problems such as aggression, self-mutilation, deliberate soiling, rocking

Developmental effects

- Delay (language, emotional maturity)
- Learning difficulties

vulvitis and no worrying features, you may choose to ask your local paediatrician specializing in CSA for an opinion. Remember there are rarely any conclusive signs, and diagnosis is usually from disclosure on careful interview.

Allegations of CSA are sometimes made as part of a custody and access dispute. This does not mean it is untrue, and a joint investigation involving the police and social services must be made for the child's sake, however unlikely you feel the abuse to be. You are not in a position to rule it out yourself.

Emotional abuse and neglect

All abuse entails some level of emotional abuse, but the latter may exist without other forms. Emotional abuse alone is not commonly the sole reason for children being placed on the at-risk register, yet its effects can be far-reaching.

Emotional abuse can broadly be described as failure to parent, encourage development, nurture and love. It may go as far as scapegoating, verbal and non-verbal rejection, criticism and ridicule. It is often chronic and may be directed at one particular child among siblings. It has severe effects on the child's behavioural and emotional development.

Emotional abuse is deliberate, rather than just poor parenting. It has long-term consequences for social and emotional development. (Box 35.6).

Emotional abuse and neglect are rarely instant diagnoses. Cases may be brought to the GP's attention by the health visitors or social workers. The abuse may affect all or just some children within the family. Children commonly present with poor growth, are socially isolated and immature, and show evidence of poor physical care.

Emotionally abused children usually present with symptoms of failure to thrive (see Box 35.6). There may be behavioural disturbances, with aggression or indiscriminate friendliness in preschool children. Growth delay may be extreme. The children may be dirty and unkempt, immature and friendless. They often do not develop sufficient maturity to make friends, a problem compounded by aggressive conduct and behavioural disturbance. They are not necessarily in immediate physical danger, so the scope for medical involvement is limited, but the GP can share concerns with the child protection team.

When emotionally abused children are taken into care there is often a dramatic improvement in their growth, development and adjustment. However, emotional abuse is notoriously difficult to prove.

Neglect may include emotional abuse but also includes failure to provide adequate physical care. It may be deliberate or occur as a result of a lack of adequate parenting skills.

Key points

- Child sexual abuse is difficult to detect and is substantially under-reported by children.

- Ongoing abuse should not be ruled out because the family are nice, the child seems happy and healthy or the story is too grotesque.

- Child sexual abuse is a major cause of morbidity.

- Child sexual abuse most often occurs in the family or household.

- Physical signs are often inconclusive, so the history from the child, taken by an expert, is very important.

- Investigation of possible child sexual abuse is a team approach involving social services, police and specialist paediatricians.

- If there is a suggestion of recent abuse, children must be seen urgently as there may be forensic evidence.

- If the suspected perpetrator may still have access to the child, referral should be urgent.

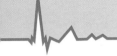

36. Management of depression

E Warren

THIS CHAPTER REVIEWS

- The presentation and prevalence of depression in primary care.
- The management of depression in primary care.
- When to refer patients.
- When to refer patients urgently.

Prevalence

Depression is one of the most common reasons for consultations in general practice, although up to half of cases are missed the first time they present. Around one in five of all adult patients consulting their GP have symptoms of depression, about a quarter of whom will have major depression.[1]

There is a wide range in severity at presentation, from mild intermittent mood disorders to major depression and psychosis. It can be difficult in the 5- or 10-minute consultation or emergency surgery to deal with such problems, and it is important for the GP to be able to detect within the standard consultation time those patients with whom more time needs to be spent then and there, however tightly booked the surgery.

Around 5% of the adult population will have an episode of major depression in any given year,[2] and there is a 17% lifetime risk.[3] Women are affected twice as often as men,[4] with the average age of presentation being 27 years.[3]

Lesser degrees of depression are more commonly seen in general practice. Around a third of people are subject to these milder depressions at some time in their lives, and a further third will have some depressive symptoms.[2]

Diagnosis

Major depression has strict diagnostic criteria, the ones in current use being derived from the Diagnostic and

Box 36.1 DSM-IV diagnostic criteria for major depression[5]

Five or more of the following:

- depressed mood for more than 2 weeks
- loss of interest in all activities (anhedonia)
- poor appetite or weight loss of more than 5%
- insomnia (over 2 hours sleep lost) or hypersomnia
- agitation or psychological retardation
- reduced libido
- fatigue or loss of energy
- diminished ability to think or concentrate, or indecisiveness
- recurrent thoughts of death/suicidal ideation/wishes to be dead or suicide attempt

Statistical Manual of the American Psychiatric Association, 4th edition (DSM-IV). These criteria were originally formulated as a research tool, but the criteria are of practical importance because the more closely an individual patient's symptoms correspond to the major depression criteria, the better is their response to antidepressant treatment of any type. DSM-IV criteria for major depression are given in Box 36.1.

Physical symptoms and 'tired all the time'

In around 25% of patients, depression gives rise to physical symptoms, but in under 10% there are only physical and no psychological symptoms.[4] However, depression makes you worry about things, and patients may well be concerned that physical symptoms represent serious illness. They will not want to feel that these symptoms are dismissed as due to nerves without proper evaluation.

Most patients' complaints of tiredness are of psychological origin.[6] Physical diagnoses, such as diabetes, hypothyroidism, polymyalgia rheumatica, congestive cardiac ▶

failure and anaemia, need to be excluded and a blood test may be neccessary. Of the non-physical reasons for tiredness, anxiety must be kept in mind; depression and anxiety commonly coexist.

However, depression should not be regarded as a diagnosis of exclusion. There are no blood tests to confirm depression, but suggesting that your patient must be depressed because you are unable to think of an alternative diagnosis is not good communication or good general practice. Use the diagnostic criteria for depression to make a positive diagnosis. In your patient's eyes things are then under control, and the management plan makes more sense.

Noticing the diagnosis

When depression is diagnosed and treated early, it is briefer in duration and less severe,[7] probably because antidepressant drugs are prescribed.[8] Some 50% of cases of depression that present to GPs are missed at the first consultation. A further 10% are picked up at subsequent consultations.[7] A number of features[9] are associated with doctors who are more likely to make a diagnosis of depression; they:

- show sympathy
- are sensitive to emotional cues
- use appropriate psychological questions and probes
- ask for clarification of the patient's complaints
- make early eye contact with the patient
- assume receptive postures.

The use of standardized questions is known to make a psychological diagnosis more likely.[4]

The Goldberg scales, developed in Manchester for GP use, correlate well with cases identified by DSM-III(R), the revised 3rd edition (Box 36.2). Using this scoring system in conjunction with an assessment of the presenting problems will give good diagnostic accuracy.

Morbidity and mortality

Depression is not pleasant for the sufferer. In addition, it is associated with increased physical morbidity and mortality. The risk of myocardial infarction is increased five-fold for patients with major depression, and two-fold for patients with lesser depressive symptoms. Hip bone density is decreased by 10% in the depressed, and there is a 40% increased risk of hip fracture over 10 years. Mortality is also markedly increased by having suffered a depressive episode in the past.[11]

Box 36.2 The Goldberg scales[10]

Score 1 for each 'yes' answer:
- Have you had low energy?
- Have you had loss of interests?
- Have you lost confidence in yourself?
- Have you felt hopeless?

If the score is 2 or more, proceed to:
- Have you had difficulty concentrating?
- Have you lost weight (due to poor appetite)?
- Have you been waking early?
- Have you felt slowed up?
- Have you tended to feel worse in the mornings?

A total score of 4 or more indicates a 50% chance of a clinically important depression

---

However, suicide is the most important complication of depressive illness. All depressed patients should be assessed for their suicidal risk. Assessing the risk with confidence can be very difficult. In practice, if you feel any doubts at all over the safety of your patient, then seek advice from a specialist colleague. If asked, most patients will readily tell you if they intend suicide – asking does not give the patient the idea. Nearly all depressed patients will have wondered what would happen if they were no longer alive, and are usually quite relieved to discuss these feelings. Suicidal thoughts are common, but if specific plans are being made (tablets collected, and so on), then the risk is significant and admission to hospital should be considered.

A support strategy

Along with any other suggested treatments, it will also be necessary to agree with your patient a programme of support while they are ill. Good practice would include:[7]

- Give advice on coping with stress (e.g. time out, avoiding confrontation).
- Be willing to listen to the problems, even if you cannot do much about them. Talking can help. Delineate problem areas. Encourage the patient's involvement. Of course a GP with an average list is effectively time limited with each patient – few GPs would feel in a position to offer regular problem-solving counselling sessions to all who might benefit.

- Recommend a self-help group if appropriate.
- Be a patient's advocate. Be prepared to support the patient's interests with other people. This might include writing to employers on the patient's behalf if the patient does not feel able to do this for themselves.
- Involve other health workers where appropriate (e.g. health visitors if a mother is postnatal or has young children). If you have ready access to a community psychiatric nurse (CPN) or counsellor, then use them. An early assessment is particularly useful. When a patient comes to you in a crisis, several weeks may be too long to wait for an assessment. In postnatal depression refer to your health visitor.
- Be prepared to see other members of the family or friends (obviously not forgetting patient confidentiality).

Medication

Current recommendations are that GPs should confine their prescribing for depression to tricyclic antidepressants (TCAs) or selective serotonin reuptake inhibitors (SSRIs).[12]

TCAs and SSRIs are equally effective in major depression.[13] Up to 65% of cases will respond partially or completely.[14] SSRIs have fewer side-effects than TCAs, and more patients taking TCAs will stop treatment because of side-effects. SSRIs are, however, considerably more expensive.[15]

SSRIs are less toxic in overdose than TCAs, but the chance of suicide is not altered by the choice of medication prescribed (including placebo).[16] A suicidal patient has other options for achieving their goal than overdosing on prescribed medication. What is important is the appropriate management of the suicidal risk.

Thirty percent of patients taking drugs for depression will stop treatment whatever they are prescribed, and a further 50% will not take their medication as prescribed.[17] Fewer than half of the population think that antidepressant medication works,[18] and 78% think it is addictive.[19] Convincing your patient that medication is a good idea is more important than the choice of medication.

Medication is commonly prescribed in general practice for degrees of depression that fall short of major depression. Its effectiveness may not be as great as in major depression, but is worth using on a 'try it and see' basis.

A number of other medicines are available that are related to TCAs but which have been modified to reduce side-effects. In addition, there are now other products that affect serotonin metabolism in completely new ways. For

example, mirtazapine (Zispin) increases central noradrenergic and serotonergic neurotransmission, while venlafaxine (Efexor) is a serotonin and noradrenaline reuptake inhibitor.

Specialist referral

Over 90% of depression is treated in general practice. Most practices are unable to offer a full range of psychiatric treatments, and this is a common reason for referral. Despite the beliefs of most patients,[19] formal counselling has little effect on depression.[8] Reasons to seek a specialist opinion are given in Box 36.3.

Follow-up

Antidepressant medication takes around 2–3 weeks to begin to work. It does not cure depression, but simply blocks the symptoms until the depression has run its course. This takes an average of 4 months, and may take up to 2 years.[1] It is therefore recommended that antidepressant medication be continued for 4–6 months after all symptoms have resolved.[12]

Depression has a high rate of relapse. After one episode the chance of recurrence is 50%, after two it is 70% and after three it is 90%.[5] In addition, one in eight depressions runs a chronic course.[7] If there is a recurrence of depression, long-term medication should be considered. ▸

Box 36.3 Reasons for referral[7]

- The diagnosis is in doubt. Is there an underlying organic cause?
- There is significant suicidal risk
- Failure of first-line treatment
- The patient is a child under 16 years of age, who may need more specialized child and adolescent psychiatry interventions, such as family therapy
- Access to additional treatment is needed
- Bipolar disorder
- Co-existing other psychiatric morbidity (e.g. alcohol dependence or eating disorder)
- The patient is unsafe to be left at home because of the severity of symptoms, psychosis or insufficient family support
- Consider referral in pregnant patients
- Consider referral in patients who reveal significant history of, for example, abuse

Most patients can be trusted to follow up their own depression. Once symptoms have resolved and medication has been stopped, patients can be asked to report back if symptoms return. Most patients will only realize in retrospect the effect the depression was having on them, and they will retain that memory for life. All depressions cause different symptoms. Your patient will be the first to know if their depression is returning. Make sure you are the second to know.

Key points

- Depression is one of the most common reasons why patients present to their GP.
- Diagnosis is based on good history taking and careful listening.
- Physical causes of somatic symptoms should be excluded.
- For typical depression the response to antidepressants is usually good.
- Recurrence rates are high.
- Always ask if the patient has contemplated suicide: find some ways of making this inquiry with which you are personally comfortable.
- SSRIs and TCAs are considered the GP drugs of choice.

References

1. Angst J. A regular review of the long term follow up of depression. BMJ 1997; 315:1143–1146.

2. Freemantle N, Long A, Mason J, et al. The treatment of depression in primary care. Effective health care, No. 5. University of Leeds/University of York/RCP; 1993.

3. Kent A. Recognising and treating depression. Monitor Weekly 1995; 8:39–42.

4. Wright AF. Depression recognition and management in general practice. London: Royal College of General Practitioners; 1993.

5. Fish D. New choices in treating depression. Practitioner 1998; 242:24–32.

6. Gambrill EC, Mead M. Tired all the time. Update 1994; 49:233–235.

7. Paykel ES, Priest RG. Recognition and management of depression in general practice: consensus statement. BMJ 1992; 305:1198–202.

8. Moore RG. Improving the treatment of depression in primary care: problems and prospects. Br J Gen Pract 1997; 47:587–590.

9. Boardman J. Detection of psychological problems by general practitioners. Update 1991; 42:1067–1073.

10. Goldberg D, Bridges K, Duncan-Jones P, et al. Detecting anxiety and depression in a general practice setting. BMJ 1988; 297:897–899.

11. Dinan TG. The physical consequences of depressive illness. BMJ 1999; 318:826.

12. British National Formulary, No. 39. London: British Medical Association/Royal Pharmaceutical Society of Great Britain; 2000.

13. Song F, Freemantle N, Sheldon TA, et al. Selective serotonin reuptake inhibitors: meta-analysis of efficacy and acceptability. BMJ 1993; 306:683–687.

14. Cowen PJ. Depression resistant to tricyclic antidepressants. BMJ 1988; 297:435.

15. Edwards JG. Long term pharmacotherapy of depression. BMJ 1998; 316:1180–1181.

16. Edwards JG. Suicide and antidepressants. BMJ 1995; 310:205–206.

17. Hale AS. Depression. BMJ 1997; 315:43–46.

18. Anon. Public more widely accept value of antidepressants. Med Monitor 1998; 11:8.

19. Priest RG, Vize C, Roberts A, et al. Lay people's attitude to treatment of depression: results of opinion poll for Defeat Depression Campaign just before its launch. BMJ 1996; 313:858–859.

37. Suicide and attempted suicide

B Lewis

THIS CHAPTER REVIEWS

- How to assess the risk of suicide.
- The recognizable risk factors.
- How risk factors can be quantified to help decision-making.
- How to manage the acute situation.
- The resources within the primary care team.
- Available external resources.

Prevalence

Suicide and attempted suicide are uncommon, but have wide-ranging effects on all involved. Deliberate self-harm and attempted suicide are more common than suicide, but such patients are at high risk of inflicting further harm on themselves and of eventually committing suicide.[1] Prevention should be a high priority.[2]

The current figures for suicide are:

- in England and Wales 12 per 100,000 people
- in inner city areas (e.g. Manchester) 14 per 100,000 people
- in the UK >5000 deaths per year (i.e. 1% total mortality).

Men commit suicide more often than women, and are more likely to use violent methods.

Assessing risk

The risk of suicide can only be assessed by getting information about the patient's current mental state and social situation, their past behaviour and any history of disturbance, and the social context of their actions (Box 37.1).

The three psychiatric conditions most commonly associated with attempted suicide are:

Box 37.1 Assessing suicide risk

Important information to obtain:
- presence of suicidal ideas and planning
- current, recent and previous mental state of the patient
- social environment and support available
- recent life events associated with an act of self-harm

Diagnostic criteria for depression:
- depressed mood or loss of interest/pleasure

Plus any four of the following for at least 2 weeks:
- feeling of worthlessness
- thoughts of suicide
- loss of energy/fatigue
- retardation or agitation
- altered appetite or weight change
- insomnia or hypersomnia
- impaired concentration

Within these, an increased risk of suicide is associated with:
- profound hopelessness and pessimism about the future
- suicidal ideation

Questions that should be asked when assessing suicidal ideation include:
- Are the ideas transient or frequent and increasing?
- Have plans been made?
- Is the means available?
- What has stopped the patient so far?
- Severity of depression: the duration, the presence of persisting biological symptoms and evidence of self-neglect

- depression
- schizophrenia and allied psychoses
- alcohol or drug misuse.

Asking questions to assess a patient's suicidal thought and intent is difficult. A common but misconceived fear is that asking questions risks 'planting' ideas in the patient's head. However, there is no evidence to support this. Organizations working with those at risk of suicide, especially the Samaritans, have extensive experience which suggests that raising the idea allows patients to vent their emotions safely. Practising the form of words you feel comfortable with is helpful and will clarify your ideas on the best way of approaching the topic.

Recent deliberate self-harm, even if not a serious attempt at suicide, is one of the most significant factors in quantifying risk. The events leading to the action should be discussed with the patient; the degree of premeditation and preparation for the act and the aftermath are important in assessing future risk. Risk is greatest if violent methods or methods very likely to succeed were used (e.g. jumping from a tall building, a large overdose).

Pointers to increased risk include: acts of self-harm in isolation, discussion of suicide prior to the act, leaving notes and messages intended to be found after death, and paying bills and apologising for perceived hurt to others (Box 37.2).

Consultation skills

Dealing with our patients' misfortune and distress is an integral part of our daily work. Attempted suicide and the

---

> **Box 37.3** The suicidal patient: important consultation skills
>
> - Attending: picking up verbal and non-verbal cues, reflecting, summarizing, respecting autonomy
> - Responding to feeling: tolerating emotions and feelings
> - Problem-solving: defining problems, exploring solutions
> - Restoring competence: applying solutions found, positive thinking, motivating change
> - Managing the relationship: treating illness, avoiding dependence

presence of suicidal thoughts may produce a variety of responses within us, ranging from anger and rejection to befriending and parenting. Understanding these emotions is a vital first step in directing efforts in an effective therapeutic way.

Sharing thoughts and feelings with colleagues when a patient commits suicide can help us to formulate our own ideas, understand our emotions, and deal with such cases effectively. The skills we use to manage patients with other mental health problems can be applied to the management of patients at risk of suicide. These skills overlap with the generic skills needed for all consultations (Box 37.3).

Management options

If the GP believes that the patient can be kept safe without admission, then urgent referral to the mental health team may be appropriate.

If the patient is willing to go to hospital, then voluntary admission is an option. Bed shortages may sometimes mean the patient cannot be admitted to the local ward and distant transfers are common, although assessment can usually be local.

Suicidal patients

In instances where the patient is considered actively suicidal but is not willing to be admitted, consider immediate intervention to place the patient in a safe environment. This will necessitate compulsory admission, usually to a psychiatry unit, using the Mental Health Act.

Not all psychiatry wards are secure, and high-risk patients who may abscond may have to be admitted to units far from their home and family. In an emergency situation

---

> **Box 37.2** Risk factors for suicide
>
> - Male and aged 30–45 years or >70 years
> - Current severe mental or physical illness
> - Social class V
> - Current substance or alcohol abuse
> - Occupation (e.g. farmer, vet, pharmacist, doctor or, especially, anaesthetist)
> - Recent loss, either bereavement or of an important relationship or employment
> - Previous attempted suicide or act of self-harm
> - Lack of social support, social isolation
> - Family history of suicide
> - Concurrent serious physical or terminal illness (including renal failure)
> - The co-occurrence of more than one risk factor greatly increases the risk
> - Hopelessness is a strong predictor of suicide potential

where the patient is actively at risk and may abscond from the GP before being assessed, it is appropriate to involve the police, who may section the patient to a place of safety (usually a police cell) while awaiting formal assessment by the duty psychiatry service. The police should also be involved if the GP cannot find the patient but receives notification from concerned relatives or friends of active suicidal intent.

Suicidal patients who are under the influence of drugs or alcohol are not sectionable, and it is necessary to involve the police in these cases. It is important to be aware that in some other unusual instances a suicidal patient may not be sectionable. The case of Diane Pretty highlighted the fact that assisting suicide is a crime, but to wish oneself dead is not always considered proof of mental disorder.

Adolescents

Acute management of adolescents who are actively suicidal can be difficult for the GP. While inpatient units for mentally ill young people do exist, compulsory admission can be very difficult. In the UK most child psychiatry departments do not provide an out-of-hours service, and the on-call adult psychiatrists will not see or admit children. Indeed, most general psychiatry wards do not accept adolescents. If the parents or carers do not feel able to keep the child safe and the paediatric ward are unable to accept the child or keep them contained, involvement of the police and the social services child protection team is one possible option to explore.

Using the healthcare team

Other members of the primary care team may have particular skills in this area. In addition, there is a whole range of non-statutory services are available in the community that can provide support during the patient's crisis and in subsequent weeks. It may be useful to find out any religious beliefs the patient may have, as religious organizations can help. Student counselling services exist on most campuses, providing a support network of fellow students or outside voluntary counsellors. The local Samaritans branch will provide support on the telephone or in person at any time, and patients should be encouraged to carry this telephone number with them to use if hopelessness or suicidal thoughts become overwhelming.

In the most serious situations, where suicidal intent is strong and supervision inadequate, voluntary admission to

hospital should be offered. It is worth finding out whether your local psychiatry department has an admissions policy and if access to the duty consultant is difficult. A session planning and formulating a protocol for this type of crisis can be time well spent and will help to avert problems.

Picking up the pieces

Despite our best efforts some patients will still carry out their threats of suicide. A successful suicide may lead to a defensive response from those who have been involved with the patient. Careful sequential analysis of the events leading up to the death can help improve reactions to future suicides. It will also help professionals explain to the family the response of the health and social services, and facilitate access to the support available.

'Significant event auditing'[3] is a process that can give structure to this type of analysis and allow it to be shared with other practices or services. Reception staff should be involved, as they may have had direct contact with the victim and be experiencing the same self-doubts and self-criticism as the medical staff.

Counselling for the bereaved can be provided in a variety of ways. As well as bereavement counselling services organized through the NHS, a number of voluntary organizations exist for supporting family and friends (e.g. Compassionate Friends, Cruse); keeping a directory in the surgery can be extremely helpful at such a stressful time.

Key points

- Suicide is most often linked to depression, schizophrenia and drug and alcohol misuse.

- Profound hopelessness and pessimism about the future should raise concerns in depressed patients.

- Always ask depressed patients about suicidal thoughts, planning and what has stopped them so far.

- Certain age, sex and demographic groups have a higher suicide rate: it is important to be aware of the 'risk factors' in this context.

- Certain occupations are also associated with higher suicide rate. The reasons for this may be in part related to occupational stresses, but possibly also in ▶

part are related to the ease of access to a suicide method.

- Not all suicides will be prevented, even by the best general practice team.

Resources

Eldrid J. Caring for the suicidal. London: Constable; 1988.

RCGP Mental Health Education Unit. Suicide awareness training pack. London: Institute of Psychiatry.

References

1. Paykel ES, Priest RG. Recognition and management of depression in general practice; consensus statement. BMJ 1992; 305:1198–1202.

2. Department of Health. Health of the nation. Key area: mental illness. London: HMSO; 1992.

3. Pringle M, Bradley CP, Carmichael CM, et al. Significant event auditing, Occasional paper 70. London: Royal College of General Practitioners; 1995.

38. Schizophrenia in primary care

A Thornett

THIS CHAPTER REVIEWS

- The presentation and diagnosis of schizophrenia.
- The current treatment of schizophrenia.
- The role of the primary care team in schizophrenia.

Prevalence

Schizophrenia is one of the most severe of the mental disorders and is likely to be a major source of distress and difficulty for patients and their families. It has a lifetime prevalence of nearly 1%, with a yearly incidence of around 3 per 10,000 adults.[1] It is found in all cultures and usually begins in adolescence or early adult life. A young age at onset is generally a poor prognostic sign.

The average GP cares for about 5–20 schizophrenic patients. Sociodemographic characteristics affect local prevalence, which is highest in urban areas.[2,3]

There is a stigma attached to the condition, often based on the inaccurate perception that sufferers are likely to be violent. In fact most are not violent, and any aggression is usually self-directed. A well-organized, properly trained general practice team can do a great deal to help patients and carers.

The National Service Framework for Mental Health requires the primary healthcare team to be able to identify and assess patients with schizophrenia, and offer effective treatments. This includes appropriate initial management and referral to the local mental healthcare team for further assessment and care.

Aetiology

Schizophrenia has a strong genetic basis, with about 10% of sufferers' children being at risk. If both parents are schizophrenic, about 50% of their children are at risk. Siblings of schizophrenics also have about a 10% risk of developing the condition. However, inheritance does not explain the illness completely, as over half of identical twins of schizophrenics do not develop the condition. Other factors must therefore be important. Problems with family relationships do not cause schizophrenia, but emotional stress within families can lead to relapses in vulnerable patients. Stressful life events, such as a bereavement or the breakdown of a relationship, can precipitate a psychotic breakdown.

Birth trauma, viral infections and social factors also influence the development and persistence of psychotic illness. Drugs such as LSD and amphetamines can produce drug-induced psychosis, which can subsequently develop into a psychotic illness indistinguishable from schizophrenia.

Clinical assessment

Diagnosis of schizophrenia is based on symptoms, and therefore requires a good history, corroborated by others, as well as a detailed assessment of the patient's mental state. It is essential to develop a good rapport with the patient when carrying out a mental state examination. The GP usually has just 10 minutes to take a history (Box 38.1), perform an examination (Box 38.2) agree a plan of management, and at the same time screen for other severe psychiatric illnesses, including suicidal risk.

Diagnosis

The ICD-10 definition of schizophrenia essentially requires a persistent history (most of the time for at least 1 month) of at least one clear symptom from 1–5 below, with usually two others in milder form, or at least two of 6–9 below.

1. Disorders of thinking (e.g. thought insertion).
2. Delusions of being controlled.
3. Hallucinatory voices.
4. Persistent delusions of other kinds (e.g. of superhuman powers or god-like identity).
5. Pressure of speech.

6. Persistent hallucinations with delusions for weeks on end.

7. Catatonic behaviour such as excitement or strange posturing.

Negative symptoms:

8. Apathy, blunting of emotional response, reduced performance.

9. Consistent change in personal behaviour, including poor self-care, loss of interest, aimlessness and social withdrawal.

The American DSM-IV, 1994, criteria are tighter and can be summarized as follows:

A. Characteristic symptoms: two or more of the following noticeable for a significant length of time during a 1-month period (less if successfully treated):

- delusions
- hallucinations
- pressure of speech

- grossly disorganized or catatonic behaviour
- negative symptoms.

B. Social or occupational dysfunction:

- of one or more areas of life for a large portion of the time.

Box 38.1 Questions for the history

- Is there a recent onset of hallucinations, delusions, unusual or disorganized speech, agitation or bizarre behaviour?
- Is there evidence of labile emotional states?
- Close relatives may ask for help with behavioural changes, including strange behaviour, withdrawal, suspiciousness or threats
- Persistent changes in ability to function at work or in personal relationships may occur before overt psychotic symptoms
- When did the presenting complaint first appear?
- Was there a precipitating factor such as losing a job, bereavement, change in relationship, physical illness or new medication? Has the patient recently stopped taking medication?
- Was the onset slow or sudden? Look for a pattern
- Judge the severity of the illness by its duration, course, effect on work and relationships and physical effects on appetite, weight, sleep, sex drive and periods
- Relevant family history may help with diagnosis
- Employment: job changes, unemployment or deteriorating relationships at work
- What is the patient's social situation?
- Is there evidence of past psychiatric illness

Box 38.2 The mental state examination

Appearance and behaviour
- Neglected or strange clothing
- Psychomotor retardation (reduced movements)
- Lack of expression of emotion (blunting of affect)

Speech
- Patients may speak in response to auditory hallucinations
- Strange use of words
- In extreme cases, there may be no logical connection between thoughts

Mood
- Depression is common
- About 10% of patients commit suicide, usually younger patients

Thought content
- A delusion is a fixed idea that is unshakeable and inappropriate to the client's society, community or religion
- Grandiose delusions are seen in mania, schizophrenia, organic disease and depression
- Ask, for example: 'Do you have any exceptional talents?', 'Do you have any special powers?', 'Are you famous or related to someone famous?'
- Delusions of guilt can be seen in depression, e.g. 'Do you blame yourself for anything?', 'Do you deserve punishment?'
- A hallucination is a perception without an object
- In delusional perception the patient expresses a delusional significance for a normal perception

Insight
- There may be a particular issue if a relative has asked you to see the patient
- Ask 'What do you think is the matter with you?', 'Is it physical or mental?', 'Do you think you are ill in any way at all?', 'Do you need treatment?'

C. Duration:

- continuous signs persist for at least 6 months, including at least 1 month of symptoms (or less if successfully treated) that meet criterion A and which may include periods of prodromal or residual symptoms.

D. Exclusions:

- the diagnosis must rule out the possibility of toxic confusional states due to drugs or organic illness.

The early or prodromal stages of schizophrenic illnesses can vary considerably. A typical presentation might start with a family's concerns that their child's personality has changed. A phase of decline in personal hygiene, loss of job and friends for no clear reason, and depressive symptoms mixed with a degree of ill-defined perplexity are all common. Anxiety, depression and emotional distress are also common.

Differential diagnosis

Other diagnoses to consider include bipolar disorder and depressive psychosis.

The presence of a toxic confusional state, such as febrile illness, temporal lobe epilepsy, cerebral lesions, hypothyroidism and systemic lupus erythematosus, precludes diagnosis of any major mental illness. Also, hallucinations associated with alcoholism, illicit drugs and medications can be confused with schizophrenia. Routine blood tests, a urine screen for drug metabolites and special investigations can be useful to exclude these conditions.

Prognosis

Prognosis depends on presentation and response to treatment. Thirty percent of patients recover to live independent lives. About half live relatively independent lives, with medication and varying levels of support. However, 20% require long-term, structured care.

Good prognostic factors include acute onset over several weeks, a supportive family, intelligence and insight, absence of negative symptoms such as flat mood and social withdrawal, onset after the age of 25 years and a good response to low doses of drugs.

Management

Approaches include drug therapy, psychological treatment and social support.

Drug treatment

About 70% of patients with psychosis show a moderate to substantial reduction in their positive symptoms (delusions and hallucinations) after treatment with antipsychotic drugs.[4] Once in remission, antipsychotic drugs substantially reduce the risk of relapse. During 1 year, 55% of patients on placebo are likely to relapse, compared with 20–25% of those on antipsychotic drugs.[4] The negative symptoms of schizophrenia (e.g. psychomotor retardation, withdrawal and lack of motivation) are less responsive to drug treatment.

The limitation of treatment with traditional antipsychotic drugs has been their side-effects. These include extrapyramidal side-effects, such as parkinsonism, akathisia (restlessness), acute dystonia and tardive dyskinesia.

The newer, atypical antipsychotic drugs such as risperidone (Risperdal), olanzapine (Zyprexa) and clozapine (Clozaril) may reduce the risk of relapse, and may also help with negative symptoms. A recent Cochrane Review has shown that clozapine has greater clinical efficacy than do traditional antipsychotics.[5]

Managing the first presentation

The patient should be referred for psychiatric assessment, urgently if neccessary. It may be appropriate to prescribe a neuroleptic unless access to a specialist is speedy and the symptoms relatively mild. If the GP does prescribe, initial medication should be one that has few side-effects so that the patient's trust is maintained. The dose can be increased gradually.

First-choice drugs include atypical antipsychotic agents, such as olanzapine 5–10 mg/day or risperidone 4–6 mg/day.[4] A more familiar drug, such as haloperidol 1.5–4.00 mg up to three times daily, may be suitable.[3]

Anti-anxiety medication may also be used in the short term in conjunction with neuroleptics to control acute agitation. Examples include diazepam 5–10 mg up to four times daily or lorazepam 1–2 mg up to four times daily.

In cases of relapse, a patient who has previously responded to a drug can restart the same medication. The dose should be the lowest possible that gives relief of symptoms.

Continuing treatment

Antipsychotic medication should be continued for at least 6 months after symptoms resolve.[3] Close supervision is usually needed to encourage patient compliance.

Depot injections, giving a slow, stable release of drugs, may be particularly useful for patients who lack insight. This type ▶

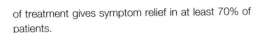

of treatment gives symptom relief in at least 70% of patients.

Treating side-effects of medication

Parkinsonian symptoms, such as tremor or akinesia, may be managed with oral antiparkinsonian drugs such as procyclidine 5 mg three times daily or orphenadrine 50 mg three times daily. Withdrawal of antiparkinsonian drugs should be attempted after 2–3 months without symptoms.

Akathisia may be managed with dosage reduction, by switching to a low-potency antipsychotic such as olanzapine or quetiapine, or with a beta blocker such as propranolol 30–80 mg/day.

If there is fever, rigidity and/or labile blood pressure, stop the antipsychotic medication and refer the patient to hospital immediately for investigation of possible neuroleptic malignant syndrome.

Psychological treatment

Psychological interventions can minimize distress and reduce the frequency of relapse. They usually centre on the development of social skills and reducing expressed emotion in the family.

Social support

Social interventions include support in the home, day care in a rehabilitation unit aimed at developing job skills and residency in a hostel or group home. A key worker can help with medication, disability benefits and housing needs.

The GP should ensure the safety of the patient, family and carers and make sure the patient's basic needs, such as meals and accommodation, are met.

Referral

All patients with schizophrenia should be referred to the mental health team. Patients should be referred urgently or admitted to hospital if:[3]

- there is serious risk of suicide, violence or neglect
- for a first episode, to confirm the diagnosis and arrange for the appointment of a key worker
- in cases of relapse, to review the effectiveness of the care plan, unless there is an established previous response to treatment and it is safe to manage the patient at home
- community treatment has failed
- there are problematic side-effects
- there are concerns about comorbid drug or alcohol use.

Advice and support

- Offer patients and carers information on the illness and its treatment and on local community or voluntary groups.
- Advise the patient and their family about the importance of continued treatment and possible side-effects.
- Avoid confrontation or criticism.
- Do not argue with psychotic thinking unless it is necessary to prevent harmful or disruptive behaviour.
- Advise acutely ill patients that they should not drive and that the DVLA should be informed.
- Encourage resumption of normal activities after symptoms improve.

Improving practice organization

There are several ways in which practices can improve their organization of care for patients with schizophrenia:

- allow longer appointment slots for patients with mental health problems
- give routine follow-up appointments for these patients
- encourage patients with chronic mental disorders to see the same team member at each visit
- keep a register of patients with severe or chronic mental illness to ensure regular follow-up and monitoring
- have a system for chasing up patients who do not attend follow-up appointments
- relieve pressure on individual doctors who have a heavy mental health workload
- have a practice policy for staff when faced with agitated or aggressive patients
- check the training and support needs of practice nurses or other members of the team who provide mental healthcare, such as giving depot injections.

Key points

- **Schizophrenia tends to be severe and long term.**
- **Positive symptoms respond well to drug treatments.**
- **Negative symptoms respond less well to drug treatments.**
- **Drug side-effects may be presented to the GP and may be controlled with additional medication or a change of therapy.**
- **Some patients do recover completely.**

- GPs may initiate treatment in mild cases while awaiting assessment.
- Admit urgently, using the Mental Health Act if necessary (see Ch. 40), if the patient's illness renders them a danger to themselves or others.

Resources

Hearing Voices Network, Dale House, 35 Dale Street, Manchester M1 2HF. Tel. 0161 834 5768. Local groups that allow people to explore their voice hearing experiences in a secure and confidential way. Information pack available.

Mental Health Drugs Helpline: provides independent advice and information for patients and carers. Tel. 020 7919 2999 (11 a.m. to 5 p.m., Monday to Friday, excluding bank holidays). Drug information website: http://www.nmhc.co.uk

Mental Health Foundation, 20/21 Cornwall Terrace, London NW1 4QL. Tel. 020 7535 7400.

MIND, Granta House, 15–19 Broadway, Stratford, London E15 4BQ. Tel. 020 8519 2122; MINDinfoLINE 0345 660 163 (outside London), 020 8522 1728 (Greater London).

National Schizophrenia Fellowship, 28 Castle Street, Kingston-upon-Thames, Surrey KT1 1SS. Tel. 020 8547 3937; advice service 020 8974 6814.

SANELine. Helpline: 0345 678000 (2 p.m. to midnight, every day).

References

1. Bamrah JS, Freeman HL, Goldberg DP. Epidemiology of schizophrenia in Salford, 1974–84. Changes in an urban community over ten years. Br J Psychiatry 1999; 159:802–810.
2. Turner T. ABC of mental health: schizophrenia. BMJ 1997; 315:108–111.
3. World Health Organization Collaborating Centre for Research and Training for Mental Health. WHO guide to mental ill health in adults. London: Royal Society of Medicine Press; 2000.
4. McGrath J, Emmerson WB. Fortnightly review: treatment of schizophrenia. BMJ 1999; 319:1045–1048.
5. Wahlbeck K, Cheine M, Essali MA. Clozapine vs 'typical' neuroleptic medication for schizophrenia. In: Cochrane Collaboration. Cochrane Library (Issue 4). Oxford: Update Software; 1998.

39. Mania

C Hallstrom

THIS CHAPTER REVIEWS

- The difference between the major psychotic illnesses.
- The presentation of mania and hypomania.
- The management of mania for the GP.

Early identification and treatment of psychotic illness will greatly improve prognosis. Cooperation between all the professionals involved will ensure optimum care for patients.

The main psychotic illnesses that a GP is likely to see in his or her practice are schizophrenia, mania and an intermediate condition known as schizoaffective psychosis. These conditions are characterized by abnormalities of thinking and abnormalities of mood and are contrasted in Box 39.1. The main distinction between mania and schizophrenia, apart from the elevation of mood seen in manic patients, is in the natural history of the condition, with periods of complete recovery.

If the patient's most prominent symptom is elevated mood, then the likely diagnosis is mania, or hypomania if the mood disturbance is not so severe. Other symptoms associated with mania include irritability, aggression, lack of insight and other disturbed behaviors, such as overspending and hypersexuality.

Schizophrenics will have negative symptoms of social withdrawal, apathy, loss of volition and a blunting of their mood, as well as positive symptoms characteristic of an overactive mind. Schizophrenia is usually associated with gradual social decline and other negative symptoms.

Prevalence of psychotic illness

Mania is less common than schizophrenia, with a lifetime prevalence of 0.8%, and it tends to have a more benign course. The patient may be in remission for many years between episodes, although the episodes become more frequent with age.

Schizoaffective illness is an intermediate condition where the clinical picture resembles schizophrenia, but strong mood abnormalities are prominent.[1] The patient

▸

Box 39.1 Common symptoms of mania, schizophrenia and schizoaffective disorder (clearly diagnostic similarities and difficulties arise)

Manic symptoms	Schizophrenia	Schizoaffective illness
Overexaggeration	Thought disorder	Any of the symptoms in either list
Elevated mood	Hallucinations	Tendency to have relapses, but periods of complete remission do occur
Overactivity	Delusions	
Lack of sleep	Paranoia	Prominent symptoms of depression and mania
Lack of insight	Suspicion	
Sexual indiscretion	Social withdrawal	
Overspending of money	Self-neglect	
Tendency have depressive phases and episodes of prolonged remission	Tendency to develop a chronic illness with residual defects	

experiences recurrent episodes, but makes a full recovery between them.

Diagnostic boundaries between the three conditions can be blurred and the diagnosis in a particular patient may change.

Presentation

Most patients will have had previous contact with psychiatric services and the diagnosis will have already been made. These patients will present in acute relapse with a series of psychotic symptoms. In mania, the patient's mood can become abnormal, with a tendency to overexaggeration, overspending and sexual indiscretion. The patient may also break the law in minor ways. These patients may have had previous depressive episodes.

Examination and investigation

The most important investigation is the history from an independent observer. A physical illness is rarely mistaken for a psychotic illness, except in the case of abnormal drug reactions (e.g. with the antimalarial mefloquine (Lariam) or steroids). Abuse of amphetamines, ecstasy, LSD and cannabis can also lead to an acute psychotic illness. Intracranial pathology, such as in epilepsy or brain tumours, and endocrine disorders can also cause behavioural changes.

Neurotransmitter abnormalities, especially dopamine overactivity, have been implicated in psychosis, and 5-HT and other excitatory amino acids may also be involved.[2] Anatomical abnormalities within the brain also have been found in patients with psychotic illness.

Physical examination of the patient may not help in diagnosis, but this is useful to assess the level of social functioning and the needs of the patient, and will help identify the intervention and care required. Questions that should be posed when assessing patients include:

- Are they able to care for themselves and can they wait for an outpatient appointment, or do they need protection from themselves or the effects of their illness?
- Do they need urgent assessment by the community mental health team or emergency admission?
- What is the risk of and level of self-neglect and the risk to their families?
- Are they about to be evicted?
- Are their relationships about to break down because of intolerable pressures on their carers?
- What is the risk of violence?

Management

Management is increasingly seen as a long-term process designed to prevent relapse and to support the patient in the community rather than in hospital. Admission to hospital is needed at times of acute relapse, especially to ensure compliance with medication and to safeguard the individual from self-harm and neglect. It is often worthwhile to admit patients briefly to focus the attention of the healthcare team on their problems, to offer their carers a period of rest, and to stabilize their mental state.

The community Care Programme Approach (CPA) should be implemented for proper aftercare, this can have a profound impact on the long-term prognosis. The CPA requires the identification of patients at risk and the appointment of a keyworker responsible for coordinating care and producing a written programme of aftercare and supervision. A list of those involved in the network of care of the patient should also be drawn up. A programme for regular review should be agreed with the patient.

Prophylactic treatment

For patients with recurrent manic illness, prophylactic lithium is traditionally prescribed. Carbamazepine and sodium valproate can also be used. Prophylaxis should be considered after only one episode of mania.

Referral of patients

There should be close liaison between the local psychiatric service and the GP. In emergencies a telephone call by the GP should bring the appropriate response, such as an early appointment, a crisis intervention or a consultation in the patient's home. Once the diagnosis and management have been established, the patient should be followed up using the CPA approach. The keyworker should be known and should be contacted if problems arise.

The patient should not be referred back to the GP without clear aftercare arrangements. If the patient's condition deteriorates, then early referral before social or psychiatric breakdown occurs is vital. Crisis prevention is much better than crisis intervention.

The Mental Health Act

The Mental Health Act of 1983 exists to enable patients to get access to treatment when their mental illness prevents them from accepting treatment. There is great confusion about when patients are sectionable and when not.

Detaining a patient depends on what is in the patient's best interests, subject to certain broad criteria being met. The criteria are:

- A mental disorder which warrants detention:
  - in the interest of the patient's own health or safety
  - to protect others
  - if informal admission is not appropriate.

If the patient is known to have a mental illness and has been treated in the past, then Section 3 of the Mental Health Act is usually applicable. Section 2 is only for assessment and treatment if the patient's diagnosis is uncertain. The social worker will advise on the most appropriate section of the Mental Health Act to use to detain a particular patient. Detention of a patient under Section 3 of the Mental Health Act imposes certain statutory obligations on the health authority for providing adequate aftercare. Proper follow-up is part of these statutory obligations.

Conclusion

Psychotic illnesses are seen as a prime responsibility of the psychiatric services. Close liaison between families, carers and the health and social services is vital to the care programme approach for the provision of a total package of care. The Mental Health Act enables patients to receive that care, and professionals should be prepared to section

patients early to enable the patient to regain control of their illness.

Key points

- **The main distinction between mania and schizophrenia, apart from the obvious elation in mood seen in manic patients, is in the natural history of the condition.**
- **If the patient's prominent symptom is an elevated mood, then the likely diagnosis is one of mania, or hypomania if it is not severe.**
- **The most important investigation is the history given by an independent observer.**
- **Management of psychotic illness is increasingly seen as a long-term process to prevent relapses and offer long-term support in the community.**
- **Professionals should be prepared to section patients early to enable the patient to regain control of their illness.**

References

1. American Medical Association. Diagnostic and statistical manual, 4th edn. Washington, DC: American Medical Association; 1994.

2. Frangou S, Murray R. Schizophrenia. London: Martin Dunitz; 1996.

40. The Mental Health Act: a guide for GPs

CH Buller and W Lewis

THIS CHAPTER REVIEWS

- The Mental Health Act legislation.
- Potential pitfalls for the GP.
- Becoming an approved doctor under the Act.

Most GPs will eventually be asked to take part in a Mental Health Act assessment on one of their patients.[1] On some occasions it is the GP who decides to initiate the procedure. In other cases the assessment is triggered by the patient's family, who may be concerned about the mental health of their relative, or opposed to their initial or continued detention in hospital.

Thus it is important for all GPs to have a basic understanding of the Mental Health Act and some of the practicalities surrounding the organization and execution of assessments. It is also a good idea to be aware of the potential problems and pitfalls (Box 40.1).

Scotland has its own mental health laws, so the following advice applies only to doctors working in England and Wales.

Mental Health Act 1983

The current Mental Health Act is the latest in a series of legislation going back to 1713, when the first laws concerned with the mentally ill were enacted (Box 40.2). It is accompanied by a Code of Practice, providing guidance for doctors, social workers and any managers who may become involved in executing duties under the act.[2]

Compared with the 1959 legislation, the 1983 Act introduced tighter provisions concerning the treatment of non-consenting detained patients, and new measures for admitting mentally disordered offenders to hospital. It also led to the creation of the Mental Health Act Commission. This organization has no powers to discharge detained

Box 40.1 The Mental Health Act: problems and pitfalls for GPs

- Always record in notes any occasions when you have considered initiating a Mental Health Act assessment on a patient, even if you decide against it
- A colleague's opinion that a patient does not meet the criteria for detention is valid at that point in time. Remember that the patient's circumstances and condition can change
- If you are to attend a Mental Health Act assessment, and you have concerns about your patient's potential for violence, you should inform the other professionals involved. It may be necessary to arrange the attendance of the police, mainly for their help in conveying the patient to hospital. This is usually arranged by the approved social worker[2]
- Do not put your home address on medical recommendations
- Check with the other professionals that you have the patient's correct full name and address
- GPs working in casualty departments must remember that Section 5(2) cannot be used to detain patients attending casualty (they are not inpatients)
- The rules for detention are different for private hospitals and nursing homes[1]

patients, but monitors their treatment and scrutinizes admission and renewal papers to make sure such patients are detained lawfully.

The current Act is divided into ten parts, and the key sections for GPs to be familiar with are:

- Part II: compulsory admission to hospital and guardianship.
- Part III: patients involved in criminal proceedings or under sentence.
- Part IV: consent to treatment.

▶

Box 40.2 History of mental health law

1713, 1744	Vagrancy Acts provided a legal basis for the apprehension and detention of mentally disordered individuals who were deemed dangerous to others
1774	The Madhouses Act aimed to ensure acceptable conditions in privately run madhouses
1808	The County Asylums Act transferred some of the responsibility of care from privately run madhouses to public asylums
1808–1890	Numerous acts dealt with the provision of care for the mentally disordered in both public and private institutions
1913, 1927	The Mental Deficiency Acts authorized separate hospitals for the 'mentally defective'. These hospitals eventually housed individuals with learning disabilities
1930	The Mental Treatment Act allowed patients to be admitted to mental hospital on a voluntary basis
1959	The Mental Health Act[3] was based on the premise that the vast majority of patients should, if possible, be cared for on an informal basis. There were, of course, also provisions for compulsory detention of patients, but for the first time this was entrusted to doctors and social workers without the involvement of a magistrate. The 1959 act also led to the creation of the Mental Health Review Tribunal, with the aim of safeguarding against inappropriate detention
1983	The latest Mental Health Act

Key terms

Approved doctor

An approved doctor is a medical practitioner who has been approved under Section 12 as having special experience in the diagnosis or treatment of mental disorder.

In practice, this approval is granted to all psychiatrists who are members of the Royal College of Psychiatrists. GPs seeking Section 12 approval are normally expected to fulfil three criteria:

- membership of the Royal College of General Practitioners
- 3 years full-time equivalent as a principal
- 6 months full-time or equivalent supervised experience of psychiatric work, including some experience of using the Act.

Doctors who satisfy the basic criteria and wish to become approved under the Act must also attend a Section 12 training course.

Even if you are not an approved doctor under the provisions of the act, you are likely to be involved in assessments and admissions of patients from your own list.

Approved social workers

An approved social worker (ASW) will have undergone a further period of training, focusing on a range of topics, including mental health legislation, the nature and treatment of mental disorder, and access to statutory, voluntary and private resources for the support of patients and their families.

When patients are admitted, under Part II of the act, it is usually the ASW who applies to the hospital. The patient cannot be detained if the ASW is not prepared to make the application, even if there are two medical recommendations supporting formal admission. The ASW must consult the nearest relative when conducting a Mental Health Act assessment on a patient, and consider alternatives to hospital admission.

Nearest relative

The Act states how the patient's nearest relative is defined, and assigns a legal role to that person. After the patient's spouse or partner, the hierarchical list includes son or daughter, father or mother, then brother or sister.

Admission orders

GPs may be contacted and asked to assess their own patients with a view to providing a medical recommendation supporting admission to hospital. The most frequently used admission orders require two medical recommendations including, where possible, one from a doctor with previous knowledge of the patient (Box 40.3).

Section 2 (assessment order)

Section 2 (assessment order) is most often used when the patient has never been in a psychiatric unit before, or where the diagnosis is unclear and an inpatient assessment is needed to formulate a plan of management.

Section 3 (treatment order)

Section 3 (treatment order) tends to be used when the diagnosis is fairly clear and the patient requires treatment

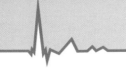

Box 40.3 Commonly used admission orders

Section 2

- Allows compulsory admission and detention for assessment, or assessment followed by treatment, for up to 28 days
- The patient cannot be admitted informally
- The patient must be suffering from a mental disorder of a nature or degree that warrants such detention
- Detention must be in the interests of the patient's health or safety or the protection of others
- Forms required include an application by an ASW or nearest relative, plus either
  - a joint medical recommendation using Form 3 or
  - two separate medical recommendations using Form 4 (no more than 5 days gap between the recommendations)
- One of the medical recommendations should be completed by an approved doctor and the other by a doctor with previous knowledge of the patient, ideally the GP

Section 3

- Allows compulsory detention for treatment for up to 6 months
- The patient must be suffering from mental illness, mental impairment, severe mental impairment or psychopathic disorder of a nature or degree that makes it appropriate for the patient to receive treatment in hospital
- Hospital treatment must be in the interests of the patient's health or safety or the protection of others
- If the patient has a psychopathic disorder or mental impairment, the medical treatment must be likely to alleviate or prevent a deterioration in the condition
- Forms required include an application by an ASW or nearest relative, plus either a joint medical recommendation, using Form 10, or two separate medical recommendations, using Form 11 (no more than 5 days gap between the recommendations)

Box 40.4 Appeals procedures

- Patients detained under Section 2 can apply to the hospital managers or to a mental health review tribunal for discharge
- Patients detained under Section 3 can apply to the hospital managers for discharge as often as they want, but only once to a mental health review tribunal in each 6-month period of detention
- The nearest relative can request discharge of the patient
- If the responsible medical officer decides to block the patient's discharge, the nearest relative can apply to a mental health review tribunal

requires only one medical recommendation plus an application by either an ASW or the nearest relative. It is designed only for genuine emergencies and should never be used for convenience.

Section 2 criteria have to be met. Also, it must be clear that there is insufficient time to get a second medical recommendation, and that it is of 'urgent necessity' for the patient to be admitted to hospital without delay.[2] Once in hospital, the patient should be assessed again as soon as possible, for either an admission or treatment order.

Section 5(2)

Section 5(2) allows the doctor in charge of an inpatient's treatment to detain them for up to 72 hours so that an assessment can be made for an admission order.

Section 7 (guardianship and supervised discharge)

The aim of guardianship (Section 7) is to make sure patients receive appropriate care in the community. The subject of a guardianship order must be over 16 years old, suffering from a mental disorder and in need of guardianship in the interests of their own welfare or for the protection of others.

Like Section 3, guardianship is initially for 6 months, renewable for 6 months and then for a year at a time. Two medical recommendations are needed, including one by an approved doctor, using Forms 19 or 20, plus an application by an ASW or nearest relative. There are specific grounds within the Act for displacing the nearest relative if they object.

for the condition. Section 2 cannot be renewed, so if the patient needs continued detention in hospital for treatment under the act, an application for Section 3 is made. Patients can appeal against detention under Section 2 or 3 (Box 40.4).

Section 4 (emergency order)

Section 4 (emergency order) allows compulsory admission and detention in hospital for up to 72 hours. The order

The guardian has the power to require the patient to reside at a specified place and attend specified locations for the purpose of medical treatment, occupation, education and training. Also, a doctor, ASW or any other person specified by the guardian can have access to the patient's residence. However, a patient under guardianship can refuse treatment.

Section 25 (supervised discharge order)

The aim of Section 25 (supervised discharge order) is to ensure appropriate aftercare for patients who have been detained in hospital for treatment, under Section 3 for example. The grounds for such an order include 'substantial risk of serious harm to the health or safety of the patient or the safety of other people, or the patient being seriously exploited, if the patient did not receive aftercare services'.

The powers granted by the order are similar to those of guardianship, except that the supervisor also has 'power to convey' the patient. However, this order conveys no additional powers to treat patients in the community against their wishes.

Being taken to a Place of Safety

Section 135

A court order can be obtained to break into a property to remove a person to a Place of Safety.

Section 136

Someone found in a public place, who appears to have a mental disorder, can be taken by the police to a Place of Safety.

Proposed changes to the Mental Health Act

The Government White Paper published in 2000 proposes changes to the Mental Health Act.[4] It includes a broad definition of mental disorder, covering any disability or disorder of mind or brain, whether permanent or temporary, which results in an impairment or disturbance of mental functioning.

Major proposed changes include a restructured compulsory admission, replacing Sections 2 and 3 as follows:

- Stage 1. Decisions to begin assessment of a patient under compulsory powers based on a preliminary examination by two doctors and a social worker or other suitably trained mental health professional.

- Stage 2. A patient will receive treatment set out in a formal care plan; the initial period of assessment and treatment under compulsory powers will be limited to a maximum of 28 days; after that continuing use of compulsory powers *must* be authorized by a new independent Mental Health Tribunal, which will obtain advice from independent experts as well as evidence from the clinical team, patient and representatives.

- Stage 3. The Tribunal will be able to make a care and treatment order authorizing the care and treatment specified in a care plan recommended by the clinical team. The first two orders will be for up to 6 months each; subsequent orders may be for periods of up to 12 months.

Other changes are:

- Care and treatment orders may also apply to patients outside hospital. This has been one of the most debated legislative issues in recent years.[5]

- Patients with long-term mental incapacity who need care and treatment for serious mental disorder to which they are unable to consent will require an assessment which includes an independent second opinion.

- They allow for the detention for assessment and treatment of those who pose a significant risk of serious harm to others as a result of a mental disorder. This will include some individuals whose risk is as a result of a severe personality disorder.

- It allows for a broader definition of mental disorder than contained in the current Mental Health Act. For example, it drops the current exclusions such as alcohol dependence. However, in order to detain a person in hospital, four criteria will have to be met:

  - the presence of a mental disorder

  - the severity of the disorder requires specialist mental health treatment and care

  - the person is at high risk of harming him- or herself or other people

  - a treatment is available.

Future developments

The recent Bournewood case[6] has exposed a gap in mental health legislation when it comes to patients who are admitted informally to hospital but lack the capacity to consent to either admission or treatment. It is likely that new legislation will be introduced in the near future to safeguard the rights of these non-detained incapacitated patients.

One of the most debated legislative issues in recent years has been compulsory treatment in the community.[5]

One of the arguments in favour of community treatment orders asserts: 'If it is moral to have a compulsory right of treatment in hospital, then improvement of patient care by moving the locus to the community does not affect that morality'.[7] However, opponents might argue that patients who are well enough to be out of hospital are also well enough to refuse treatment. Whether a community treatment order, in whatever form, is included in new mental health legislation will be of interest.

Key points

- The most frequently used admission orders are Sections 2 and 3.

- Section 2 allows for compulsory admission and detention for assessment or assessment followed by treatment of mental disorder for up to 28 days.

- Section 3 allows compulsory detention for up to 6 months and tends to be used where the diagnosis is clear and the patient requires treatment for that condition.

- Section 4 is for use only in an emergency when it is of 'urgent necessity' for the patient to be admitted to hospital without delay. Section 4 allows compulsory admission and detention in hospital for up to 72 hours.

- The Mental Health Act may be changing soon, and the effect of the proposed changes will be to widen the spectrum of patients who may be detained under the Act, and to make treatment orders dependent on the recommendations of a new independent body.

References

1. Department of Health. Mental Health Act 1983. London: HMSO; 1983.

2. Department of Health. Mental Health Act 1983. Code of Practice. London: HMSO; 1983.

3. Department of Health. A review of the Mental Health Act 1959 (the consultative document). London: HMSO; 1976.

4. Draft Bill on Proposed Reform of the Mental Health Act. Available at: http://www.doh,gov.uk/mentalhealth/draftbill2002/index.htm

5. Turner T. Compulsory treatment in the community: some debating issues. Psychiatr Bull 1994; 18:657–659.

6. Eastman N, Peay J. Bournewood: an indefensible gap in mental health law. BMJ 1998; 317: 94–95.

7. Eastman N. Mental health law: civil liberties and the principle of reciprocity. BMJ 1994; 308:43–45.

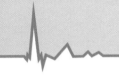

41. Tired all the time

F Machado

THIS CHAPTER REVIEWS

- How to assess the patient who is tired all the time.
- How to exclude organic disorders.
- Chronic fatigue syndrome.

Prevalence

Consultations that begin with the words 'I'm tired all the time, doctor' often produce a Pavlovian response of despair in the GP. The term 'heartsink' comes to mind. Fatigue, however, is a common symptom that can indicate important organic disease requiring investigation and treatment.

Although fatigue is very common, few patients see their doctors about it. It is estimated that 400 episodes of fatigue result in one consultation.[1] On average, 13 out of 1000 registered patients present to their GP each year with fatigue as the main complaint.[2]

There have been relatively few studies on patients presenting with fatigue in primary care. Only 2% are referred to secondary care, so data from specialist fatigue clinics will represent a different population of patients to those seen in general practice (Table 41.1).[3] Even so, only 2.7% of patients attending a dedicated fatigue clinic had a physical cause for the problem (Table 41.2), and two-thirds also had a psychiatric diagnosis.[4]

Causes of fatigue

Almost any disease process, whether physical or psychological, can cause tiredness. A prospective study of adults presenting with fatigue in four UK general practices in a variety of settings found that a physical cause for the problem was identified through standard investigations in only 9% of patients (see Table 41.1).[3] Three-quarters of the patients with fatigue had symptoms of emotional ▸

Table 41.1 Physical causes of fatigue in 19 patients in general practice[3]

Diagnosis	No. of patients
Anaemia	8
Hypothyroidism	3
Infection	3
Glandular fever	3
Diabetes mellitus	1
Carcinomatosis	1

Table 41.2 Medical diagnosis of 405 patients presenting with fatigue in a dedicated clinic[4]

Diagnosis	No. of patients
Obstructive sleep apnoea	5
Periodic hypersomnia	2
Nocturnal limb movements	2
Temporal lobe epilepsy	2
Hypothyroidism	2
Hypopituitarism	1
Polymyalgia rheumatica	2
Systemic lupus erythematosus	1
Asthma	2
Pulmonary sarcoidosis	1
Anaemia	1
Infections (Lyme disease, cytomegalovirus, hepatitis, Epstein–Barr virus)	7
No medical diagnosis	377

distress – twice as many as in a control group matched for age and sex.

Assessment

When a patient presents complaining of being tired all the time, it is tempting to reach for the pathology request form. However, empathetic listening and appropriate examination will do more to define the possible causes, and identify appropriate investigations and management. Most patients presenting with fatigue have an underlying emotional cause, so it is important to ask about any psychological symptoms.

The nature of the patient's fatigue can give clues to its origin. Fatigue on exertion that goes away with rest suggests an organic cause, such as anaemia. Associated symptoms, such as shortness of breath on exertion, may mean further investigation is needed.

Marked weight loss, anorexia or other 'alarm' symptoms also call for investigation. Fatigue that never goes away and is worst in the morning suggests the patient may be depressed.

The onset of symptoms and their duration may also provide clues. A short history and an abrupt onset may suggest a postviral aetiology or the onset of diabetes. A protracted history may be more in keeping with an emotional cause, and has implications for the prognosis.

Asking about the patient's sleeping pattern may uncover a history of unrefreshing sleep or early morning waking, indicating possible depression. However, a history from the patient's partner of snoring, possible apnoeic episodes and daytime somnolence suggests that referral for assessment of sleep disorder should be considered.

The GP may be able to identify the patient's underlying fears and concerns by asking what they think is the cause of their tiredness. Underlying depression is often unrecognized by the GP; but tiredness is the most common symptom. It is important to ask about other symptoms of depression, and to ask patients directly whether they feel low. Symptoms of anxiety or stress may indicate other psychological problems, such as panic disorder. This may be revealed by asking about conditions at home and work. It may not be easy to convince some people that their tiredness indicates a psychological cause, but simply raising the issue may lead the patient to consider this and to discussion at a later date.

Iatrogenic causes for tiredness, such as beta blockers, should be considered.

Examination

Most patients with fatigue believe there must be a physical cause. A normal examination may go a long way to reassuring the patient that no physical cause underlies their fatigue. During the physical examination, the GP should pay particular attention to:

- posture, affect, expression
- evidence of weight loss
- pallor
- signs of tonsillitis and mucosal pigmentation
- any cervical lymphadenopathy or goitre
- chest, cardiovascular and abdominal signs, if examination is indicated.

Investigations

In a general practice study, one-third of patients with fatigue had one or more abnormal results in a standard set of investigations. However, the doctors judged that abnormal results were clinically important in only 9% of the study group.[3] The most common clinically important abnormality was a low haemoglobin.

Other investigations should be tailored to the patient's complaint. It is important not to overinvestigate. Ten percent of patients seen in a dedicated chronic fatigue clinic were found to have somatization disorder after repeated normal investigations. It has been suggested that viral tests do not help in the management of longstanding fatigue.[4]

Management and prognosis

If a physical cause for the symptoms is identified, this should be managed as indicated. Patients need to be reassured that no physical cause is found in most cases. However, the incidence of anxiety and depression is twice that of patients presenting to the GP with problems other than fatigue. Discussion of the role of social and emotional problems in fatigue, and appropriate treatment, should improve the patient's symptoms.

Just over half the patients presenting with fatigue have symptoms that still persist 6 months later. A history of anxiety or depression is associated with a three-fold risk of symptoms persisting. Patients should be warned that their fatigue may persist, and that any associated emotional symptoms may prolong the recovery.

A history of fatigue for a short period of time with no anxiety or depression improves the prognosis, so such patients can be offered reassurance.

Referral

Referral may be needed for patients with either physical or psychological problems. Reasons for referral include:

- chronic, disabling fatigue with no identified cause
- suspected sleep disorders (for sleep study investigation)
- suspected chronic fatigue syndrome.

Chronic fatigue syndrome

The incidence of chronic fatigue syndrome is about 7 per 100,000. It is a diagnosis of exclusion, as there are no pathognomonic, clinical or laboratory findings.

It is usually defined as severe disabling fatigue with a combination of symptoms that prominently feature self-reported disturbances in concentration, memory and sleep, as well as musculoskeletal pain.

The common features of chronic fatigue syndrome are:

- Persisting or relapsing fatigue for >6 months, affecting family, work and leisure activity. Patients rest excessively, fearing exercise will make them worse.
- Other common symptoms, present or fluctuating for >6 months, include:
  - migratory arthralgias and muscles pains
  - impaired memory and concentration
  - post-exertion exhaustion
  - headache present or fluctuating
  - malaise
  - unrefreshing or disturbed sleep
  - sore throat with tender lymph nodes
  - multiple, often vague, symptoms, including abdominal pain, bloating, constipation, diarrhoea, irritability, depression, anxiety, panic attacks, weight loss, palpitations, jaw pain, chest pain, sweating, shortness of breath and paraesthesia
  - initial presentation may be flu-like, but persist
  - few patients report psychological symptoms, and those that do report them as secondary to their physical symptoms (this is in contrast to most patients with depression, who report mood disturbance high on their list of symptoms)
- Patients fear underlying sinister pathology.

Clearly there is considerable overlap with depression, but mood changes are not invariable in chronic fatigue. Where the do occur they do not necessarily precede the tiredness, which is the dominant feature, and may be a consequence of it.

A report from three royal colleges advises a biopsychological approach to management.[5] Patients may resist this approach, and their supervision may be beyond the primary healthcare team. Referral to a dedicated clinic may be needed, where the patient will be assessed by physicians and psychiatrists with an interest in chronic fatigue syndrome.

Fibromyalgia is a similar and to some extent overlapping condition, in which muscle pains and tenderness predominate, but many of the same symptoms are found.

Key points

- **Fatigue is a common symptom, but only a few patients will see their GP about it.**
- **In about 1 in 10 patients there is a physical cause, which needs to be identified.**
- **In most patients there is a psychosocial cause which needs to be addressed.**
- **The vast majority of patients are managed in primary care, but some need referral.**
- **Chronic fatigue syndrome requires a biopsychological approach that may be difficult to provide in primary care.**
- **Patients with a short history and no emotional symptoms have a better prognosis than do patients with a long history and accompanying psychological problems.**
- **A holistic approach is needed to prevent overinvestigation and reinforcement of a possible somatization disorder.**

References

1. Morrell DC, Wale CJ. Symptoms perceived and recorded by patients. J R Coll Gen Pract 1976; 26:398–403.
2. Morrell DC. Symptom interpretation in general practice. J R Coll Gen Pract 1972; 22: 295–309.
3. Risdale L, Evans A, Jerrett W, et al. Patients with fatigue in general practice: a prospective study. BMJ 1993; 307:103–106.

4. Llewelyn MB. Assess the fatigued patient. Br J Hosp Med 1996; 55:125–129.

5. Joint Working Group of the Royal Colleges of Physicians, Psychiatrists and General Practitioners. Chronic fatigue syndrome. London: Royal College of Physicians; 1996.

NEUROLOGY

42. Understanding epilepsy

RJ Simister and JS Duncan

THIS CHAPTER REVIEWS

- The definition and prevalence of epilepsy.
- How to assess a patient presenting with seizures.
- How patients with epilepsy are investigated.
- What advice to give patients with epilepsy.
- When to refer patients.
- Contraception and pregnancy in epilepsy.

Definition

Epilepsy is the occurrence of two or more unprovoked epileptic seizures of cerebral origin. It is not a single disease, but a manifestation of underlying brain dysfunction arising from many different possible causes. Single seizures and those occurring during an acute illness should not be classified as epilepsy.

Epidemiology

There are 20–70 new cases of epilepsy per 100,000 population each year in the UK.[1] About 0.5% of the population have active epilepsy,[2] and the lifetime prevalence of a single non-febrile seizure is 2–5%.[3]

About half of those who develop epilepsy do so before the age of 15 years. There is a growing prevalence in older people, due to demographic shifts and the increase in degenerative cerebrovascular disease.

The prevalence is slightly higher in males and in lower socioeconomic groups.

Aetiology

The aetiology is unknown in about two-thirds of cases. Most individuals with epilepsy probably have a polygenic susceptibility. However, there are several common identified aetiologies:[3]

- cerebrovascular disease, 15% of cases
- cerebral tumour, 6% of cases
- alcohol-related, 6% of cases
- post-traumatic, 2% of cases.

Refractory epilepsy is most commonly due to hippocampal sclerosis, malformations of cortical development, cerebral lesions and low-grade gliomas. Infectious causes are common in other parts of the world.

Diagnosis

Epileptic seizures are paroxysmal events. They take many different forms, but they are usually stereotyped in the individual patient.

The diagnosis is clinical, based largely on the history given by the patient and a witness of a typical seizure. Ask about the circumstances of seizures, pattern of occurrence, preceding symptoms, duration, evolution, observed behaviour during and after the seizure, and the time to recovery. Atypical or unusual features may indicate an alternative diagnosis.

Neurological examination is necessary and may indicate the underlying aetiology. Cardiovascular examination may indicate an alternative diagnosis.

GP investigations may include:

- full blood count
- urea and electrolytes
- liver function tests
- glucose
- bone profile
- electrocardiogram.

Classification of seizure types

Generalized seizures

In generalized seizures there is widespread involvement of the cerebral cortex from outset. These are subdivided further into:

- Tonic–clonic seizures: loss of consciousness; tonic phase with cyanosis; subsequent clonic convulsion with stertorous breathing; perhaps incontinence and tongue injury; slow recovery with a desire to sleep before complete recovery.
- Absences: sudden cessation or slowing of activity with (typical absence) or without (atypical absence) characteristic electroencephalogram (EEG) pattern.
- Epileptic myoclonic jerks: usually sudden flexion movements of the upper limbs without loss of consciousness.

Partial seizures

In partial seizures there is focal cortical onset with or without later spread. The location of seizure onset may be indicated by description.

Automatisms or semipurposeful release phenomena (e.g. lip smacking and swallowing) or more complex behaviours (e.g. vocalization or wandering) may occur in partial seizures or prolonged absences.

The GP taking the history must consider the differential diagnoses and other possible causes of a first seizure.

Differential diagnosis

Events which are not true seizures are:

- Syncope: brief, small, irregular secondary anoxic movements may occur. Forms include vasovagal, micturition and postural syncopy.
- Cardiac disorders, such as arrhythmias, aortic or mitral stenosis and cardiomyopathies.
- Metabolic or endocrine disorders, such as hypoglycaemia, phaeochromocytoma and porphyria.
- Neurological disorders, such as transient ischaemic attack, cataplexy, narcolepsy, and basilar migraine.
- Psychological or psychiatric features, such as hyperventilation, panic attacks and non-epileptic attack disorder.

All patients with a possible diagnosis of epilepsy should be referred to a specialist, usually a neurologist, for evaluation and advice on treatment.

Status epilepticus

Status epilepticus is serial seizures without recovery in between. It is a medical emergency, requiring prompt general supportive and specific anti-epileptic treatment.[4]

Common causes are drug withdrawal or non-compliance, alcohol withdrawal, intracranial infection and tumour.

Investigations

Investigations are only occasionally needed to establish the diagnosis, but they do help with classification and management.

A routine awake EEG will show epileptiform changes in only one-third of patients with epilepsy. The yield can be increased by repeating recordings in sleep or after procedures such as hyperventilation. Occasionally, the EEG may be diagnostic, but it cannot be used in isolation to confirm or exclude epilepsy.

Magnetic resonance imaging (MRI) is best practice in all patients who develop epilepsy, with the exception of clear-cut benign paediatric epilepsy syndromes. It is particularly important for patients with partial seizures, generalized seizures starting in the first year of life or in adulthood, focal neurological symptoms or signs and recent loss of seizure control. MRI identifies the relevant underlying abnormalities in 70% of patients.[5]

Further investigations in specialist centres include prolonged EEG monitoring, telemetry and neuropsychological testing.

Treatment

Treatment is usually needed once epilepsy has been diagnosed. The aim is to prevent seizures with minimum side-effects. Treatment is usually prolonged, so in the UK, treatment is not usually given after a single unprovoked seizure unless the risk of recurrence is thought to be high. Any precipitating factors should be avoided. If there is an underlying condition this may need to be treated independently.

Drug therapy

Anti-epileptic drug choice depends on the classification of the epilepsy and the requirements of the patient. Treatment is initiated at low dosage and increased gradually to an effective level, minimizing side-effects and promoting compliance. All patients started on anti-epileptic drugs must be kept under review.

Phenytoin, carbamazepine and barbiturates are associated with an increased incidence of osteomalacia in chronic usage, and the patient may be at a higher risk of osteoporosis.[6,7]

The long-term risks of anti-epileptic drugs are poorly quantified. Barbiturates, phenytoin, valproate and vigabatrin have chronic adverse effects. The risk associated with newer drugs is less clear.

Management of young and old

Treatment of epilepsy in childhood should be undertaken by paediatricians or paediatric neurologists.

There is a second peak of epilepsy incidence in old age, when it is most likely to be caused by cerebrovascular disease. It may also be a feature of cerebral tumours and progressing dementia. Only low doses of drug treatment may be tolerated by older patients, and interactions with concomitant medication are common.

Stopping drugs

Withdrawal of treatment can be considered if the patient is free of seizures for at least 3 years. However, there is no guarantee that the individual will remain seizure-free after withdrawal, so the decision must be informed.

The risk of relapse is highest in the first year, being about 40% on withdrawal and 20% if treatment is continued but this will vary with the underlying aetiology, epilepsy syndrome, and the severity and duration of the epilepsy before remission.

Patients should be advised to stop driving and avoid potentially unsafe activities such as unsupervised swimming for 6 months after withdrawal.

Contraception and pregnancy

Carbamazepine, oxcarbazepine, phenytoin, barbiturates and topiramate all induce hepatic microsomal enzymes and thus enhance the metabolism of oestrogens. An oestradiol content of at least 50 µg/day is needed, and any breakthrough bleeding implies that the dose is ineffective. Depot preparations such as Depo-Provera 150 mg every 12 weeks are a useful alternative.

Valproate has been associated with an increased chance of polycystic ovary syndrome, reproductive dysfunction and insulin intolerance in some young women.[8,9] Alternative treatments should be considered.

Preconception measures are essential for women with epilepsy who are planning to have a family. No anti-epileptic drug is considered entirely safe in pregnancy. Valproate is more teratogenic than the other agents, but there is still insufficient experience with the newer drugs. If possible, patients should discuss medication with their specialist before trying to conceive. Joint consultant care through pregnancy is advised.

The baseline risk of malformation is about 3%. Treatment with a single antiepileptic drug may increase this to 7–8%, and the risk becomes progressively higher with multiple therapy.[10] However, the risk of malformation must be balanced against the dangers to mother and baby of continued seizures.

Folate supplements (5 mg/day) reduces the risks of spina bifida and should be prescribed throughout pregnancy.[11] Vitamin K_1 (phytomenadione) 20 mg/day orally should be prescribed during the last month.[10]

Breast-feeding is generally recommended.[11] Several anti-epileptic drugs achieve significant levels in breast milk, but the baby will have already been exposed during the pregnancy.

Surgery

Potentially curative surgery is performed to remove seizure foci or interrupt pathways of seizure spread. Up to 3% of patients with chronic medically refractory epilepsy may be potential candidates for surgery.[12]

Lifestyle advice

All patients with epilepsy must stop driving. They are legally obliged to inform the DVLA and surrender their licence. The license is reissued once the patient has been seizure free, whether on or off medication, for specified periods. The licence is reissued once the patient has been seizure-free, whether on or off medication, for specified periods. For a Group 1 licence it is necessary to be seizure-free for 1 year, or to have had seizures only during sleep for 3 years. Public service vehicle and heavy goods licenses cannot be re-obtained unless the patient is seizure free while off all medication for 10 years.

Patients should be advised against unsupervised bathing or swimming and exposure to open heat, unguarded heights, waterfronts and other circumstances in which a seizure might lead to injury. Showers are a safer alternative to bathing, and microwave cooking may be more appropriate than preparing meals at a conventional stove.

Nursing mothers should not bathe babies alone, and should sit on the floor when feeding their babies. However, patients should be encouraged to lead as normal lives as possible, despite their all-pervading diagnosis.

Nurse specialists can provide important information and support, and local patient support groups are invaluable.

Prognosis

Some 70% of cases of epilepsy remit, usually over a period of years.[1] After a first seizure, the risk of recurrence is greatest in the first few months. About one-third of patients with a single unprovoked seizure have a further seizure within 5 years, and about three-quarters with two unprovoked seizures have further seizures.[13] Patients with congenital abnormalities or underlying structural abnormalities are least likely to remit.

Epilepsy is associated with an increased standardized mortality ratio (SMR). Because of the mortality associated with the underlying causes, the SMR is highest in the first year after diagnosis.[14] It is also increased by epilepsy-related accidents, suicide, non-cerebral cancers and sudden unexpected death in epilepsy (SUDEP).

SUDEP is defined as a non-traumatic, unwitnessed death in an individual with epilepsy who has been previously well, with no cause established even after post mortem. The incidence of SUDEP is 1 per 200 each year in refractory epilepsy, and is probably seizure-related. Effective treatment of epilepsy may reduce this risk.[15]

Referral

Ideally, all patients with epilepsy should be seen by specialists to confirm the diagnosis and advise on management. Re-referral may be necessary if there is a relapse or a change in seizure control.

Key points

- The diagnosis of epilepsy is based around a full description of a typical seizure from the patient and a witness.
- An awake EEG is positive in only one-third of cases.
- First seizures require assessment and investigation.
- Optimized seizure control improves mortality and morbidity.
- High-dose combined oral contraceptives are necessary for patients on some types of anti-epilepsy medication.
- Antiepileptics are associated with an increased risk of foetal malformation.
- All patients should be reviewed by a specialist.

Resources

British Epilepsy Association. Freephone helpline 0808 800 5050. Website: http://www.epilepsy.org.uk

National Society for Epilepsy. Helpline 01494 601400. Website: http://www.epilepsynse.org.uk

References

1. Sander JWAS. Some aspects of prognosis in the epilepsies: a review. Epilepsia 1993; 34:1007–1016.

2. Goodridge DM, Shorvon SD. Epileptic seizures in a population of 6000. 1. Demography, diagnosis and classification, and the role of hospital services. BMJ 1983; 287:641–644.

3. Sander JWAS, Hart YM, Johnson AL, et al. National general practice study of epilepsy: newly diagnosed epileptic seizures in the general population. Lancet 1990; 336:1267–1271.

4. Shorvon S. The management of status epilepticus. J Neurol Neurosurg Psychiatry 2001; 70:1122–1127.

5. Li LM, Fish DR, Sisodiya SM, et al. High resolution magnetic resonance imaging in adults with partial epilepsy or secondary generalised epilepsy attending a tertiary referral unit. J Neurol Neurosurg Psychiatry 1995; 59:384–387.

6. Feldkamp J, Becker A, Witte OW, et al. Long-term anticonvulsant therapy leads to low bone mineral density – evidence for direct drug effects of phenytoin and carbamazepine on human osteoblast-like cells. Exp Clin Endocrinol Diabetes 2000; 108:37–43.

7. Stephen LJ, McLellan AR, Harrison JH, et al. Bone density and antiepileptic drugs: a case–controlled study. Seizure 1999; 8:339–342.

8. Isojarvi JIT, Laatikainen TJ, Pakarinen AJ, et al. Polycystic ovaries and hyperandrogenism in women taking valproate for epilepsy. N Engl J Med 1993; 329:1383–1388.

9. Isojarvi JI, Laatikainen TJ, Pakarinen AJ, et al. Obesity and endocrine disorders in women taking valproate for epilepsy. Ann Neurol 1996; 39:579–584.

10. Duncan JS, Shorvon SD, Fish DR. Clinical epilepsy. Edinburgh: Churchill Livingstone; 1995. p 267–282.

11. Crawford P. CPD – education and self-assessment: epilepsy and pregnancy. Seizure 2001; 10:212–219.

12. Duncan JS, Shorvon SD, Fish DR. Clinical epilepsy. Edinburgh: Churchill Livingstone; 1995, p 349–371.

13. Hauser WA, Rich SS, Lee Ju R-J, et al. Risk of recurrence after two unprovoked seizures. N Engl J Med 1998; 338:429–434.

14. Cockerell OC, Johnson AL, Sander JW, et al. Mortality from epilepsy: results from a prospective population based study. Lancet 1994; 344:918–921.

15. Sperling MR, Feldman H, Kinman J, et al. Seizure control and mortality in epilepsy. Ann Neurol 1999; 46:45–50.

43. Headache

- The symptoms and signs that differentiate headaches with sinister causes.
- The necessary examination.
- Investigations and their rationale.
- The diagnosis of migraine.
- The treatment and prophylaxis of migraine.
- Migraine and the oral contraceptive pill.
- The treatments for non-migraine headaches.
- The nature and management of medication-misuse headache.

While most cases of headache do not have a sinister cause, the GP should be alert to the possibility and recognize that patients' worries need to be addressed before agreeing a management plan.

Headache is a symptom, and a non-specific one at that. We all suffer from headaches at some time and many people treat themselves. However, some patients do come to their GP complaining of headaches; some are looking for treatment, some for a diagnosis, some for reassurance, some for a combination of outcomes.

The GP needs to be able to offer the patient some idea of why the headache has arisen, what can be done about it and, in the case of chronic headaches, ways of preventing the pain in future. Thus the management of a patient with headache depends on the patient's concerns and expectations as well as the underlying cause of the condition.

Aetiology

As the word 'headache' can mean so many different things it is important first of all to clarify what the patient is complaining of. The classic format for taking a pain history is useful here, asking about:

- main site
- radiation
- character
- severity
- onset
- duration
- course
- pattern
- aggravating factors
- relieving factors
- associated symptoms.

The GP needs to decide whether the headache is primary or secondary (Box 43.1). The site of the pain is a useful discriminating factor (Table 43.1). Are there any other associated symptoms? Does the patient have any idea what might be causing the headache? Many patients equate headaches with raised blood pressure, and this belief should be explored.

The diagnosis may be apparent from the history, which should include lifestyle factors, family history, recent stressful events, trigger factors and occupation. There are certain symptoms and signs that suggest a sinister cause for a headache and these should be asked about (Box 43.2). A short accelerating history is a cause for concern. Neurological symptoms such as diplopia, changes in mood or motivation, and attacks of disturbed consciousness suggest a cerebral tumour. However, the number of patients who are diagnosed as having a tumour is very small.

Examination and investigations

The choice of examination depends on the history and possible diagnosis. It may include the ears and the eyes, the temples in the elderly and neck movement. The skin should be inspected for signs of a shingles rash.

If there are worrying symptoms, the GP should carry out a neurological examination. Minor degrees of imbalance, unilateral weakness, loss of sensation or unequal reflexes suggest a space-occupying lesion in the brain.

The fundi should be examined. Papilloedema is a rare sign of raised intracranial pressure; many patients do not develop it regardless of how high their pressure rises.

As patients often expect to have their blood pressure measured, this can be done, with the appropriate explanation. If the blood pressure is high this becomes an added complication in the consultation, as it is unlikely to be causing the headache, although it may be secondary to the pain and subsequent anxiety.

If a secondary headache is suspected, the GP should arrange the appropriate investigations. An erythrocyte sedimentation rate (ESR) is necessary if temporal arteritis is a possibility in patients over the age of 50 years.

Box 43.1 Causes of headache

Primary causes
- Migraine
- Tension-type headache
- Cluster headache
- Idiopathic stabbing headache
- Exertional and postcoital headache
- Medication-misuse (analgesic) headache

Secondary causes
- Systemic infection
- Head injury
- Drug-induced headache, including alcohol
- Subarachnoid haemorrhage
- Vascular disorders
- Brain tumour
- Trigeminal neuralgia
- Shingles
- Carbon monoxide poisoning

Referred causes
- Temporomandibular joint
- Cervical spine
- Sinuses/middle ear
- Glaucoma
- Teeth

If there are signs of systemic illness, urea and electrolytes and liver function tests may be indicated as renal and liver dysfunction can precipitate headaches. If a brain tumour is suspected, the patient should be referred urgently to a neurologist and for computed tomography scanning.

Patients with secondary headaches will need specialist treatment, either immediately (for brain haemorrhage or meningitis) or urgently (for brain tumour).

Common headaches

Migraine

Some patients use the word 'migraine' synonymously with headache, but it is a specific condition, characterized by episodic headaches and associated features that may include (Figs 43.1 and 43.2):

- pulsation
- aura (in about 30% of cases)
- nausea
- photophobia
- aggravation by movement
- a unilateral site.

These features help to distinguish migraine from tension-type headache. Migraine attacks last 4–72 hours. According to some neurologists, migraine is common and if it is not diagnosed regularly in general practice it is being missed.[1] Asking patients to keep headache diaries for 1–3 months often helps to clarify the diagnosis. Headaches that are one sided, throb and are associated with nausea are highly likely to be migraines.

Most migraine sufferers are between 25 and 55 years of age and will have about 1–2 attacks each month.[2]

A first attack of migraine can be extremely worrying for both patient and doctor. Unilateral headache, vomiting and photophobia can also suggest meningitis, a condition about which there is much information in the media. Check for true neck stiffness (which means the neck is stiff on passive, not active, flexion; i.e. the doctor cannot flex the patient's neck).

Attacks may occur frequently, leading to loss of schooling, days off work and interference with family and social life.

Patients can often identify trigger factors (Box 43.3), and a headache diary is particularly useful for this. Avoiding identified trigger factors is not always easy, especially as some patients seem to be susceptible to a great many different triggers.

Table 43.1 Types of headache and sites

Condition	Site
Tension headache	Bilateral, generalized or occipital, often band like
Migraine	Unilateral, throbbing, nausea common, sometimes preceded by aura
Cluster headache	Unilateral, severe, eye, nose, cheek, headaches cluster in time rather than place, common in young men
Subarachnoid or other intracranial haemorrhage	Bilateral, generalized or occipital, may be altered consciousness level; always consider in anticoagulated patients
Cranial arteritis	Unilateral with scalp tenderness
Trigeminal neuralgia	Unilateral, distribution in branches of nerve, sharp, stabbing
Postherpetic neuralgia	Unilateral, distribution in branch of nerve
Swim-goggle headache	Band across forehead after wearing tight hat band or goggles
Sinusitis	Worse on leaning forwards, associated with nasal symptoms
Raised intracranial pressure	Worse on waking and sitting up, worse on coughing, straining, bending forwards; never goes
Meningitis (viral, bacterial or other)	Severe headache with true photophobia, passive neck stiffness and vomiting, altered consciousness may be a feature, pyrexia is not necessarily present

Box 43.2 Worrying symptoms and signs in patients with headache

- Headache present on waking
- Pain increases with actions that raise intracranial pressure (e.g. coughing, straining)
- Associated neurological symptoms and/or signs
- Sudden onset of severe headache
- Severe headaches of recent onset, particularly in patients over 50 years of age
- Recent change in nature or increase in frequency of headache
- Pain refractory to treatment
- Headache in children (although acute headache is a common feature of pyrexia or cervical lymphadenopathy in school-age children)

Treatment of acute migraine

Treatment may be specific, that is anti-migraine medication, or non-specific, such as simple analgesia and anti-inflammatory drugs.

Aspirin or paracetamol combined with an anti-emetic, such as metoclopramide, are useful in mild attacks, being safe and well tested over the years. The addition of a gastric-motility drug not only helps with the patient's vomiting but also helps the absorption of the painkiller by increasing oesophageal motility and gastric emptying. Analgesics need to be taken as soon as possible.

Specific anti-migraine treatment

This includes two classes of compounds: ergotamine and the 5-HT$_1$ agonists (triptans). Ergotamine is rarely used nowadays because of its side-effect profile and because it was superseded by sumatriptan, in 1991.

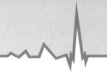

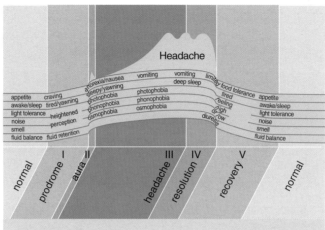

Figure 43.1 The five phases of the migraine attack: prodrome, aura, headache, resolution and recovery. Adapted with permission from Blau & Drummond, *Migraine*, Office of Health Economics, London, 1991.

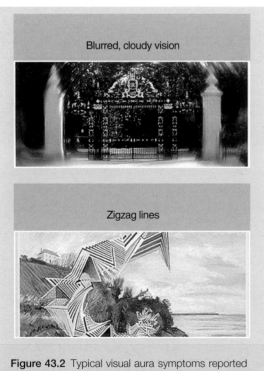

Figure 43.2 Typical visual aura symptoms reported by patients.

Box 43.3 Trigger factors for migraine

- Food (e.g. chocolate, red wine, cheese, coffee, citrus fruit, monosodium glutamate)
- Dehydration (e.g. post-exercise or lack of food)
- Lack of sleep or 'lie-ins' at weekend
- Stress (headache typically comes after rather than during stress)
- Sexual intercourse
- Environment (e.g. too hot, too cold, smells, noise)
- Hormonal (e.g. menopause, premenstrual syndrome, the contraceptive pill)

The triptans, given orally, work quickly and reliably and relieve acute attacks of migraine in about 50–70% of patients. The drugs also come in intranasal and self-administered subcutaneous formulations. They should be taken as soon as a patient is aware that symptoms are developing. Sometimes a second dose is needed to relieve the headache fully; a second dose can also be taken if the headache returns within 24 hours.

Five triptans are now licensed in the UK. All have similar efficacy, but there are differences between them in speed of onset and tolerability. Only sumatriptan is available in injectable and intranasal forms, which work quicker than the oral route. Subcutaneous sumatriptan is the only triptan licensed in the UK for the treatment of cluster headaches.

Side-effects of the triptans include tiredness, dizziness, nausea, neck and shoulder stiffness and a sensation of heaviness in various parts of the body.[3] They are contraindicated in patients with ischaemic heart disease or uncontrolled hypertension.

Evidence suggests that the usual stepwise within-attacks approach to care is not as effective as either a stepwise across-attacks strategy or a stratified care approach (Box 43.4).[4] If a patient reports a change in the pattern of headaches this should be investigated, as rarely migraine is symptomatic of an underlying brain condition such as a tumour or vascular lesion.

Opiates

Opiates are not a good choice for migraine, particularly if attacks are frequent. They are short acting and thus several doses are often required, which may result in analgesic-overuse headache.

Prevention of migraine

The aim of preventive treatment is to reduce the frequency and severity of attacks with the fewest possible side-effects. The first step is to identify trigger factors and to try and avoid them.

The need for prophylactic treatment should be discussed with patients and the decision to take daily medication made in partnership between doctor and patient. Such medication is really only required if migraine attacks are frequent, disabling and/or not responsive to acute treatment.

As there is no ideal drug, the different options and their benefits and side-effects need to be explained. Prophylactic treatment is given for a definite period, usually 2–3 months, and then reviewed. It should result in a 50% reduction in the frequency of attacks.

- Pizotifen (Sanomigran) can lead to weight gain.
- Propranolol has well-recognized side-effects, including tiredness, poor peripheral circulation and impotence. It is contraindicated in patients with asthma.
- Amitriptyline (Lentizol, Triptafen), calcium channel blockers and sodium valproate may also be of use.[5,6]

Migraine and the combined oral contraceptive pill

There are important factors to consider when prescribing the contraceptive pill for women with a history of migraine.

Box 43.4 Strategies for treatment of acute attacks of migraine

- **Stepwise care within attacks.** Each migraine attack is treated first with simple analgesia/antiemetic and only with triptans if first-line medication fails
- **Stepwise care across attacks.** Patients who do not respond to first-line medication in at least two of the first three attacks are switched to a triptan for attacks four to six
- **Stratified care.** Treatment is decided on the basis of the severity of an individual attack and previous response to medication

The pill may increase the frequency and severity of attacks, while some women develop migraine for the first time while taking it. If the migraine has associated focal features, the pill should be stopped and the patient advised about alternative forms of contraception. Migraine in young women raises their risk of ischaemic stroke and this risk is further increased if they take the pill, smoke or have hypertension.[7]

Tension headaches

Daily or frequent headaches occurring in patients who can carry on with their usual activities are not characteristic of migraine. Such headaches, in the absence of significant additional symptoms and signs, are most likely to be tension headaches. Of course, some individuals can suffer from tension headache and migraine at different times.[8]

Tension headaches are caused by muscular contraction and may be precipitated by such things as too much caffeine, tiredness and changes in lifestyle, as well as stress. They can be relieved by exercise.

Chronic daily headache

Chronic daily headache is defined as a primary headache that occurs on most days for a period often longer than 6 months. Again, muscle tension is a feature. Women are ffected twice as often as men are.[9] Chronic daily headache is often precipitated by the overuse of analgesics (see below) as well as by head and neck injuries. The condition is best treated by physiotherapy to the neck if appropriate, avoiding painkillers and, if necessary, prescribing antidepressants or antiepileptic medication.

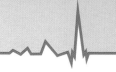

Medication-misuse headache

Medication-misuse headache, or analgesic headache, is an unusual condition in that a treatment aggravates the symptoms for which it is given. Patients who start taking over-the-counter analgesics for their tension headaches may find that eventually such preparations fail to work. They then ask for stronger painkillers. If they are prescribed higher dose codeine their headaches may increase in severity, and a vicious cycle ensues.

Any analgesics may aggravate tension headache and migraine when taken daily. Ideally, neither centrally acting analgesics nor compound preparations should be used to treat these problems. The frequency and severity of the headaches improves after daily painkillers are stopped, but this may take several months.

The mechanism of this type of headache is uncertain, as the analgesics induce headaches only in patients who suffer from headaches already and not in patients who take regular analgesics for other conditions such as rheumatoid arthritis.[10]

The treatment of medication-misuse headache involves a careful explanation to the patient of the aetiology of their pain and psychological support as the drugs are withdrawn. Painkillers are stopped for at least 4–6 weeks.

Patients who take regular analgesics to treat migraine may find that the analgesia causes a rebound headache. Sumatriptan taken instead helps break the cycle.[11]

The triptans themselves can cause drug-induced headaches, especially if they are used too frequently or inappropriately.[12]

Addressing patient concerns

A patient who seeks a doctor's help for headaches often has an underlying worry about the cause of the problem. Thus it is important to ask about the patient's ideas and concerns as well as what they hope to achieve in the consultation. Some patients may feel that labelling what is to them a severe pain as a simple tension headache is not satisfactory, and they should be offered a clear explanation of why the doctor has made this diagnosis.

Those patients who are convinced that they have a brain tumour may be expecting an x-ray or brain scan. The reasons why such investigations are not needed should be discussed.

Key points

- **The diagnosis of headache is made after careful history taking and appropriate examination.**
- **Various symptoms and signs suggest a more sinister cause of headache.**
- **Migraine is characterized by unilateral throbbing headache and associated factors.**
- **The introduction of triptans has led to a decrease in the number of patients requiring prophylaxis.**
- **Regular use of analgesics can precipitate analgesic-overuse headache.**

Resources

Information and leaflets for migraine sufferers. Website: http://www.psych.fullerton.edu/king/migraine

Journal of the American Medical Association, migraine pages. Website: http://www.ama-assn.org/special/migraine/migraine.htm

References

1. Goadsby PJ, Olesen J. Fortnightly review: diagnosis and management of migraine. BMJ 1996; 312:1279–1283.

2. Von Korff M, Stewart WF, Simon DJ, et al. Migraine and reduced work performance: a population-based diary study. Neurology 1998; 50:1741–1745.

3. Dowson A. Migraine. Pharm J 2000; 265:519–523.

4. Lipton RB, Stewart WF, Stone A, et al. Stratified versus step care strategies for migraine. The disabilities in strategies of care (DISC) study: a randomised trial. JAMA 2000; 284:2599–2605.

5. Dowson AJ, Gruffydd-Jones K, Hackett G, et al. Migraine management guidelines. Migraine in primary care advisers. London: Synergy Medical Education; 2000.

6. Anon. Managing migraine. Drug Ther Bull 1998; 36:41–44.

7. Chang CL, Donaghy M, Poulter N. Migraine and stroke in young women: case–control study. BMJ 1999; 318:13–18.

8. Sharff L, Turk DC, Marcus DA. Triggers of headache episodes and coping responses of headache diagnostic groups. Headache 1995; 35:397–403.

9. Solomon S, Lipton RB, Newman LC. Clinical features of chronic daily headache. Headache 1992; 32:325–329.

10. Olesen J. Analgesic headache. BMJ 1995; 310: 479–480.

11. Drucker P, Tepper S. Daily sumatriptan for detoxification from rebound. Headache 1998; 38:687–690.

12 Limmroth V, Kazarawa Z, Fritsche G, et al. Headache after frequent use of serotonin agonists zolmitriptan and naratriptan. Lancet 1999; 353:378.

GASTROENTEROLOGY

44. Dyspepsia

A Cooper

Box 44.1 Causes of dyspepsia[1]

- Non-ulcer dyspepsia, 60% of cases
- Gastro-oesophageal reflux disease, 15–25% of cases
- Peptic ulcer disease, 15–25% of cases
- Gastric cancer, 2% of cases

The management of dyspepsia occupies a great deal of professional time in both primary and secondary care. Each year in the UK up to 40% of adults experience symptoms of dyspepsia.[1] Although most treat themselves with over-the-counter medication,[2] about 10% of patients seek help from their GP annually and 10% of these are referred for specialist opinion.[1] Once diagnosed, nearly 40% of dyspeptic patients consult their GP more than four times a year.[2]

One of the main reasons why people with dyspeptic symptoms consult their GP is fear of cancer. However, gastric cancer is rare, being found in less than 2% of endoscopies.[3] Evidence from Sweden suggests a causal relationship between gastro-oesophageal reflux and oesophageal adenocarcinoma.[4] However, most dyspepsia is not life-threatening, although the symptoms affect quality of life and can be disabling. In one survey, 2% of respondents reported absence from work because of their symptoms.[2] Patients should be given a sympathetic hearing, careful diagnosis and appropriate treatment.

Definition

Dyspepsia is characterized by episodic epigastric pain, heartburn (retrosternal burning), fullness, bloating, nausea and vomiting arising from the upper gastrointestinal (GI) tract. It is in many cases a symptom of an underlying condition, such as gastro-oesophageal reflux disease (GORD), peptic ulcer disease (PUD) and gastric cancer (Box 44.1). Most patients with dyspepsia have no abnormalities on endoscopy and so are described as having functional, or non-ulcer, dyspepsia.

Aetiology

In most patients GORD is the result of abnormally prolonged exposure of the distal oesophagus to acid and pepsin from the stomach. This is the result of a defect in the oesophageal sphincter, although oesophageal sensitivity may be a factor in some patients.[5]

Most cases of PUD are caused by infection with *Helicobacter pylori* (90% of duodenal ulcers, 70% of gastric ulcers). Most of the remaining patients have PUD induced by use of aspirin and non-steroidal anti-inflammatory drugs (NSAIDs).[3]

The cause of non-ulcer dyspepsia remains uncertain. Acid secretion is usually normal. However, gastric and duodenal sensation is disturbed, and delayed gastric emptying is present in some patients. Other patients have anxiety disorder or depression, although this may be an effect rather than a cause of their dyspepsia.

Factors contributing to dyspepsia include being overweight, excessive alcohol consumption, smoking, and a diet high in fat and spicy foods. However, we should be wary of stereotyping our patients. One analysis drew attention to the fact that the patients included in randomized controlled studies of GORD were predominantly >40 years old, non-obese and non-smokers.[6]

Differential diagnosis

In managing dyspepsia the main challenge is to distinguish those patients with a serious, underlying condition who require referral to secondary care. A detailed history and examination should help to differentiate dyspepsia from other possible causes of the patient's symptoms, such as angina.

The history should also identify patients with GORD, where the cardinal symptom is frequent heartburn (retrosternal or epigastric burning radiating up towards the throat) relieved temporarily by antacids and precipitated by food or lying down. Up to 60% of people with upper GI symptoms report both heartburn and epigastric pain or discomfort, but GORD remains the likely diagnosis if heartburn is the predominant symptom.[3]

PUD is harder to diagnose. The classic ulcer symptoms of postprandial epigastric pain or night pain may also be reported by patients with non-ulcer dyspepsia.[3] Endoscopy remains the gold-standard investigation to confirm PUD, but GPs can use indirect breath testing for *H. pylori* to diagnose most patients.[3] Breath test kits are now available on prescription, but 'near-patient' blood tests are no longer recommended, due to poor performance.

A detailed drug history should reveal the remaining aspirin- or NSAID-induced cases, and if the patient is on other prescribed medication consider whether GI upset could be iatrogenic (Box 44.2). Remember over-the-counter medications; most patients are unaware that analgesics can cause PUD.[2]

Differential diagnoses of the cause of upper GI pain include angina and hepatic pain due to congestive cardiac failure, together with pain from other abdominal organs, including

the pancreas, gall bladder and bowel, and pain from the abdominal wall itself. Irritable bowel syndrome may co-exist with dyspepsia, although it is also important to remember that Crohn's disease may affect any part of the GI tract.

Management

Helicobacter eradication

For patients <45 years old presenting with a recurrence of epigastric pain with no alarm symptoms a 'test and treat' strategy for *Helicobacter* is recommended.

If a positive test is found, eradication with triple therapy of a proton pump inhibitor (PPI), clarithromycin and amoxycillin (metronidazole if allergic to penicillin) for 1 week is recommended.

Antacids and alginates

Antacids neutralize acids in the stomach, while alginates reduce acid contact with the oesophagus by forming a protective raft over the stomach contents. It is tempting to start newly presenting patients on treatment with these drugs, but many will have already tried self-treatment with over-the-counter medication for at least 6 months before consulting their GP.[2]

Antacids are no better than placebo in non-ulcer dyspepsia, although the response can be as high as 60%. In any event, the decision to seek medical help undoubtedly correlates with the severity of symptoms (people with moderate or severe dyspepsia are more likely than those with mild symptoms to visit their GP[2]) and it is more appropriate in most patients to start treatment with an acid-suppressing drug.

Proton pump inhibitors and H_2-receptor antagonists

Acid suppression is greater with PPIs than with H_2-receptor antagonists, and the increasing use of these undoubtedly effective drugs led the National Institute of Clinical Excellence (NICE) to issue guidance on the use of PPIs in the treatment of dyspepsia in July 2000 (Box 44.3). NICE recommends that the least expensive appropriate PPI should be used at the lowest dose that will maintain symptom control.

In GORD, the aim of treatment is relief of symptoms followed by PPIs to maintain symptom relief and healing. This is undertaken with regular follow-up to ensure continuing adherence to treatment.

Box 44.2 Likely non-analgesic causes of iatrogenic dyspepsia[3]

- Antibiotics (macrolides, metronidazole)
- Colchicine
- Corticosteroids
- Digoxin
- Gemfibrozil
- Iron
- Levodopa
- Niacin
- Oestrogens
- Oral steroids
- Quinidine
- Theophylline

Box 44.3 NICE guidance on the appropriate use of PPIs in dyspepsia[1]

Peptic ulcer disease
- In *H. pylori*-positive patients:
  - eradication therapy (PPI + clarithromycin + amoxycillin)
  - use metronizadole if allergic to amoxycillin
  - do not use long-term acid suppression therapy
- In *H. pylori*-negative patients or those remaining symptomatic after eradication therapy:
  - use lowest dose of a PPI that provides effective symptom relief
- In NSAID-induced peptic ulcer disease:
  - if possible withdraw the NSAID
  - if NSAID therapy must continue, co-prescribe an acid suppressant (usually a PPI)
  - step down to a maintenance dose when the ulcer has healed

Severe GORD or proven pathology (Barrett's oesophagus, oesophageal ulceration)
- Maintain on full dose of PPI

Complicated oesophagitis (stricture, ulcer, haemorrhage)
- Control symptoms with a healing dose of a PPI
- Then step down to the lowest dose of PPI that maintains control of symptoms

Mild GORD symptoms and/or no proven pathology, non-ulcer dyspepsia, mild dyspeptic symptoms
- Try antacids, alginates or H_2-receptor antagonists, then step up to a PPI if necessary
- Do not routinely use a PPI
- For acid-related symptoms use an antacid or the lowest dose of acid suppressant that controls symptoms
- Treat on either a step-up or a step-down basis
- Do not treat with a long-term PPI in the absence of a confirmed clinical diagnosis

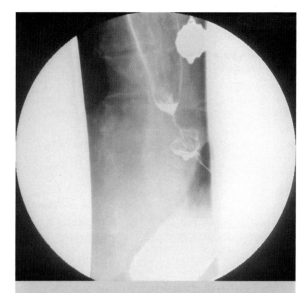

Figure 44.1 The changes seen at endoscopy are erythema of the oesophageal mucosa, erosions and ulceration immediately proximal to the gastro-oesophageal junction. Reproduced from Cullen & Chapman, *Update*, 10 June 1999.

Box 44.4 Alarm symptoms warranting referral for endoscopy in patients of all ages[1,3,7]

- Unintentional weight loss
- Anorexia
- Iron-deficiency anaemia
- Gastrointestinal bleeding
- Recent onset of persistent symptoms
- Persistent vomiting
- Previous gastric surgery
- Epigastric mass
- Dysphagia (barium studies are the best investigation for dysphagia)

Endoscopy

Sixty to ninety percent of people with early gastric cancer present with initial symptoms of dyspepsia.[3] The disease is potentially curable if caught early. The risk of gastric cancer is, however, extremely low in patients aged <55 years presenting with new-onset dyspepsia, so current advice is to reserve referral for endoscopy (Fig. 44.1) for those aged >55 years and for any patient with alarm symptoms (Box 44.4).[1,3]

Endoscopy is inappropriate in patients:[7]
- with a known duodenal ulcer who have responded symptomatically to treatment
- aged <45 years who are asymptomatic after a single episode of dyspepsia

- who have undergone a recent satisfactory endoscopy for the same symptoms.

There is general agreement that immediate endoscopy is not recommended for newly presenting patients aged <45 years without alarm symptoms, but endoscopy in patients aged 45–55 years is controversial. The Dyspepsia Management Guidelines, published in 1996, recommend the age of 45 years as the cut-off for endoscopy in patients with recent-onset dyspepsia without alarm symptoms.[7] According to NICE, however, the cost-effectiveness of endoscopy in the 45–55 year old age group is 'equivocal'.[1]

This issue will presumably be resolved when NICE publishes its clinical guidelines on the primary management of dyspepsia, as the appropriate use of endoscopy is specifically included in the scope of the document.[8] This is currently expected in March 2004.

Lifestyle modification

Most patients need effective and appropriate pharmacological treatment from the range of drugs currently available.

There is little objective evidence that lifestyle is the predominant factor in the pathogenesis of GORD, and lifestyle measures are not recommended as primary therapy, although they may have a strong placebo effect in making patients feel more in charge of their symptoms.[5]

However, dyspepsia is still regarded by the general public as a lifestyle condition caused by unhealthy diet, alcohol, smoking and stress,[2] and patients increasingly ask their GP about non-pharmacological treatment.

It is reasonable for patients to avoid specific foods that they feel exacerbate their symptoms, although exclusion of food groups, such as gluten or milk products, should not be encouraged without evidence of true intolerance. While coffee exacerbates symptoms in some patients with non-ulcer dyspepsia, smoking and alcohol appear to have no effect.

Clearly, drugs causing dyspepsia should be withdrawn or substituted where possible and advice offered about over-the-counter analgesics.

Key points

- Most patients have self-medicated with antacids for some time before seeing the GP. Antacids are no better than placebo in non-ulcer dyspepsia, but placebo helps in 60% of cases.

Ideas for audit
- What is the ratio of patients on a treatment versus a maintenance dose of PPIs?
- How many patients with a past history of PUD are still being treated for dyspepsia? Have they been tested and treated for *H. pylori*?

- Patients under the age of 45 years with suspected ulcer disease should be tested for *Helicobacter pylori* and if positive have 'eradication therapy' before referral for an endoscopy.
- Patients over 55 years old with new-onset disease and patients with alarm symptoms should be referred for endoscopy.
- NICE guidelines are awaited for management of 45–55-year-old patients, as endoscopy in this group (with new onset but no alarm symptoms) is controversial.
- Proton pump inhibitors are better acid suppressors than H_2-receptor antagonists.
- Dietary and lifestyle advice is less important than commonly thought.
- While gastric cancer often presents with dyspepsia, less than 2% of dyspepsia is due to gastric cancer.

References

1. National Institute for Clinical Excellence. Guidance on the use the proton pump inhibitors in the treatment of dyspepsia. Technology appraisalgGuidance No. 7. London: NICE; 2000.
2. Penston JG, Pounder RE. A survey of dyspepsia in Great Britain. Aliment Pharmacol Ther 1996; 10:83–89.
3. Talley NJ, Phung N, Kalantar JS. ABC of the upper gastrointestinal tract. Indigestion: when is it functional. BMJ 2001; 1323:1294–1297.
4. Largergren J, Bergstrom R, Lindgren A, et al. Symptomatic gastroesophageal reflux as a risk factor for esophageal adenocarcinoma. N Engl J Med 1999; 340:825–831.
5. Dent J, Brun J, Fendrick AM, et al. An evidence-based appraisal of reflux disease management – the Genval Workshop Report. Gut 1999; 44(suppl 2):S1–S16.
6. Anon. Treatment effectiveness and costs in reflux disease. Bandolier 2000; 77:77–72.

7. British Society for Gastroenterology. Dyspepsia management guidelines. London: British Society for Gastroenterology; 1996. Available at: www.bsg.org.uk/pdf_word_docs/dyspepsia.pdf

8. National Institute for Clinical Excellence. Scope for the development of a clinical guideline on the primary management of dyspepsia. London: NICE; 2001.

45. Inflammatory bowel disease

D Morris

THIS CHAPTER REVIEWS

- The presenting features of inflammatory bowel disease.
- The investigation and diagnosis of Crohn's disease and ulcerative colitis.
- The treatment of acute exacerbations of inflammatory bowel disease.
- The maintenance treatments for inflammatory bowel disease.
- Long-term management issues.

Definition

The term inflammatory bowel disease (IBD) encompasses both Crohn's disease and ulcerative colitis. Inflammation of the gut mucosa (Figs 45.1 and 45.2), with periods of relapse and remission, is a feature common to both Crohn's disease and ulcerative colitis, but the extent of disease varies between the two conditions.[1,2]

The underlying causes of IBD remain unknown; however, there is an increased incidence within families. Smoking increases the risk of developing Crohn's disease, but appears to be protective against ulcerative colitis.[3] Concerns have been raised that measles infection or vaccination might predispose to Crohn's disease, but the ▸

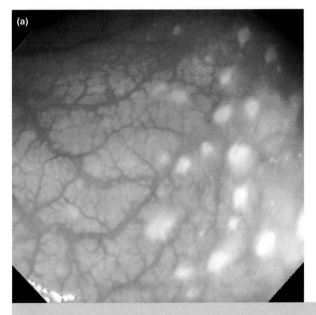
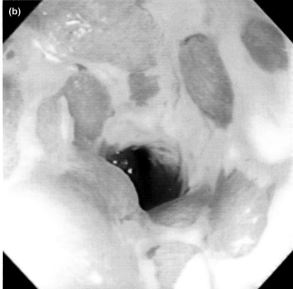

Figure 45.1 Crohn's disease. Colonoscopic appearances of (a) aphthoid ulcers typical of Crohn's disease and (b) cobblestone appearance. Reproduced with permission from Kumar & Clark, *Clinical Medicine*, 5th edn, Saunders, 2002.

incidence has not increased since the introduction of measles vaccination, and review of the available evidence does not support this hypothesis.[4]

Prevalence

In the UK, ulcerative colitis has a prevalence of around 1 in 600 people, more than double that of Crohn's disease, which is approximately 1 in 1500 people. Therefore, the average GP list of 2000 would include four or five patients with IBD.[5]

Presentation

Although symptoms can occur at any age, onset is most common in young adults. The key pathological differences between Crohn's disease and ulcerative colitis are summarized in Box 45.1.

Crohn's disease

Patients with Crohn's disease of the ileum present with abdominal pain, weight loss, diarrhoea, anorexia and fatigue. Onset may be insidious or with acute abdominal

pain. Failure to thrive may be apparent in children. Tenderness and a mass in the right iliac fossa may be found on examination.

Over half of patients with Crohn's disease will have evidence of perianal disease (skin tags, fissures, fistulae and abscesses) and up to a quarter of cases of Crohn's disease present with a colitis clinically similar to ulcerative colitis. Aphthous ulceration of the mouth may also be present. Strictures can lead to colicky abdominal pain and ultimately to intestinal obstruction. The bladder and vagina may also be affected, through fistulae to adjacent inflamed bowel.

Ulcerative colitis

Bloody diarrhoea is more typical of ulcerative colitis. There is frequency and urgency of defaecation, and incontinence is not uncommon. Abdominal pain is frequently left-sided in ulcerative colitis, reflecting rectosigmoid involvement. As with Crohn's disease, there is fatigue, weight loss and fever.

Occasionally extra-intestinal manifestations of IBD can be the presenting feature. The possibilities are listed in Box 45.2.

Investigation

A number of investigations help in the diagnosis.

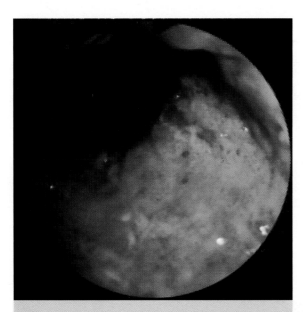

Figure 45.2 View of colonic epithelium at colonoscopy, revealing the inflammatory changes of ulcerative colitis. Reproduced with permission from Swash, *Hutchison's Clinical Methods*, 21st edn, Saunders, 2001.

Box 45.1 Differences in pathology between Crohn's disease and ulcerative colitis

Crohn's disease
- Can affect any part of the gut
- The terminal ileum is commonly involved
- Perianal disease is common
- There is transmural inflammation of the gut wall (strictures, perforation, fistulae and abscesses are possible)
- Areas of diseased and normal bowel alternate ('skip' lesions)

Ulcerative colitis
- Disease is limited to the colon
- Disease spreads proximally from the rectum
- The perianal area is spared
- There is superficial inflammation of the gut mucosa and submucosa
- A continuous length of bowel is affected

Box 45.2 Extra-intestinal manifestations of inflammatory bowel disease

- Peripheral arthritis
- Ankylosing spondylitis
- Sacroiliitis
- Sclerosing cholangitis
- Iritis, episcleritis
- Erythema nodosum
- Pyoderma gangrenosum

Box 45.3 Differential diagnosis of colitis in IBD

- Infectious colitis
- Ischaemic colitis
- Diverticulitis
- Drug-induced colitis (e.g. antibiotics, NSAIDs)
- Colorectal carcinoma
- Irritable bowel syndrome

Stool culture

Stool culture is done to exclude infection from agents such as *Salmonella*, *Shigella* and *Campylobacter* spp.

Blood tests

- The erythrocyte sedimentation rate and C-reactive protein are inflammatory markers that are raised in active IBD.
- A full blood count may demonstrate anaemia and raised white cell and platelet counts.
- Serum ferritin, vitamin B_{12} and folate may all be reduced, reflecting malabsorption.
- Liver function tests may show hypoalbuminaemia in patients with widespread disease.

Lower gastrointestinal endoscopy

This is the key investigation in IBD. While sigmoidoscopy with biopsy is useful in rectosigmoid disease, colonoscopy allows identification of the extent of inflammation and permits serial biopsies through to the terminal ileum.

Radiological investigation

- A double-contrast barium enema is an alternative investigation of the lower bowel. Proximal disease can be studied using a barium follow-through test.
- Abdominal ultrasound can be useful for locating abscesses.
- Computed tomography and magnetic resonance imaging abdominal scans can give important anatomical information, delineating masses, fistulas and abscesses.

- A radiolabelled leucocyte scan can be used to identify the site of intestinal inflammation and possible abscess formation.

Diagnosis

Diagnosis is based on the clinical picture and the bowel investigations. Differentiating between Crohn's disease and ulcerative colitis can be difficult, particularly with Crohn's disease of the colon, but it is important in directing acute and maintenance medical therapy and surgical treatment.

The differential diagnosis of Crohn's disease is wide and includes other causes of chronic diarrhoea and malabsorptive conditions (e.g. coeliac disease) (Box 45.3). Tuberculosis of the terminal ileum can mimic Crohn's disease and is most likely to be found in Asian immigrants.

Management

Management of IBD is directed towards settling acute attacks and maintaining remission with appropriate medication. For patients whose disease is not controlled by medication, surgery may be needed, and in the long term there is the issue of surveillance for colorectal carcinoma.

Acute treatment

The choice of medical intervention depends on the severity of IBD and the area of bowel affected.[6]

Mild-to-moderate proctitis or distal colitis affecting the rectosigmoid colon can be treated with local corticosteroids or aminosalicylates. Topical steroid foams, suppositories and enemas are commonly used. Examples include Colifoam (hydrocortisone), Entocort enema (budesonide) and Predfoam (prednisolone) and these are typically used ▸

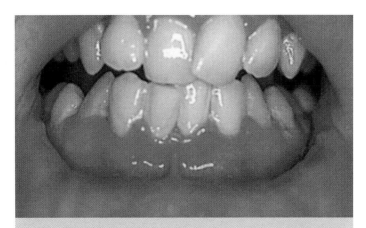

Figure 45.3 The patient shown suffered from Crohn's disease and had been treated with long-term azathioprine. The ulcerative stomatitis resolved when the drug was withdrawn. Reproduced from Bailie, *Update*, 7 May 1999.

for 2 weeks, with subsequent dosage reduction. They are less expensive but no more effective than the aminosalicylates.[5]

More extensive IBD, affecting proximal areas of the gut, requires oral therapy. Oral corticosteroids are preferable to oral aminosalicylates. For both ulcerative colitis and Crohn's disease, prednisolone 20–40 mg/day should be started and, depending on improvement, the dose titrated downward over 8 weeks or so. Early specialist review should be arranged.

An alternative steroid for Crohn's disease of the ileum or ascending colon is enteric-coated budesonide (Entocort, Budenofalk) which, again, can be used orally for 8 weeks in reducing dosages. Although budesonide is probably less effective than prednisolone, it has the advantage of causing less systemic side-effects.[7,8] Budesonide is poorly absorbed and also undergoes extensive first-pass metabolism in the liver, and so has significantly less bioavailability.

Severe cases of IBD require hospital admission, often for intravenous corticosteroid therapy. Attention to fluid balance and electrolytes is needed, and parenteral nutrition may be necessary. A low residue diet is employed and in Crohn's disease an elemental diet (consisting of peptides or protein feeds) can be given either orally or a via nasogastric tube, either in addition to or instead of steroids. Preparations are unpalatable and expensive.[9]

Should Crohn's disease not respond to steroid treatment (or if withdrawal of steroids leads to relapse) then immunosuppressants such as azathioprine (Fig. 45.3), 6-mercaptopurine or methotrexate may be tried.[10] In exceptional cases, cyclosporin may be used to induce remission in IBD, as a last option before surgery.[11]

Metronidazole is an effective treatment for perianal and fistulating Crohn's disease and, again, may avoid the need for corticosteroids.

Infliximab (Remicade) is a monoclonal antibody directed against tumour necrosis factor-α, a pro-inflammatory cytokine, which drives IBD. It is licensed for use in severe active Crohn's disease refractory to treatment with corticosteroids and immunosuppressants and is also useful in the treatment of persistent perianal fistulas.[12] Infliximab is given by infusion and can be rapidly effective in this resistant group of patients. In addition to hypersensitivity reactions, there is concern that use of infliximab may predispose to opportunistic infections (including reactivation of tuberculosis) and possibly malignancy (particularly lymphoma).

Toxic megacolon and unresponsive colitis are indications for surgery in ulcerative colitis. Surgery for strictures, abscesses and fistulas may be needed in Crohn's disease.

Maintenance of remission

There is good evidence that 5-aminosalicylates (5-ASAs) are effective in maintaining remission in ulcerative colitis.[13]

The evidence supporting their use in Crohn's disease is weaker. Sulfasalazine (Salazopyrin) is the prototype molecule and, while the newer 5-ASA derivatives have similar efficacy, they do appear to have fewer side-effects.[13] A drug such as mesalazine (Asacol, Pentasa, Salafalk), may be used in Crohn's disease because it has activity within the ileum.

Sulfasalazine may cause reversible azoospermia, and all 5-ASAs can suppress bone-marrow activity. Therefore, patients on treatment who develop a sore throat, purpura or bleeding should stop the drug and have an immediate full blood count. Nephritis is also possible, and periodic urea and electrolytes and urine dipstick tests are advised.

Steroids are not suitable for long-term maintenance treatment of IBD because of their unacceptable side-effect profile.[5]

Azathioprine and 6-mercaptopurine are effective in maintaining remission in Crohn's disease and are useful steroid-sparing agents.[14] Regular full blood counts are recommended to monitor for bone-marrow depression. To a lesser extent, the thiopurines may be used for maintenance therapy in ulcerative colitis when 5-ASAs do not prevent relapse, and in patients who relapse when corticosteroid treatment is withdrawn.[13]

Antidiarrhoeal agents, such as loperamide or codeine, may be appropriate in Crohn's disease, but should be avoided in ulcerative colitis where there is a risk of inducing toxic megacolon. With terminal ileal disease or right hemicolectomy, cholestyramine (Questran) can relieve diarrhoea resulting from loss of bile-salt absorption.

It is crucial that patients with Crohn's disease stop smoking as, at the 5-year follow-up, the relapse risk is 30% lower in non-smokers than in smokers.[1] NSAIDs are best avoided as they may trigger relapse of IBD.

Malabsorption is a feature of IBD, particularly of Crohn's disease, and consideration needs to be given to provision of food supplements, fat-soluble vitamins and vitamin B_{12} injection in those with ileal resection, and prophylaxis against osteoporosis.

Relapse

If medical treatment fails to maintain remission, surgery should be considered. In ulcerative colitis the procedure of choice is proctocolectomy with ileal pouch–anal anastomosis, as this avoids an ileostomy and prevents disease recurrence. A common problem with this procedure is 'pouchitis' (inflammation of the ileal reservoir).

Referral

All suspected new cases of IBD need to be referred to a specialist. Patients with increasingly severe abdominal pain and stool frequency, passage of blood rectally, fever, tachycardia and marked abdominal tenderness need emergency referral.

With moderate exacerbations of IBD treatment may be initiated in general practice and early outpatient review arranged.

In patients with longer disease duration, consider the possibility of colorectal cancer if new symptoms such as weight loss and rectal bleeding start. These patients need urgent referral.

GPs need to be aware of possible extra-intestinal complications (e.g. eye disease) and refer appropriately.

Follow-up

The GP is the first port of call for exacerbations of IBD. GPs also have responsibility for repeat prescription of maintenance treatments and for monitoring blood test results for patients taking immunosuppressants.

Usually, patients with controlled IBD are seen routinely in specialist clinics once or twice yearly. A recent study suggested that patients with IBD preferred open-access clinics rather than routine booked outpatient appointments and this could be achieved without loss of quality of care and with savings of secondary care resources.[15]

Specialist nurses have an important role in providing information and support to patients, particularly those with ileostomy or colostomy. Patients should be given information about the National Association for Colitis and Crohn's disease (see Resources).

Patients with extensive colitis of longer duration are most at risk of colorectal cancer and, because symptoms may be thought to be due to IBD itself, colonoscopic surveillance is practiced.[16]

Key points

- Smokers are at increased risk of Crohn's disease.
- Ulcerative colitis is over twice as common as Crohn's disease.
- Key clinical features of Crohn's disease are abdominal pain (often in the right iliac fossa), weight loss, loose stool and failure to thrive in children. Anaemia is frequently present.

- Ulcerative colitis is characterized by abdominal pain (often left-sided), bloody diarrhoea and urgency of defaecation.

- Extra-intestinal features such as arthritis, iritis and sclerosing cholangitis may be present in both ulcerative colitis and Crohn's disease.

- Colonoscopy with biopsy is the gold-standard investigation in inflammatory bowel disease. Disease activity is reflected in inflammatory markers.

- Moderate disease of the rectosigmoid colon can be treated with local corticosteroid applications. More extensive disease requires oral steroids and early specialist review. Severe disease needs emergency hospital admission.

- 5-Aminosalicylate preparations are the most important drugs in maintaining remission in ulcerative colitis and, to a lesser extent, in Crohn's disease.

- Patients with extensive colitis of long duration are at risk of developing colorectal cancer. Colonoscopic surveillance is employed in such cases.

- Surgery may be required when medical treatment fails. For ulcerative colitis, proctocolectomy with ileal pouch–anal anastomosis can effectively eliminate the disease.

Resources

National Association for Colitis and Crohn's Disease (NACC), 4 Beaumont House, Sutton Road, St. Albans, Herts AL1 5HH. Tel. 01727 844296. E-mail: nacc@nacc.org.uk

References

1. Rampton DS. Management of Crohn's disease. BMJ 1999; 319:1480–1485.

2. Ghosh S, Shand A, Ferguson A. Ulcerative colitis. BMJ 2000; 320:1119–1123.

3. Thomas GAO, Rhodes J, Green JT. Inflammatory bowel disease and smoking; a review. Am J Gastroenterol 1998; 43:144–149.

4. Metcalf J. Is measles infection associated with Crohn's disease? BMJ 1998; 316:166.

5. Inflammatory Bowel Disease. MEREC Bull 1999; 10:45–48.

6. British Society of Gastroenterology. Guidelines in gastroenterology 4: inflammatory bowel disease. London: British Society of Gastroenterology; 1996.

7. Bar-Meir S, Chowers Y, Lavy A, et al. Budesonide versus prednisolone in the treatment of active Crohn's disease. Gastroenterology 1998; 115:835–840.

8. Controlled-release budesonide in Crohn's disease. Drug Therapeut Bull 1997; 35: 30–31.

9. Griffiths AM, Ohlson A, Sherman PM, et al. Meta-analysis of enteral nutrition as primary therapy of active Crohn's disease. Gastroenterology 1995; 108:1056–1067.

10. Feagan BG, Rochon J, Fedorak R, et al. Methotrexate for the treatment of Crohn's disease. New Engl J Med 1995; 332:292–297.

11. Stack WA, Long RG, Hawkey CJ. Short and long-term outcome of patients treated with cyclosporin for severe acute ulcerative colitis. Aliment Pharmacol Ther 1998; 12:973–978.

12. Bell S, Kamm M. Infliximab: a new era in Crohn's management? Prescriber 2000; 11:38–47.

13. Maintenance drugs for inflammatory bowel disease. Drug Therapeut Bull 2001; 39:91–95.

14. Bouhnik Y, Leman M, Mary JY, et al. Long-term follow-up of patients with Crohn's disease treated with azathioprine or 6-mercaptopurine. Lancet 1996; 347:18–24.

15. Williams JG, Cheung WY, Russell IT, et al. Open access follow up for inflammatory bowel disease: pragmatic randomised trial and cost-effectiveness study. BMJ 2000; 320:544–548.

16. Pinezowski D, Ekbom A, Baron J, et al. Risk factors for colorectal cancer in patients with ulcerative colitis: a case-control study. Gastroenterology 1994; 107:117–120.

46. Irritable bowel syndrome

JE Thistlethwaite

THIS CHAPTER REVIEWS

- The symptoms of irritable bowel syndrome.
- The aetiology of irritable bowel syndrome.
- Making a diagnosis.
- When to refer patients.
- Drug treatment.
- The role of dietary manipulation.
- Psychological approaches to management.

Box 46.1 Symptoms associated with IBS

- Pain eased after bowel motion
- Looser stools at onset of pain
- Abdominal distension
- Feeling of incomplete emptying
- Indigestion
- Tiredness
- Headache
- Frequency of urination
- Back pain

Presentation

A syndrome is a collection of symptoms with a characteristic pattern. The word is usually applied to a condition that is likely to have a multifactorial aetiology and consequently a variety of management options.

The symptoms of irritable bowel syndrome (IBS) include abdominal discomfort, bloating and variable bowel patterns. There may be diarrhoea, constipation or both in an alternating pattern. Such gastrointestinal symptoms are present in up to a quarter of the population.[1] Other symptoms patients may complain of are listed in Box 46.1.

Definition

As the symptoms are so common, an international working party in Rome in 1992 defined the criteria by which the diagnosis of IBS should be made (Box 46.2).[2] A positive diagnosis of the condition is preferable to the common process of diagnosing it by exclusion. By applying the criteria it is hoped that many patients will avoid unpleasant and expensive investigations.

The Rome criteria are not without their critics.[3] The criteria relate solely to the presenting symptoms, rather than the cause of the problem in individual patients. Like the other 'syndromes' (e.g. premenstrual, chronic fatigue), IBS is difficult to manage and does not fit well into a biomedical

Box 46.2 Diagnostic criteria for irritable bowel syndrome[2]

At least 3 months of continuous or recurrent symptoms of:

- Abdominal pain or discomfort, which is relieved by defaecation and/or associated with a change in frequency of stool and/or associated with a change in the consistency of stool

Two or more of the following on at least a quarter of occasions or days:

- Altered bowel frequency (>3 bowel movements/day <3 bowel movements/week)
- Altered form of stool (lumpy/hard or loose/watery)
- Altered passage of stool (straining, urgency, feeling of incomplete evacuation)
- Passage of mucus
- Bloating or feeling of abdominal distension

model of cause and treatment. IBS also has a great impact on the lives of sufferers, leading to problems with personal relationships, libido and employment.[4]

IBS has been defined as a functional bowel disorder. 'Functional' in this context means a variable combination of ▶

chronic and recurrent gastrointestinal symptoms not explained by structural or biochemical abnormalities.[5] This definition indicates the possible role of stress in the aetiology of IBS.

Aetiology

Most of us will have experienced an alteration in bowel habit as a result of stress or lifestyle changes. The need to defaecate before examinations is common, and is a reminder that our bowel function is linked to our emotions. The colonic response to acute stress includes delayed gastric emptying and increased colonic transit time. Patients with IBS appear to have gastrointestinal tracts that are more sensitive to mechanical, chemical and emotional stimuli, and are more reactive, often leading to exaggerated motor responses such as diarrhoea.[6] A difference in the way that IBS sufferers process visceral stimuli in the central nervous system has also been demonstrated.[7]

An episode of gastroenteritis greatly increases the risk of developing IBS,[8] and has been shown to be a factor in its aetiology in about 20% of cases.[9]

There is continuing debate as to whether food intolerance plays a part in the development of IBS. A systematic review of the literature has failed to find conclusive proof of this.[10]

Some women also report cyclical IBS-type symptoms linked to their periods. IBS may also be precipitated by having a hysterectomy,[3] suggesting a hormonal trigger to the syndrome.

It appears that both central and peripheral components are important in the pathogenesis of IBS, and this has led to the development of the concept of the brain–gut axis.[11] This concept proposes that the brain and the gut nervous system act together to produce the symptoms of IBS. Neurotransmitters implicated in the process include 5-hydroxytryptamine (5-HT) and opioid peptides, among others.

Only a small proportion of patients with symptoms of IBS seek medical advice, but about half of those who do also have symptoms of depression, anxiety or both.[5] The question is whether IBS causes psychological symptoms or whether the affective disorder precipitates IBS. The brain–gut axis model suggests that the answer is a mixture of the two. Certain life events can trigger IBS in the same way that they may trigger migraine or more overt psychological conditions. However, it is important to remember that not all patients with IBS have an affective disorder.

Box 46.3 Red flag symptoms/signs in patients with gastrointestinal symptoms

- Onset of symptoms after the age of 40 years
- Weight loss
- Rectal bleeding
- Anaemia
- Raised erythrocyte sedimentation rate

Diagnosis

GPs will use a variety of clues, including the Rome criteria, to make a diagnosis of IBS. The patient's age, sex, family history and past medical history should all be taken into account.

Worrying symptoms raising the possibility of inflammatory bowel disease (IBD) and malignancy are listed in Box 46.3. Patients with any of these symptoms should be referred for further investigation.

Many patients will have had symptoms for several months or even years before seeking medical advice, and it is important to find out why the patient is consulting now. Have the symptoms changed? Has a family member or friend been diagnosed as having cancer? Has the patient's life changed in some way so that the symptoms can no longer be endured? Patients with longstanding IBS whose symptoms change also need reassessment.

As life events and psychological factors are so important in the aetiology of IBS, the patient's psychosocial history must be explored. However, the predominant physical nature of the symptoms means that patients are often concerned about the possibility of a serious underlying bowel condition, and these concerns should be allayed. Asking about possible life stresses may lead patients to conclude that their physical symptoms are being downplayed, and they may be reluctant to have such symptoms attributed solely to stress.

Physical examination should include an abdominal and rectal examination. The results will be normal in IBS.

A full blood count and an erythrocyte sedimentation rate measurement are useful, to exclude anaemia due to rectal bleeding and inflammation. Women with symptoms of IBS and symptoms suggestive of pelvic pathology, such as bloating combined with pelvic pain, dyspareunia and/or urinary frequency, also need a bimanual vaginal examination. Ovarian cancer is difficult to diagnose and a high index of suspicion is required.

If, after a full evaluation of the clinical picture, the GP is happy to diagnose IBS and the patient is happy with the diagnosis, treatment may begin in primary care. Many referrals to secondary care are made not because of uncertainty with the diagnosis,[2] but because of the patient's dissatisfaction with the explanation offered. IBS is implicated in 20–50% of referrals to hospital gastroenterologists.[5]

Management

Once a diagnosis of IBS has been made, management should be tailored to the individual patient. Considering the brain–gut axis model, the most successful therapies are those that aim to break cycles within this axis. Possible treatment strategies are listed in Box 46.4.

Explanation

The first step is to help the patient to understand the diagnosis. The GP next needs to find out what the patient hopes to gain from treatment. Some patients may be content with a diagnosis and the knowledge that nothing more sinister is happening. They may already have some idea of the best way to tackle the symptoms from trial and error over the years.

Drug treatment

Drug treatment controls symptoms, rather than tackling underlying causes. Antispasmodic and antidiarrhoeal agents are helpful to a limited extent. Patients with constipation-dominant IBS may find that laxatives increase their bloating and abdominal pain.

There is interest in agents that act on 5-HT receptors. One such 5-HT receptor antagonist, alosetron, has shown great promise in the treatment of diarrhoea-predominant IBS in women; however, it was withdrawn in the USA because of a series of cases of ischaemic colitis.[11]

Dietary treatment

Many patients ask how they may control their symptoms by manipulating their diet. Some will have already found that certain foods trigger symptoms, although there is no conclusive evidence that food intolerance plays a role in the aetiology of IBS.

Common foods implicated by patients include dairy products, coffee, wheat, onions, citrus fruit and yeast. Proper assessment of dietary triggers requires the patient to keep a food diary and to note any change in symptoms relative to changes in food intake. Many GPs feel ill equipped to offer more than basic advice on diet, and so referral to a dietician may be helpful if such a resource is available locally.

The mainstay of dietary treatment in the past has been manipulation of the amount of fibre ingested, in particular bran. High-fibre diets, while relieving constipation,[12] do not achieve symptomatic improvement in the majority of patients with IBS.[13] This may be because fibre in food is composed of non-starch polysaccharides (NSPs) that can be divided into soluble and insoluble fractions.[14] Bran is an insoluble NSP.

Box 46.4 Treatment strategies for irritable bowel syndrome

All patients
- Explanation and reassurance
- Shared decision making about management

Constipation-dominant IBS
- Dietary fibre, preferably soluble
- Bulk laxatives
- Stool softeners

Diarrhoea-dominant IBS
- Antimotility drugs
- Antidiarrhoea drugs
- Reduce caffeine intake

Abdominal pain and spasm
- Antispasmodics
- Antidepressants

Other therapies
- Cognitive behavioural therapy
- Hypnotherapy
- Homeopathy
- Acupuncture
- Psychotherapy

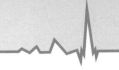

> **Box 46.5** Dietary sources of soluble fibre
>
> - Oats
> - Barley
> - Rye
> - Pulses
> - Apricots
> - Bananas
> - Cherries
> - Clementines
> - Figs
> - Grapefruit
> - Plums
> - Prunes
> - Satsumas

Soluble NSPs, such as found in cereals other than wheat, delay gastric emptying and increase colonic fermentation, resulting in increased faecal bulking.[15] They may therefore be more helpful in the management of IBS than wheat bran. Other sources of soluble NSPs are listed in Box 46.5.

Caffeine in large amounts can stimulate colonic motor activity as much as a meal does.[16] Patients with IBS who drink a lot of coffee or cola should therefore be advised to reduce their intake.

Psychological treatment

Treatments such as hypnotherapy and cognitive behavioural therapy are useful in certain patients,[17] particularly where there is a psychological component to the condition or following an obvious life-event trigger. Cognitive–behaviour therapy in particular helps patients to develop coping strategies for their symptoms,[18] but is time-consuming and may not be locally available for this indication.

Antidepressants may also alleviate symptoms after discussion with the patient about why this line of management is being suggested.

Complementary treatment

A lot of patients with IBS try complementary therapies. Acupuncture and homoeopathy are popular in the UK. Relaxation therapy and biofeedback techniques are also being explored as alternatives to drug treatment.

Conclusion

IBS is a fascinating problem and a challenge for the GP to diagnose and manage. By gaining an understanding of the way in which the brain and gut interact to produce the clinical picture in an individual patient, hopefully a management plan can be negotiated between clinician and sufferer.

Key points

- IBS is a common problem, but many sufferers do not seek medical advice.

- The symptoms are very variable, but usually include alteration in bowel habit and bloating.

- The aetiology of IBS is not clearly understood, but the brain–gut axis model is helpful in explanation and treatment.

- IBS should be a positive diagnosis rather than one of exclusion, based on a careful history and assessment of the patient.

- Drug treatment tends to treat the symptoms rather than the underlying cause and is often not successful in the long term.

- Dietary manipulation may be helpful in individual cases, but there are no hard and fast rules.

- A psychological approach to management is helpful in certain cases.

Resources

Website: http://www.ibsnetwork.org.uk. Information, support and education for those with IBS and their families. Based at Northern General Hospital, Sheffield. Lots of links to other IBS sites.

Website: http://www.ibs-research-update.org.uk. Explanation of symptoms and guidelines for management. Charity based at the Central Middlesex Hospital.

References

1. Jones R, Lydeard S. Irritable bowel syndrome in the general population. BMJ 1992; 304:87–90.

2. Thompson WG, Creed F, Drossman DA, et al. Functional bowel disease and functional abdominal pain. Gastroenterology Int 1992; 5:75–91.

3. Read NW. Irritable bowel syndrome: the GP's role. Update 1999; 58:1182–1190.

4. Silk DB. Impact of irritable bowel syndrome on personal relationships and working practices. Eur J Gastroenterol Heptol 2001; 13:1327–1332.

5. Farthing MJG. Fortnightly review. Irritable bowel, irritable body or irritable brain? BMJ 1995; 310:171–175.

6. Rogers J, Henry MM, Misewicz JJ. Increased segmental activity and intraliminal pressures in the sigmoid colon of patients with the irritable bowel syndrome. Gut 1989; 30:634–641.

7. Chang L, Munakata J, Mayer EA, et al. Perceptual responses in patients with inflammatory and functional bowel disease. Gut 2000; 47:634–641.

8. Rodriguez LAG, Ruigomez A. Increased risk of irritable bowel syndrome after bacterial gastroenteritis: cohort study. BMJ 1999; 318:497–505.

9. Neal KR, Hebden J, Spiller R. Prevalence of gastrointestinal symptoms six months after bacterial gastroenteritis and risk factors for development of irritable bowel syndrome: postal survey of patients. BMJ 1997; 314:779–787.

10. Burden S. Dietary treatment of irritable bowel syndrome; current evidence and guidelines for future practice. J Hum Nutr Dietet 2001; 14:231–241.

11. Bose M, Farthing MJG. Irritable bowel syndrome: new horizons in pathophysiology and treatment. Br J Surg; 88:1425–1426.

12. Can PA, Read NW, Holdsworth CD. What is the benefit of coarse wheat bran in patients with irritable bowel syndrome? Gut 1984; 25:168–173.

13. Rees GA, Tevan M, Davis GJ. Dietary fibre modification and the symptoms of irritable bowel syndrome. J Hum Nutr Dietet 1994; 7:179–189.

14. Englyst HN, Bingham SA, Runswick E, et al. Dietary fibre (non-starch polysaccharides) in fruit, vegetables and nuts. J Hum Nutr Dietet 1988; 1:247–286.

15. Friedman G. Diet and the irritable bowel syndrome. Gastroenterol Clin N Am 1991; 20:313–324.

16. Rao SS, Welcher K, Zimmerman B, et al. Is coffee a colonic stimulant? Eur J Gastroenterol Heptol 1998; 10:113–118.

17. Guthrie E, Creed F, Dason DJ, et al. A controlled trial of psychological treatment for the irritable bowel syndrome. Gastroenterology 1991; 100:450–457.

18. Van Dulmen AM, Fennis JF, Bleijenberg G. Cognitive–behavioural group therapy for irritable bowel syndrome: effects and long-term follow-up. Psychosom Med 1996; 58:508–514.

47. Peptic ulcer

E Warren

THIS CHAPTER REVIEWS

- The diagnosis and investigation of peptic ulcer.
- The management of patients presenting with dyspepsia.
- Testing for and treating *Helicobacter pylori*.

Prevalence

Each year, about 50 patients per 10,000 consult their GPs because of peptic ulceration, but the figure is gradually falling.[1] It is probable that the prevalence of peptic ulcer is genuinely in decline.

One in 20 patients will have a peptic ulcer during their life. Duodenal ulcers are most likely at the age of 40–50 years in men and 50–60 years in women. Gastric ulcers peak at the age of 50–60 years in men and 60–70 years in women. A GP can expect to see eight new cases of duodenal ulcer and two new cases of gastric ulcer each year.[2]

Between 15% and 20% of patients with dyspepsia who undergo gastroscopy will have evidence of peptic ulcer or duodenitis.[1]

Presentation and diagnosis

Peptic ulceration typically causes localized epigastric pain that is clearly related to eating. Food either makes it worse or better. Relief is obtained, even if only briefly, by taking antacids or after acid vomiting. The pain often occurs at night.

It is a relapsing and remitting disease, causing symptoms for 2–4 weeks, followed by a remission of 3–6 months.[2] Clinically, there is localized epigastric tenderness. Patients are often able to put the tip of a finger on a precise spot where the pain is worst.

Cancer should be suspected if there is evidence of anaemia, weight loss and copious vomiting, although a severe ulcer with pyloric stenosis can also produce such symptoms. Urgent investigation is required.

If left alone, a peptic ulcer will tend to relapse and remit for 10–25 years and then resolve.[2]

Indigestion and dyspepsia

Patients present with indigestion. The term is in widespread use – patients generally use it to refer to a problem they see as a commonplace annoyance, rather than something particularly serious. Patients often use the term 'indigestion' to rationalize symptoms that have a more serious cause.

Dyspepsia, the medical equivalent term, is not well defined. In one of its guidelines, the National Institute for Clinical Excellence states that dyspepsia refers to 'a broad range of symptoms related to dysfunction of the upper gastrointestinal tract from the oesophagus to the duodenum, including retrosternal or epigastric pain, fullness, bloating, wind, heartburn, nausea and vomiting'.[3]

The prevalence of dyspepsia is not changing.[4] Patients with dyspepsia account for 3–4% of general practice consultations and the loss of 1.5 million working days each year.[2,4] However, three-quarters of patients with dyspepsia treat themselves and do not attend a doctor.[5]

History

The GP should listen to the patient's description of the symptoms. The site of any pain, any association of the pain with eating or hunger, and relief or not with antacids are all important clues. Further questions may reveal nausea or vomiting, heartburn or abdominal distension. There may be associated lower gastrointestinal symptoms.

The reason for attending now may be significant. Most individuals with dyspepsia do not consult a doctor and so those who do must have a reason. Patients with severe symptoms are probably more likely to attend, but there is a considerable overlap in symptom severity between those who do and those who do not seek medical help.

265

What does this patient want?

Most GPs assume their patients attend for medicines and a cure. This is only partly true. Many want an explanation and perhaps some advice on treatment, after which they will happily return to self-management. Some expect investigation, especially if they think their dyspepsia signifies a serious disease or might lead to serious disease.

Abdominal examination helps only slightly, but it will be expected. Its main value is to localize the pain and make sure there are no masses.

Investigation

Most patients with dyspepsia can be safely treated symptomatically, at least for a time. Investigation is needed to secure a fuller diagnosis, but is also used to rule out stomach cancer. If a gastric cancer is present, its prognosis is no worse after 4–6 weeks of symptomatic treatment.[4] Investigation should be considered if treatment fails to control symptoms, or if symptoms recur after 6 weeks of treatment.

Gastroscopy is the investigation of choice. It has a sensitivity of over 90% for upper gastrointestinal cancer, and a complication rate of under 1%.[4] Most GPs can refer to open-access gastroscopy services. Gastroscopy reveals no abnormality in 30–40% of cases, whether the referral is open access or from a specialist outpatient clinic.[6] Barium meal is an alternative for patients who are unable to tolerate gastroscopy, but it has a much higher false-positive rate for abnormalities.[4]

Some patients prefer to tolerate their symptoms or continue with symptomatic treatment rather than undergo gastroscopy. Their beliefs and wants should be respected, but the decision should be informed. The GP should explain why the procedure is recommended, and make a full record if the offer is still declined.[7]

Some clinical features of dyspepsia may suggest that early referral or gastroscopy is a better idea than a trial of 6 weeks' symptomatic treatment.

The British Society of Gastroenterology has published guidelines on the features that might indicate cancer and other serious pathology (Box 47.1).[8] The guidelines also suggest which patients should be offered gastroscopy even if symptomatic treatment has been effective.

GPs deal with 80% of cases of dyspepsia without referral.[5] Some patients ask for further investigation whether there are indications or not. This wastes resources, causes anxiety because of the wait for results and the inevitable false-positive and false-negative results, and reinforces

---

Box 47.1 Dyspepsia: indications for early gastroscopy[8]

- Unintentional weight loss
- Iron-deficiency anaemia
- Gastrointestinal bleeding
- Dysphagia and pain on swallowing
- Previous gastric surgery
- Persistent vomiting
- Epigastric mass
- Suspicious barium meal results
- Previous gastric ulcer
- Use of NSAIDs
- Epigastric pain sufficient to hospitalize patient
- Recent-onset after the age of 45 years
- Troublesome symptoms in patients <45 years old who test positive for *Helicobacter pylori* on non-invasive testing

---

inappropriate health-seeking behaviour. However, a normal gastroscopy reduces GP attendances for dyspepsia by two-thirds, and even an abnormal result reduces attendances by a third.[6]

National Institute of Clinical Excellence (NICE) guidelines on gastroscopy, particularly for the age group 45–55 years with new dyspepsia but no other alarm symptoms, are currently awaited (see Ch. 44).

Management

Symptomatic treatment through acid suppression is the most appropriate strategy. Antacids neutralize acids in the stomach, while alginates reduce acid contact with the oesophagus by forming a protective raft over the stomach contents, but neither are significantly more effective that placebo, so are not usually the appropriate sole treatment where ulcer is suspected.[9]

Acid suppression is greater with proton pump inhibitors (PPIs) than with H_2-receptor antagonists, and the increasing use of these undoubtedly effective drugs led NICE to recommend that the least expensive appropriate PPI should be used at the lowest dose that will maintain symptom control.[9]

Helicobacter pylori infection

Helicobacter pylori is a small, curled, highly mobile, Gram-negative bacillus that lives in human gastric mucus (Fig. 47.1). ▶

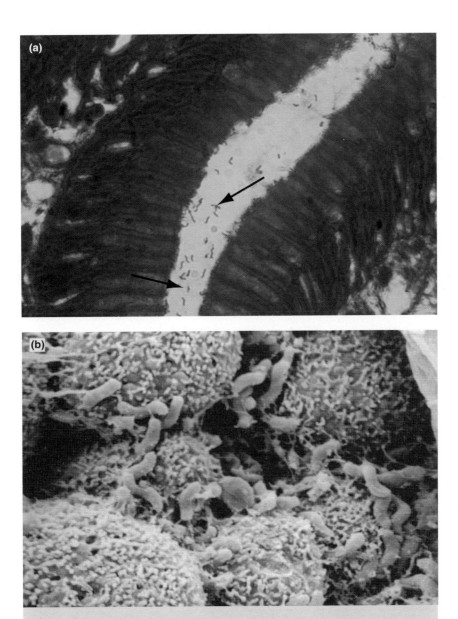

Figure 47.1 *Helicobacter pylori* infection. (a) Organisms (arrowed) are shown on the gastric mucosa (cresyl fast violet (modified Giemsa) stain). Courtesy of Dr Alan Phillips, Department of Paediatric Gastroenterology, Royal Free Hospital. (b) Scanning electron microscopy, showing the spiral-shaped bacterium. Reproduced with permission from Kumar & Clark, *Clinical Medicine*, 5th edn, Saunders, 2002.

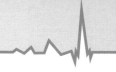

It is found in 20% of 20 year olds, 50% of 50 year olds and so on, and over 70% of infected people are asymptomatic.[10]

H. pylori is responsible for 95% of duodenal ulcers found in people who do not take non-steroidal anti-inflammatory drugs (NSAIDs) and eradication can proceed without testing.[11] Overall, 15% of infected people will develop peptic ulcer or gastric cancer in the long term.[10]

There is good evidence that eradicating H. pylori in patients suffering from gastric or duodenal ulcer and not taking NSAIDs speeds ulcer healing and reduces recurrence. However, despite evidence implicating H. pylori as a cause of stomach cancer, there is no proof that eradication decreases an individual's risk.[11]

H. pylori can be identified invasively at gastroscopy or non-invasively in tests of blood, faeces or breath. All methods offer up to 95% specificity and sensitivity.[10]

Gastric ulcer versus duodenal ulcer

All gastric ulcers should be biopsied to exclude cancer. As it is difficult to distinguish gastric from duodenal ulcers without gastroscopy, it makes sense to investigate all patients with a suspected peptic ulcer and to test for H. pylori at the same time.

The best treatments for H. pylori consist of a PPI plus two out of amoxycillin, clarithromycin or a nitroimidazole such as metronidazole. These regimens are up to 90% effective.[11]

Four weeks after treatment, if symptoms persist, a non-invasive test for H. pylori will show whether the eradication attempt has been successful. Eradication failure may be due to poor adherence to treatment or to treatment failure, which is often due to resistance to metronidazole. An alternative regimen using the other drugs is then required.

Gastric ulcers take longer to heal, and the British Society of Gastroenterology recommends a further 2-month course of antisecretory medication.[8] Continued treatment may also be needed in other cases if the symptoms are not fully resolved.

Surgery

In 1958, 25% of ulcer sufferers ended up having surgery, but this is rarely needed now.[2] Where surgery is needed, it is usually because of a complication of the ulcer. Surgery is still the best treatment for perforation, and is sometimes needed for a bleeding ulcer. Pyloric stenosis may be the result of a long-standing ulcer, and will need surgical release.

Referral and follow-up

Reasons to refer to a specialist include:

- cancer suspected or proven
- diagnostic uncertainty
- treatments not available outside hospital
- failure of treatment, symptoms persisting
- patients' wishes
- management problem, sharing responsibility.

Some patients have continuing symptoms, but at lower severity. Some have other gastrointestinal problems as well as the ulcer, and they may need continued acid suppression with a PPI or another agent. The risk of recurrence, however, is very much reduced if H. pylori has been eradicated.

Issues for the primary care trust

The local primary care trust has a responsibility to:

- encourage appropriate prescribing
- ensure availability of gastroscopy and non-invasive H. pylori testing
- provide urgent hospital access for suspected cancer.

Key points

- **The prevalence of dyspepsia is unchanged, but the prevalence of peptic ulcer is declining.**
- **As it is difficult to distinguish gastric from duodenal ulcers without gastroscopy, it makes sense to investigate all patients with a suspected peptic ulcer and test for H. pylori at the same time.**
- **H. pylori should be eradicated in patients with peptic ulcer. Tests for the organism are 95% sensitive and eradication is 90% successful.**

References

1. Logan R, Delaney B. ABC of the upper gastrointestinal tract. Implications of dyspepsia for the NHS. BMJ 2001; 323:675–677.

2. Jones CTA. Peptic ulcers and dyspepsia. Update 1993; 47:227–233.

3. National Institute for Clinical Excellence. Guidance on the use of proton pump inhibitors in the treatment of dyspepsia. London: TSO; 2000.

4. Brown C, Rees WDW. Dyspepsia in general practice. BMJ 1990; 300:829–830.

5. Lee J, O'Morain C. Managing dyspepsia in the community. Int J Gastroenterol 1997; Mar:13–17.

6. Hungin APS, Thomas PR, Bramble MG, et al. What happens to patients following open access gastroscopy? An outcome study from general practice. Br J Gen Pract 1994; 44:519–521.

7. Jones R. Patient education needed on causes of dyspepsia. Med Monit 1996; 8:26–27.

8. British Society of Gastroenterology. Dyspepsia management guidelines. London: British Society of Gastroenterology; 1996.

9. Galmiche JP, Letessier E, Scarpignato C. Treatment of gastro-oesophageal reflux disease in adults. BMJ 1998; 316:1720–1723.

10. Logan RPH, Walker MM. ABC of the upper gastrointestinal tract. Epidemiology and diagnosis of *Helicobacter pylori* infection. BMJ 2001; 323:920–922.

11. Harris A, Misiewicz JJ. ABC of the upper gastrointestinal tract. Management of *Helicobacter pylori* infection. BMJ 2001; 323:1047–1050.

48. Gastroenteritis

M McGhee

Box 48.1 Common causes of gastroenteritis

- Idiopathic (culture negative), 50% of cases
- *Campylobacter* sp., 25% of cases
- *Salmonella* sp., 15% of cases
- *Shigella* sp., 5% of cases
- *Clostridium difficile*, 5% of cases
- Other, 5% of cases

Prevalence and presentation

Gastroenteritis is characterized by diarrhoea and abdominal pain, usually of short duration, which may be accompanied by nausea and/or vomiting. It is vital to distinguish gastroenteritis from acute appendicitis, in which the abdominal pain is more severe, or colitis, the diarrhoea is more chronic.

In a random sample of adults in the UK, 2–4% of men and women had experienced diarrhoea in the preceding 2-week period.[1] Some 14% had consulted their doctor because of their symptoms and 27% had taken some sort of medication.[2]

Aetiology

A change in diet, for example when people go abroad on holiday, can cause a sudden change in bowel habit.

Viruses are the most common cause of gastroenteritis, while bacteria can be invasive or produce toxins. The most common infective causes in the UK are listed in Box 48.1.

Rarer disorders should be considered in individuals who have just returned from travel abroad. Possible bacterial

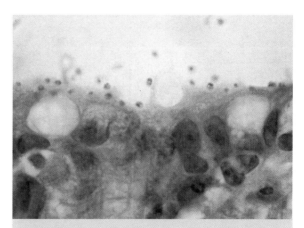

Figure 48.1 Small bowel biopsy from a patient with diarrhoea caused by *Cryptosporidium*, showing intermediate forms of cryptosporidia (small pink dots) on the surface of the mucosa. Reproduced with permission from Roitt & Brostoff, *Immunology*, 6th edn, Mosby, 2001.

infections include *Salmonella typhi* and *Salmonella paratyphi* (enteric fever).

Diarrhoea may also indicate a parasitic infection such as *Cryptosporidium* sp. (Fig. 48.1), *Giardia lamblia* (Fig. 48.2), *Entamoeba histolytica* and *Leishmania* sp.

Diagnosis

Take an accurate history. Risk factors include (Table 48.1):

- recent foreign travel
- eating unusual food such as take-away meals
- family or close friends similarly affected.

The incubation period of some bacteria can give a clue as to the possible cause.

Botulism is rare, the most common source being fermented canned foods. Characteristics are gastroenteritis and

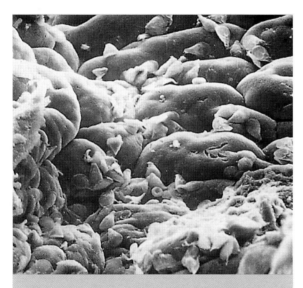

Figure 48.2 Innumerable *Giardia lamblia* parasites can be seen swarming over the mucosa of the jejunum of a patient with CVID. Reproduced with permission from Roitt & Brostoff, *Immunology*, 6th edn, Mosby, 2001.

symmetrical bilateral neurological symptoms, beginning at the cranial nerves and descending, causing paralysis.

Causes and consequences of gastroenteritis are listed in Table 48.2. Erythema nodosum may occur in patients infected with *Yersinia enterocolitica* or *Campylobacter* sp.

Rare severe consequences of gastroenteritis include dehydration, particularly in the young and old, and septicaemia in immunocompromised, elderly or hyposplenic patients.

Reactive arthritis can occur after gastroenteritis caused by *Y. enterocolitica* or *Campylobacter* sp. and can be confused with Crohn's disease and ulcerative colitis.

Investigations

Most cases of gastroenteritis require no investigation: the diagnosis can only be confirmed by stool culture. Stool culture may be appropriate if:

- diarrhoea has persisted for >5 days;
- the patient is systemically unwell
- there is bloody diarrhoea
- the patient lives in an institution or works with susceptible people
- the individual has been handling food regularly, for example at work.

A full blood count, including a white cell count and a platelet count, may be helpful in prolonged cases, especially if colitis is suspected.

Patients who have had persistent diarrhoea for more than 3 weeks should be referred for sigmoidoscopy, to exclude colitis and malignancy.

Stool examination for viruses by electron microscopy may be helpful in children or if there is an outbreak of culture-negative diarrhoea.

Table 48.1 Sources of gastroenteritis

Organism	Incubation time (h)	Possible food source
Bacillus cereus	1–5	Fried or reheated rice
Staphylococcus aureus	2–6	Unrefrigerated meat or milk
Vibrio parahaemolyticus	12–18	Crabs and shellfish
Clostridium perfringens	8–22	Cooled stewed meat
Salmonella sp.	12–24	Undercooked poultry, eggs
Clostridium botulinum	18–36	Canned food

Table 48.2 Severe infections causing gastroenteritis

Symptoms	Infection
Bloody diarrhoea	*Shigella* sp., *Campylobacter* sp., *Escherichia coli*
Colicky abdominal pain	*Campylobacter* sp.
Vomiting	*Bacillus cereus*
Systemic upset (e.g. fever or headache and myalgia)	*Shigella* sp., *Campylobacter* sp., *Yersinia enterocolitica*

Table 48.3 Drug therapy for gastroenteritis

Infection	Treatment
Campylobacter sp.	Antibiotics are rarely indicated, but ciprofloxacin may be useful if the diarrhoea is prolonged or abdominal cramps are severe
Shigella sp.	Sometimes treated with antibiotics (amoxycillin or ciprofloxacin) if the patient is unwell
Salmonella sp.	Should not be treated with antibiotics unless the patient is systemically unwell and requires admission to hospital for ciprofloxacin or trimethoprim
Cryptosporidium sp.	No treatment required, except in immunocompromised patients
Giardia lamblia	Metronidazole or tinidazole

Treatment

Often the most important consideration in treatment is ensuring adequate fluid replacement. Clear fluids should be consumed. Carbonated soft drinks such as cola are highly nutritious and provide a well-balanced source of fluid replacement in the short term in those only moderately unwell. Dioralyte or Rehidrat may be beneficial, especially in young children or the elderly.

Antidiarrhoeal drug therapies such as loperamide (Imodium) should be avoided in the short term as they may delay excretion of the causative agent, but may be appropriate if the diarrhoea is prolonged. Loperamide should not be prescribed for children because of the potential risk of paralytic ileus which can be fatal.

Antiemetics, such as domperidone (Domperamol) or metoclopramide (Gastrobid Continus), should also be avoided if possible, but may be necessary if symptoms are prolonged.

Treatments for infectious causes of gastroenteritis are listed in Table 48.3. The risk of cross-infection may be reduced by good personal hygiene (e.g. using personal hand towels and eating utensils).

Notifying the authorities

Cases of suspected food poisoning should be reported to the local health authority who will investigate any possible source of infection. *Salmonella* sp., *Shigella* sp. and *Vibrio cholerae* are notifiable infections.

Follow-up

Most patients with gastroenteritis do not require follow-up, but infants and the elderly can become dehydrated quickly and should have a check up. The local microbiologist and consultant in communicable diseases are invaluable sources of advice and help in a difficult or protracted case. ▸

Key points

- Gastroenteritis is common in general practice and usually does not require investigation or medication.
- The young and elderly can become acutely ill more quickly.
- Antibiotics are very rarely necessary or required.
- The most important consideration is ensuring adequate fluid replacement.
- Gastroenteritis caused by food poisoning or *Salmonella* sp., *Shigella* sp. or *Vibrio cholerae* infection is a notifiable disease.
- Rare but serious cases of diarrhoea can occur in the patient returning from travel abroad and these patients should be referred to a specialist unit dealing with infectious diseases.

Resources

NHS Executive. Referral guidelines for suspected cancer. Available at: http://www.doh.gov.uk/cancer/proforma.htm

References

1. Dunnell K, Cartwright A. Medicine takers, prescribers and hoarders. London: Routledge and Kegan Paul; 1972.
2. Wadsworth MEJ, Butterfield WJH, Blaney R. Health and sickness; the choice of treatment. London: Tavistock; 1971.

49. Coeliac disease in adults

G Rubin

THIS CHAPTER REVIEWS

- The risk factors for coeliac disease.
- When to suspect coeliac disease.
- The changing presentation of coeliac disease.
- The complications of untreated coeliac disease.
- The management of coeliac disease.

Prevalence

Coeliac disease is a chronic, potentially life-threatening inflammatory condition affecting the intestinal mucosa. It is triggered by a reaction to gluten and may also be referred to as gluten-sensitive enteropathy or non-tropical sprue.

Coeliac disease is significantly underdiagnosed in the UK and may affect as many as 1 in 300 people.[1,2] For every individual with a confirmed diagnosis, another two remain undiagnosed: what we see is just the tip of the iceberg.

Untreated coeliac disease is associated with long-term health risks, including osteoporosis[3] and gastrointestinal malignancy. However, most sufferers are able to lead normal lives if they stick strictly to a gluten-free diet.[4]

While coeliac disease was once regarded as a disease of childhood, it is now thought mainly to affect adults. More than 85% of newly diagnosed patients joining the Coeliac Society in 1998 were adults.

Pathology: the gut

In coeliac disease, damage is caused to the small intestine by exposure to gluten, the group of proteins found in wheat. Similar proteins found in other cereals, such as rye and barley, have the same effect. The case against oats remains undecided, but most coeliac patients can tolerate a moderate amount of oats.

When a gluten-sensitive individual is exposed to gluten, an immune response is triggered. This leads to inflammatory changes in the mucosa villi. Long-term exposure results in villous atrophy and hyperplasia of the crypts of Lieberkühn (Fig. 49.1). As the villi flatten and reduce the gut's surface area, the ability to absorb nutrients is reduced. The disease affects the mucosa of the proximal small intestine, with damage gradually lessening towards the distal small intestine.

Presentation

The classic symptoms of coeliac disease are malabsorption and diarrhoea, which were first described by Samuel Gee in 1888.[5] Today's coeliac patient is less likely to be a child presenting with these symptoms than an adult with less defined and more varied symptoms.

Many doctors still associate coeliac disease with the classic symptoms described by Gee. However, results of serological assays[6] have shown that only a small proportion of patients present with these clinically overt symptoms.[2] As well as the classic and atypical forms, there are silent and latent forms of coeliac disease.[7] This disease should be considered in individuals presenting with:

- anaemia
- unexplained diarrhoea
- chronic fatigue or 'tired all the time'.

Borderline or intermittent anaemia is one of the most common presentations in older patients with coeliac disease.[2]

The incidence peaks between 30 and 45 years of age, and the average age of diagnosis is 44 years.[1] Men and women are equally likely to be affected.[2] However, twice as many women as men have the diagnosis confirmed, probably because they are more likely to consult their GP frequently.[8]

In children, symptoms usually become apparent on weaning. Coeliac disease should be considered if a child who was previously well on milk begins to lose weight, refuse food, suffer from diarrhoea, irritability and, occasionally, generalized oedema when cereals are

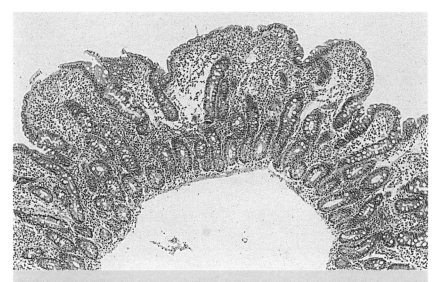

Figure 49.1 Coeliac disease. Jejunal biopsy from a patient with coeliac disease, showing severe villous atrophy and crypt elongation (hyperplasia). Reproduced with permission from Underwood, *General and Systematic Pathology*, 3rd edn, Churchill Livingstone, 2000.

introduced into the diet. Children may also suffer vomiting and abdominal pain, and, uncommonly, constipation, hypotonia and abdominal distension.

Older children may present with short stature, iron-deficiency anaemia and behavioural problems. This presentation is characteristic of children in the UK whose families originate from the northern part of the Indian subcontinent.[9]

There has been a decline in the number of children diagnosed with coeliac disease. This may be the result of recent guidelines on weaning, which recommend that gluten should not be introduced before the age of 6 months.

Risk factors for coeliac disease are listed in Box 49.1.

Diagnosis

Endomysial antibody (EMA) testing should be performed if coeliac disease is suspected. The results will be negative in the 2% of sufferers who are immunoglobulin A (IgA) deficient, so GPs should request an IgA level at the same time; indeed many laboratories will do this as a matter of course.

If the initial diagnosis is uncertain, patients may be given another EMA test following 6 weeks on a normal gluten-containing diet, which includes four slices of bread per day.

If the EMA test is positive, the diagnosis should be confirmed by a biopsy of the small intestine. However, if this is not done and the patient adheres to a gluten-free diet for several weeks, any biopsy will be normal, leading to a quandary about when to commence treatment.

Serial measurements of EMA are a reliable way of monitoring compliance to the gluten-free diet.

Risks of undiagnosed coeliac disease

Untreated coeliac disease may cause life-threatening complications. It is strongly associated with osteoporosis, and there is a two-fold increase in the risk of gastrointestinal malignancy. However, if patients follow a diet that excludes all gluten, the mucosal damage may be reversed and the gut returns to normal or near-normal function, with long-term risks significantly reduced.

Osteoporosis

Coeliac patients absorb nutrients less efficiently, and so may suffer from nutritional deficiencies. As many as 50% of coeliac patients suffer from osteoporosis as a result of calcium deficiency. Up to 20% have a five-fold increase in fracture risk.[2] One reason for this is that peak bone mass is

Box 49.1 Risk factors for coeliac disease

- Family history of coeliac disease
- Osteoporosis
- Insulin-dependent diabetes mellitus
- Down's syndrome
- Infertility
- Dermatitis herpetiformis
- Undefined neurological disorders
- Autoimmune and thyroid disease
- Muscle pain

achieved in early adulthood, while the average age for coeliac diagnosis is 44 years. These coeliac patients therefore have a lower starting point for bone density.

Patients should boost their daily calcium intake by up to 1500 mg with calcium and vitamin D supplements, in conjunction with a gluten-free diet, to protect against further bone loss and to increase bone mineral density.[10] Patients should be advised on managing osteoporosis, including the importance of regular, weight-bearing exercise.

The National Osteoporosis Society has produced a patient fact sheet to increase awareness of the links between coeliac disease and osteoporosis (see Resources).

Cancer

A study of 210 patients diagnosed with coeliac disease followed up over 21 years found that those who did not stick strictly to a gluten-free diet had, on average, a two-fold increase in their overall risk of cancer.[11]

Those in the strictly gluten-free group showed no significant increase in their risk of cancer, but those on a normal diet had a two-fold risk of developing gastrointestinal cancer, including cancer of the mouth, pharynx and oesophagus. The relative risk of enteropathy-associated T-cell lymphoma was 77.8.

Patients diagnosed with coeliac disease after the age of 60 years have a significantly increased risk of lymphoma or small intestine adenocarcinoma.[12]

Type 1 (insulin-dependent) diabetes mellitus

As many as 1 in 50 people with type 1 diabetes mellitus may also have coeliac disease.[4] The two conditions share a

similar genetic background: both are associated with a high frequency of HLA-DR3 genotypes.[8]

Individuals with diabetes are advised to follow a diet rich in complex carbohydrates, so those who also have coeliac disease should be provided with gluten-free alternatives to foods such as pasta and bread.

Patients with type 1 diabetes mellitus should be tested for coeliac disease every few years, even if their initial screening is negative, as it is possible for a later test to be positive.[13,14]

This is also true of diabetic children, in whom growth fall-off and increased frequency of hypos should raise strong suspicions. It is likely that 1 in 40 diabetic children develop coeliac disease.

Down's syndrome

The prevalence of coeliac disease is up to 43 times greater in children with Down's syndrome, but they may not have any gastrointestinal symptoms. The average prevalence of villous atrophy in Down's syndrome is estimated at 4.7–16.9% at any age.

Management

The only treatment for coeliac disease is a strict gluten-free diet for life.[15] To help individuals with this disease to find suitable foods, the Coeliac Society (see Resources) produces a regularly updated list of naturally gluten-free foods and specially made gluten-free foods.

Regular follow-up gives the primary care team the chance to encourage dietary compliance, provide patient-centred care, and discuss the risks and benefits of treatment at different stages of life. Patients may also need additional support at times of physical or emotional stress.

Bone mineral density should be measured using dual-energy x-ray absorptiometry (DEXA) at the time of diagnosis, to rule out osteoporosis. DEXA should then be carried out again in women at the menopause, in men at the age of 55 years and if a fragility fracture occurs.

Key points

- Coeliac disease should no longer be regarded as rare, as prevalence in adults is at least 1 in 300.
- As many as two-thirds of sufferers are undetected.
- In children, coeliac disease may often become apparent at weaning, when cereals are introduced

and when a child who was previously well fails to thrive.

- Coeliac disease should be considered in patients with iron or folate deficiency anaemia, chronic fatigue, 'tired all the time' or unexplained diarrhoea.
- The clinical picture of coeliac disease has changed considerably, and it is now most commonly seen in adults who present with ill-defined gastrointestinal symptoms.
- Patients with coeliac disease should switch to a gluten-free diet. If patients strictly follow the diet for life, the risk of complications, notably gastrointestinal malignancy and osteoporosis, can be minimized.
- Risk factors include a family history of coeliac disease, insulin-dependent diabetes mellitus, osteoporosis, Down's syndrome, infertility, thyroid disease or an undefined neurological disorder.
- Treatment is a gluten-free diet, which must be followed strictly and permanently to avoid the risk of long-term complications.

Resources

Coeliac Society, PO Box High Wycombe, Buckinghamshire HP11 2HY. Tel. 01494 437278; fax 01494 474349.

Decision points in the management of adult coeliac disease in primary care: Available at: http://www.ocsg.org.uk/html/pub_coeliacDisease.html

Fact sheet on osteoporosis and coeliac disease: The National Osteoporosis Society. Tel. 01761 471771.

Primary Care Society for Gastroenterology, c/o East Oxford Health Centre, Cowley Road, Oxford OX4 1XD.

References

1. Catassi C, Ratsch I-M, Fabiani E, et al. Coeliac disease in the year 2000: exploring the iceberg. Lancet 1994; 343:200–203.

2. Hin H, Bird G, Fisher P, et al. Coeliac disease in primary care: case-finding study. BMJ 1999; 318:164–167.

3. Shaker JL, Brickner RC, Findling JW, et al. Hypocalcemia and skeletal disease as presenting features of coeliac disease. Arch Intern Med 1997; 157:1013–1016.

4. Page SR, Lloyd CA, Hill PG, et al. The prevalence of coeliac disease in adult diabetes mellitus. Q J Med 1994; 8:748–751.

5. Gee S. On the coeliac disease. St Bart Hosp Rep 1888; 24:17–20.

6. Unsworth DJ, Brown DL. Serological screening suggests that adult coeliac disease is underdiagnosed in the UK and increases the incidence by up to 12%. Gut 1994; 35:61–64.

7. Fergusson A, Arranz E, O'Mahony S. Clinical and pathological spectrum of coeliac disease – active, silent, latent, potential. Gut 1993; 34:150–151.

8. Shanahan, F, McKenna R, McCarthy CF, et al. Coeliac disease and diabetes mellitus: a study of 24 patients with HLA typing. Q J Med 1982; 51:329–335.

9. British Society of Gastroenterology. Guidelines for the management of patients with coeliac disease. London: British Society of Gastroenterology; 1996.

10. Primary Care Society for Gastroenterology. Decision points in the management of adult coeliac disease in primary care. Oxford: Primary Care Society for Gastroenterology; 1999.

11. Holmes GKT, Prior P, Lane MR, et al. Malignancy in coeliac disease – effect of a gluten free diet. Gut 1989; 30:333–338.

12. Freeman H. Neoplastic disorders in 100 patients with adult coeliac disease. Can J Gastroenterol 1996; 10:163–166.

13. Maki M, Huupponen T, Holm K, et al. Seroconversion of reticulin autoantibodies predicts coeliac disease in insulin diabetes mellitus. Gut 1995; 36:239–242.

14. Saukkonen T, Savilanti E, Reijonen H, et al. Childhood Diabetes in Finland Study Group. Coeliac disease: frequent occurrence after clinical onset of insulin-dependent diabetes mellitus. Diabetic Med 1996; 13:464–470.

15. Trier JS. Coeliac sprue. In: Sleisenger MH, Fordtran JF, eds. Gastrointestinal diseases. Pathophysiology, diagnosis, management, vol 1. Philadelphia: WB Saunders; 1993.

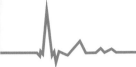

Index

Note: Page references in *italics* refer to figures; those in **bold** refer to tables

Index

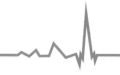

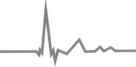

Index

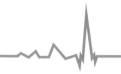

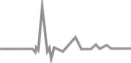

Index

Index

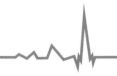

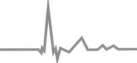

Index

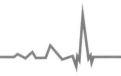

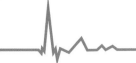

Index

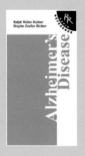
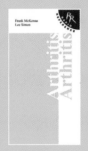
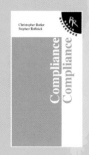
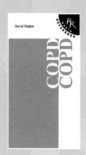
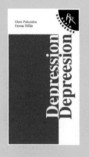
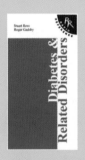
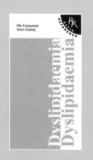
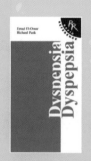
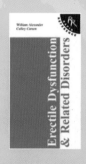
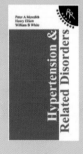
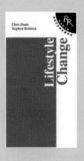
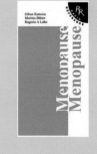
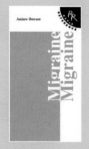
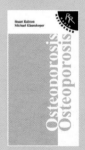
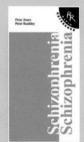
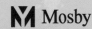